ECG
for
Medical Diagnosis

ECG *for* Medical Diagnosis

SK Apu
MBBS D-Card
Assistant Professor
Department of Cardiology
Mymensingh Medical College and
Hospital (MMCH)
Mymensingh, Dhaka, Bangladesh

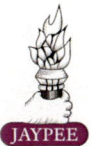

JAYPEE BROTHERS MEDICAL PUBLISHERS
The Health Sciences Publisher
New Delhi | London

Jaypee Brothers Medical Publishers (P) Ltd.

Headquarters
EMCA House
23/23-B, Ansari Road, Daryaganj
New Delhi 110 002, India
Landline: +91-11-23272143,
+91-11-23272703
+91-11-23282021, +91-11-23245672
E-mail: jaypee@jaypeebrothers.com

Corporate Office
Jaypee Brothers Medical Publishers (P) Ltd.
4838/24, Ansari Road, Daryaganj
New Delhi 110 002, India
Phone: +91-11-43574357
Fax: +91-11-43574314
E-mail: jaypee@jaypeebrothers.com

Overseas Office
JP Medical Ltd.
83, Victoria Street, London
SW1H 0HW (UK)
Phone: +44-20 3170 8910
E-mail: info@jpmedpub.com

EU GPSR Authorised Representative
Logos Europe, 9 rue Nicolas Poussin
17000, La Rochelle, France
Phone: +33 (0) 6 67 93 73 78
E-mail: Contact@logoseurope.eu

Website: www.jaypeebrothers.com
Website: www.jaypeedigital.com

© 2017, Jaypee Brothers Medical Publishers

The views and opinions expressed in this book are solely those of the original contributor(s)/author(s) and do not necessarily represent those of editor(s) of the book.

All rights reserved. No part of this publication may be reproduced, stored or transmitted in any form or by any means, electronic, mechanical, photocopying, recording or otherwise, without the prior permission in writing of the publishers.

All brand names and product names used in this book are trade names, service marks, trademarks or registered trademarks of their respective owners. The publisher is not associated with any product or vendor mentioned in this book.

Medical knowledge and practice change constantly. This book is designed to provide accurate, authoritative information about the subject matter in question. However, readers are advised to check the most current information available on procedures included and check information from the manufacturer of each product to be administered, to verify the recommended dose, formula, method and duration of administration, adverse effects and contraindications. It is the responsibility of the practitioner to take all appropriate safety precautions. Neither the publisher nor the author(s)/editor(s) assume any liability for any injury and/or damage to persons or property arising from or related to use of material in this book.

This book is sold on the understanding that the publisher is not engaged in providing professional medical services. If such advice or services are required, the services of a competent medical professional should be sought.

Every effort has been made where necessary to contact holders of copyright to obtain permission to reproduce copyright material. If any has been inadvertently overlooked, the publisher will be pleased to make the necessary arrangements at the first opportunity.

Inquiries for bulk sales may be solicited at: jaypee@jaypeebrothers.com

ECG for Medical Diagnosis

First Edition: **2017, Reprint: 2025**

ISBN: 978-93-86322-91-3

Printed at: Samrat Offset Pvt. Ltd.

Dedicated to

*My wife Shelley Dutta
and
My daughter Asmita Shaily Mum*

Preface

ECG is a simple, useful and practical diagnostic test for cardiac diseases. ECG helps physicians to make the correct diagnosis, evaluate myocardial function and monitor the efficacy of treatment.

Now-a-days, a proper clinical diagnosis is impossible without ECG. So, this is a widespread application not only in cardiology but also in other branches of medical sciences.

This book, in short, describes most of the available changes in ECG pattern in different heart ailments along with possible interpretations which are helpful for medical students and practicing physicians.

Many doctors and medical students have given helpful advices and valuable suggestions. I am grateful for their help. I cordially invite constructive criticism from readers so that any error can be corrected in future edition.

SK Apu

Acknowledgments

I would like to express my deep appreciation and gratefulness to Professor Md Shamsul Haque, MD (Cardiology), Former Head, Department of Cardiology, Mymensingh Medical College and Hospital (MMCH), for his hearty inspiration, guidance and constructive criticism.

I am also grateful to Professor CN Sarker, Former Professor of Medicine; Dr M Saiful Bari, Associate Professor and Head; Dr Mirza Nazrul Islam, Associate Professor, Department of Cardiology, MMCH, for their encouragement and valuable suggestions in preparing the book.

I express my thanks to Professor Motiur Rahaman, Principal and Head, Department of Surgery, MMCH, for his encouragement and valuable support.

I am grateful to my colleagues, doctors and students, who helped me by providing advice, corrections and motivation:

- Dr Ranjan Kumar Majumder, Assistant Professor, Department of Cardiology, MMCH;
- Dr MA Bari, Assistant Professor, Department of Cardiology, MMCH;
- Dr RC Debnath, Assistant Professor, Department of Cardiology, MMCH;
- Dr AKM Sazidur Rahman Siddique, Assistant Professor, Department of Cardiology, MMCH;
- Dr Gobinda Kumar Paul, Assistant Professor, Department of Cardiology, MMCH;
- Dr Towhidul Ahsan Khan, Assistant Professor, Department of Cardiology, MMCH; and
- Dr Hari Mohon Pandit.

I also express my gratitude to Professor AKM Mohibullah, Professor of Cardiology and Director, National Institute of Cardiovascular Diseases (NICVD), Dhaka; Professor Mohosin Khalil, MMCH, Professor Mansoor Khalil, Principal, MMC; Professor Amal Kumar Basak; Drs Md Shamsuzzaman; Md Salehuddin; Md Nasiruddin; Harun-or-Rashid; MA Taher; Biplob Podder, and Zakir, for their encouragement in preparing the book. My thanks to all MD (Cardiology) and D. Card students, Registrar and Assistant Registrar for helping this book.

My special thanks to Shri Jitendar P Vij (Group Chairman) and Mr Ankit Vij (Group President) of M/s Jaypee Brothers Medical Publishers (P) Ltd, New Delhi, India, who have worked for the timely publication of the book.

I am always grateful to Professor Mannan Faridi for his great help in computer composing and graphic designing of the book.

I would like to express my gratitude to my wife, Shelley Dutta and daughter, Asmita Shaily Mum, for their support, sacrifice and encouragement.

Contents

1. **Introduction** 1
   Definition *1*
   What to Look for in the ECG? (How to Report an ECG?) *1*
   Clinical Value of the Electrocardiogram *2*

2. **Anatomy and Physiology** 3
   Anatomy of the Heart *3*
   Coronary Circulation *4*
   Conductive System of the Heart
   (Junctional Tissues of the Heart) *6*
   Sequence of Heart Activation *8*
   Properties of Cardiac Cells *8*
   Nerve Supply of the Heart *8*

3. **Electrocardiographic Leads** 10
   Definition *10*
   Types of Leads *10*
   Electrode Placement of the Standard Leads *11*
   Representation of the Surface of the Heart by Electrode *15*
   R-wave Progression *17*

4. **Essential Basic Electrocardiogram Principles** 18
   The Basic Action: Depolarization and Repolarization *18*
   Recording Depolarization and Repolarization *20*

5. **Normal Electrocardiogram** 22
   Basic Shape of the Normal Electrocardiogram *22*
   Various Forms of the QRS Complex *25*
   Electrocardiogram Paper *26*
   Calibration *26*
   Normal Electrocardiogram Measurements *27*
   Making a Recording *28*
   Heart Rate Determination *28*
   Standardization of Electrocardiogram *30*

6. **Axis and Vectors** 32
   Axis *32*
   Vector *33*
   QRS Axis *33*
   Relation of ECG Leads to Axis Leads *34*
   Axis Leads and Corresponding Degrees *34*
   Determination of QRS Vector *35*
   Determination of Mean QRS Axis *36*
   Axis Deviation *38*
   Rapid Estimation of Mean QRS Axis *40*

7. **Abnormalities of Wave Intervals and Segments** 42
   Normal P-wave *42*
   Abnormal P-wave (Clinical Significance) *42*

Normal and Pathological Q-wave 44
Normal and Abnormal R-wave 45
Normal and Abnormal QRS Complex 46
Normal and Abnormal T-wave 48
Juvenile T-wave Pattern 52
Normal and Abnormal U-wave 52
Normal and Abnormal P-interval 53
QT Interval: Normal and Abnormal 54
Normal and Abnormal ST Segment 56
Early Repolarization (High Take Off) Syndrome 61
Rhythm of the Heart 62
Normal Variants in Electrocardiogram 62

8. Hypertrophy 63
Atrial Hypertrophy 63
Right Atrial Hypertrophy 63
Left Atrial Hypertrophy 64
Both Right and Left Atrial Hypertrophy (P-Tricuspidale) 65
Ventricular Hypertrophy 67
Left Ventricular Hypertrophy 67
Overload Concept of Left Ventricular Hypertrophy 71
Systolic Overload (Pressure Overload) of Left Ventricular Hypertrophy 73
Diastolic Overload (Volume Overload) of Left Ventricular Hypertrophy 73
Biventricular Hypertrophy 74

9. Arrhythmias: Disorders of the Cardiac Rhythms 76
Arrhythmias 76
Normal Sinus Rhythm 80
Sinus Bradycardia 82
Sinus Arrhythmia 83
Pacemaker Sites of the Heart 85
Ectopic Beat 86
Atrial Extrasystoles (AES) or Atrial Premature Contraction (APC) or Atrial Premature or Ectopic Beats 87
Junctional Premature Contraction 88
Nodal Rhythm (Junctional Rhythm) 88
Wandering Atrial Pacemaker (Wandering Pacemaker) 89
Multifocal Atrial Tachycardia 91
Accelerated Junctional Rhythm 92
Supraventricular Tachycardia (SVT) or Paroxysmal Atrial Tachycardia (PAT) 93
Atrial Tachycardia 97
Normal Ranges and Variations in the Adult ECG 100
An Approach to Interpretation of ECG 102
Nonconducted (Blocked) Atrial Premature Contraction 105
Atrial Tachycardia Associated with Atrioventricular Block 106
Atrial Tachycardia with Aberrant Ventricular Conduction (AVC) 106
Atrial Flutter 107
Atrial Fibrillation 111

Ashman Phenomenon *117*
Ventricular Extrasystoles (VES) or Ventricular Premature Contraction (VPC) or Ventricular Ectopic *118*
Patterns of Ventricular Premature Complex or Ventricular Extrasystole *120*
Ventricular Tachycardia *125*
Nonsustained Ventricular Tachycardia *127*
Sustained Ventricular Tachycardia *127*
Accelerated Idioventricular Rhythm *131*
Torsades de Pointes *133*
Ventricular Flutter *135*
Ventricular Fibrillation *135*
Ventricular Parasystole *138*
Chaotic Ventricular Rhythm *139*
Ventricular Escape Rhythm *139*
Ventricular Standstill (Arrest) or, Cardiac Standstill or Asystole *140*

10. Heart Block — 142
Definition *142*
Classification *143*
Causes of Heart Block *143*
Classification by Degree *143*
Classification by Site/Location *144*
Sinoatrial Block *144*
Sinus Arrest or Sinus Pause or Sinus Standstill *145*
AV Block: First Degree *146*
Atrioventricular Block: Second Degree [Mobitz Type I (Wenckebach)] *147*
AV Block: Second Degree (Mobitz Type II Atrioventricular Block) *148*
Atrioventricular Block: Third Degree (Complete Heart Block) *150*
Stokes-Adams Syndrome (Attack) *153*
Atrioventricular Dissociation (AV Dissociation) *154*
Complete Right Bundle Branch Block *155*
Incomplete Right Bundle Branch Block *156*
Complete Left Bundle Branch Block *157*
Incomplete Left Bundle Branch Block *158*
Left Anterior Fascicular Block or Left Anterior Hemiblock *158*
Left Posterior Fascicular Block or Left Posterior Hemiblock *160*
Intermittent Bundle Branch Block *161*

11. Myocardial Ischemia, Injury, Infarction — 163
Basic Presentation *163*
Insufficient Myocardial Perfusion *164*
Location or Site of Myocardial Ischemia or Infarction *166*
Myocardial Ischemia *168*
Electrocardiographic Phase of Myocardial Infarction *172*
Evolution of Acute MI *173*
Types of MI: Minnesota Criteria *188*
Acute Coronary Syndromes *190*

12. Drugs and Electrolytes Effects   195
Digitalis Effect *195*
Digitalis Toxicity (Digoxin Toxicity) *195*
Quinidine Effects *196*
Potassium Effect *197*
Potassium Effect: Hypokalemia *199*
Calcium Effect *201*
Hypermagnesemia *202*
Hypomagnesemia *202*
ECG Changes Associated with Electrolyte Disturbances *203*

13. Miscellaneous Conditions   204
Hypothermia *204*
Cerebrovascular Accident Pattern *204*
Pericarditis *205*
Pericardial Effusion *207*
Chronic Obstructive Pulmonary Disease *207*
The S_1, S_2, S_3 Syndrome *208*
Pre-excitation Syndromes *209*
Sick Sinus Syndrome (Bradycardia Tachycardia) *214*
Pulmonary Embolism *216*
Dextrocardia *218*
Hyperthyroidism *220*
Hypothyroidism *220*
Electromechanical Dissociation *220*
Early Repolarization Pattern *221*
Juvenile T-wave Pattern *221*
Cardiomyopathy *222*
Ventricular Aneurysm *223*
Emphysema *224*

14. Congenital Heart Diseases   226
Ventricular Septal Defect *226*
Atrial Septal Defect *227*
Patent Ductus Arteriosus *228*
Tetralogy of Fallot *228*
Ebstein's Anomaly *229*
Pulmonary Stenosis (Congenital) *230*

15. Pacemakers and Exercise Tolerance Test   232
Pacemakers *232*
Exercise Tolerance Test (ETT), or Exercise Testing *236*

16. Echocardiogram Interpretation and Diagnosis   239
ECG Interpretation-1 *239*
ECG Interpretation-2 *242*
ECG Diagnosis-1 *250*
ECG Diagnosis-2 *258*

Glossary   *265*

Suggested Reading   *273*

Index   *275*

Abbreviations

ACS	Acute coronary syndrome
AES	Atrial extrasystole
AF	Atrial fibrillation
APC	Atrial premature contraction
AR	Aortic regurgitation
AS	Aortic stenosis
ASD	Atrial septal defect
AV block	Atrioventricular block
AV junction	Atrioventricular junction
AV node	Atrioventricular node
B.D. or b.d.	Twice daily
BP	Blood pressure
CHB	Complete heart block
COPD	Chronic obstructive pulmonary disease
CPR	Cardiopulmonary resuscitation
CVA	Cerebrovascular accident
DC shock	Direct current shock
Dig. toxicity	Digitalis toxicity
ECG	Electrocardiogram
HCM	Hypertrophic cardiomyopathy
HR	Heart rate
IHD	Ischemic heart disease
IM	Intramuscular
Inj	Injection
IV	Intravenous
JPC	Junctional premature contraction
LAD	Left axis deviation
LAFB	Left anterior fascicular block
LAH	Left atrial hypertrophy
LAHB	Left anterior hemiblock
LBBB	Left bundle branch block
LGL syndrome	Lown-Ganong-Levine syndrome
LPFB	Left posterior fascicular block
LPHB	Left posterior hemiblock
LVH	Left ventricular hypertrophy
MAT	Multifocal atrial tachycardia
MR	Mitral regurgitation
MS	Mitral stenosis
mV	Millivolt
PAT	Paroxysmal atrial tachycardia
PDA	Patent ductus arteriosus
q.d.s	Four times daily
RAD	Right axis deviation
RAH	Right atrial hypertrophy

RBBB	Right bundle branch block
RVH	Right ventricular hypertrophy
SA block	Sinoatrial block
SA node	Sinoatrial node
SBE	Subacute bacterial endocarditis
SC	Subcutaneous
SOS	If necessary
SVT	Supraventricular tachycardia
Tab.	Tablet
t.d.s.	Three times daily
TOF	Tetralogy of Fallot
VAT	Ventricular activation time
VES	Ventricular extrasystole
VPC	Ventricular premature contraction
VF	Ventricular fibrillation
VSD	Ventricular septal defect
VT	Ventricular tachycardia
WPW syndrome	Wolff-Parkinson-White syndrome

1

Introduction

DEFINITION

Electrocardiography: It is a diagnostic procedure that graphically records the conduction, magnitude and duration of the electrical current generated by the heart.

Electrocardiograph: It is an instrument utilized to record the surface electrocardiogram (ECG). So, this is a sophisticated galvanometer, a sensitive electromagnet, which can detect and record changes in electromagnetic potential. It consists of:
- *The electrodes:* Located on the patient
- *The cables:* Attached to the electrodes
- An amplifier
- A galvanometer
- *The write of mechanism:* Effected through the galvanometer.

Electrocardiogram (ECG): It is a graphic recording of the electrical potentials or activity produced by cardiac tissue. By the placement of electrodes on selected areas of the body we usually record 12 views of the electrical activity. All four chambers of the heart are represented on this recording.

ECG is a graphic recording of electrical activity of the heart during the various events of cardiac cycle as recorded by placing the suitable electrodes on the surface of the body connecting them with a suitable galvanometer.

Willem Einthoven (1860-1927): Dutch physiologist and physician whose application of the string galvanometer to recording of the electrical activity of the heart lead to the development of clinical electrocardiography.

Augustus Desiré Waller (1856-1922): English physiologist who obtained the first ECG in man using a capillary electrometer.

WHAT TO LOOK FOR IN THE ECG?
(HOW TO REPORT AN ECG?)

1. Name   :   Mr Hassan
2. Age   :   45 yrs
3. Date   :   14th June 2013

4.	Rate	:	110/min
5.	Rhythm	:	Sinus and regular
6.	P-wave	:	Tall and peaked in II, V_1
7.	P-R interval	:	0.28 sec, and constant
8.	QRS complex	:	
	Width	:	0.16 sec in V_1
	Height	:	Tall R in V_1
	Configuration	:	Normal or deep Q in II, III, aVF
9.	ST segment	:	Coved or raised or depression in 1, avL
10.	T-wave	:	Inverted in II, III aVF
11.	U-wave	:	Prominent in leads V_3 – V_6
12.	The cardiac axis	:	–30°
13.	Comments	:	• Sinus tachycardia • P-pulmonale • First degree heart block • Acute myocardial infarction • Right bundle branch block
14.	Additional remarks	:	Suggest exercise tolerance test (ETT)

CLINICAL VALUE OF THE ELECTROCARDIOGRAM

The ECG is of diagnostic value in the following clinical circumstances:
- Atrial and ventricular hypertrophy/chamber enlargement/tachycardia or bradycardia
- Myocardial ischemia and infarction
- Pericarditis
- Systemic diseases that affect the heart
- Determination of the effect of cardiac drugs, especially digitalis and certain antiarrhythmic agents
- Disturbances in electrolyte balance, especially potassium (hypokalemia or hyperkalemia)
- Evaluation of function of cardiac pacemakers
- Analysis of abnormal rhythm.
- Arrhythmias
- Block—first degree block, sinoatrial (SA) block, bundle branch block
- Low voltage—in myxoedema, hypothermia, emphysema
- Exercise ECG to see coronary artery disease

2

Anatomy and Physiology

ANATOMY OF THE HEART (FIG. 2.1)

The heart is a highly specialized muscular organ that contracts rhythmically, pumping the blood through the circulatory system. It consists of four chambers.

1. The right atrium
2. The left atrium   (Upper chamber)
3. The right ventricle
4. The left ventricle   (Lower chamber)

Right and left atrium are separated from each other by interatrial septum, and right and left ventricles are separated by an interventricular septum. The atria communicate with the ventricles through the atrioventricular orifices. The orifice between the right atrium and right ventricle is known as tricuspid orifice which is guarded by the tricuspid valve. The orifice between left atrium and left ventricle is known as mitral orifice which is guarded by mitral or bicuspid valve.

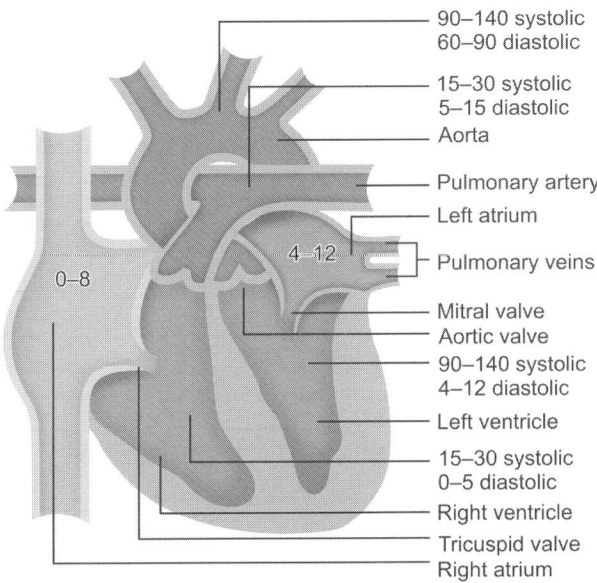

Fig. 2.1 Heart with normal resting pressures in mm Hg

The upper chambers are thin walled and propel blood to the right and left ventricles, respectively. The lower chambers are thick walled. The right ventricle pumps blood into the lungs (pulmonary circulation). The left ventricle pumps blood into body (systemic circulation).

A normal heartbeat consists of contraction of both atria followed by contraction of both ventricles. The orderly process of contraction is initiated and maintained by the hearts electrical forces which are recorded the electrocardiogram (ECG).

Layers of the Heart Wall

- Epicardium
  - External layer of the heart
  - Coronary arteries
  - Blood capillaries lymph capillaries
  - Nerve fibers, nerves and fat are found

- Myocardium
  - Middle and thickest layer of the heart
  - Responsible for hearts pumping action
- Endocardium
  - Innermost layer of the heart
  - Lines hearts inner chambers
  - Valves, chordae tendineae and papillary muscles
  - Continuous with innermost layer of arteries, veins, and capillaries of body

CORONARY CIRCULATION

The coronary arterial system (Fig. 2.2) consists of:
- *Right coronary artery (RCA)*: Starts from anterior aortic sinus
  - SA nodal branch
  - Conus branch
  - Right ventricular branch
  - Right marginal branch
  - Posterior descending (PD) branch
  - AV nodal branch.
- *Left coronary artery (LCA)*: Starts from left posterior aortic sinus
  - Left main artery (LMA)
  - Left circumflex (LCX) artery
  - Left anterior descending (LAD) artery
  - Obtuse marginal branches—from LCX
  - SA nodal branch—from LCX
  - AV nodal branch—from LCX
  - Diagonal branch—from LAD
- *Right coronary artery supplies:*
  - Right atrium and right ventricle
  - Posteroinferior 1/3rd of the interventricular septum
  - Posterior left ventricular wall

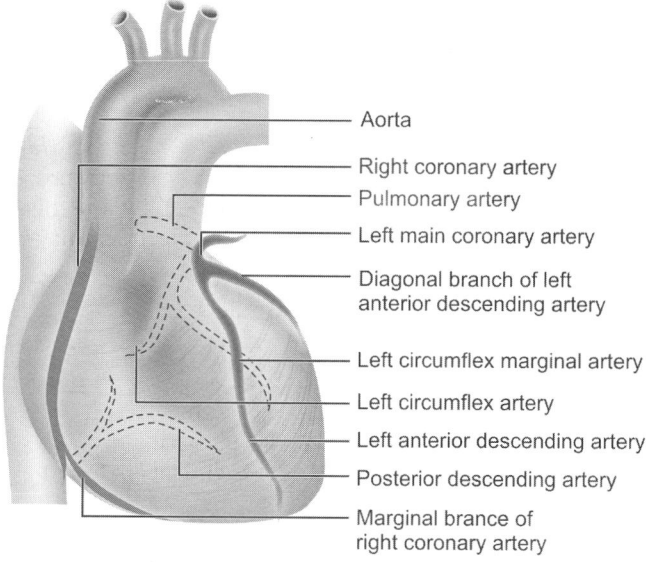

Fig. 2.2 The normal coronary arterial anatomy

- SA node (65%) and AV node (35%)
- Bundle of His (before bifurcation).
- Left coronary artery supplies:
  - Left atrium and left ventricle
  - Anterosuperior 2/3 of the interventricular septum
  - Anterior left ventricular wall
  - Left bundle branch and most of right bundle branch
  - SA node (80%), AV node (20%).

Coronary Arteries

Coronary artery and its branches	Portion of myocardium supplied	Portion of conduction system supplied
Right CA Posterior descending	Right atrium right ventricle	SA node (60%)
Right marginal	Inferior surface of LV (85%). Posterior surface of LV (85%)	AV node (85–90). Proximal portion of bundle of His. Part of posterior-inferior fascicle of LBB.
Left CA Anterior descending (LAD)	Anterior surface of LV. Part of lateral surface of LV. Most of the interventricular septum	Most of RBB. Anterior superior fascicle of LBB. Part of posterior-inferior fascicle of LBB.
Left circumflex A (LCX)	Left atrium. Part of lateral surface of LV inferior surface of LV (15%). Posterior surface of LV (15%)	

CONDUCTIVE SYSTEM OF THE HEART (JUNCTIONAL TISSUES OF THE HEART) (FIG. 2.3)

The normal site of impulse formation in the heart is SA (sino-atrial) node. The atria are then depolarized. The impulse then spreads thought the AV (atrioventricular) node and bundle of His to the left bundle branch (LBB) and right bundle branch (RBB) and then to the ventricular muscle through the Purkinje fibers, leading to ventricular depolarization.

Atria Conducting System (Table 2.1)

Primary pacemaker of the heart (SA node) is located in the upper part of the right atrium SA node initiates 60–100 beats/min. The impulses travel thought 3 main internodal conduction pathways named anterior, middle and posterior, in and around both atria and in a pathway called 'Bachmann's bundle' leading to the left atrium. Stimulation of the slower-conduction muscle cells of both atria produces P wave in the ECG. The P wave represents electrical excitation of the atrial muscle cells.

Electrical impulses enter the AV node junction which acts as a way station, a delay area where impulses from both atria are slowed down. This delay gives time for the atria to contract and propel (kick) their contents into their respective ventricles.

Ventricular Conducting System

After the brief delay in the AV node, the impulses proceed down in the bundle of His which divides into two pathways: RBB, which traverses the right ventricles, and LBB, which

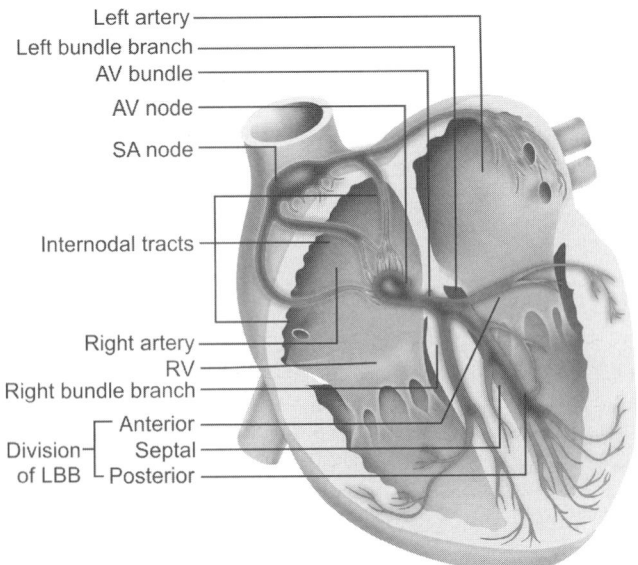

Fig. 2.3 The conductive system of the heart

Anatomy and Physiology

Table 2.1 | Summary of the conduction system

Structure	Location	Function	Intrinsic pacemaker
SA node	RT atrial wall just inferior to opening of superior vena cava (SVC)	Primary pacemaker initiates impulse that is normally conducted throughout the LT and RT atria	60–100 bpm
AV node	Floor of the RT atrium immediately behind the tricuspid valve and near the opening of the coronary sinus	Receives impulse from SA node and delays relay of the impulse to the bundle of His	
Bundle of His	Superior portion of interventricular septum	Receives impulse from AV node and relays to RT and LT bundle branch	40–60 bpm
RT and LT bundle branches	Interventricular septum	Impulse from bundle of His and relays it to Purkinje fibers	
Purkinje fibers	Ventricular myocardium	Impulse from bundle branch and relays to ventricular myocardium	20–40 bpm

traverses left ventricles. Automatic firing rate of bundle of his is 40–60 beats/min.

The LBB divides into anterior and posterior fascicles which supply the anterior superior and posterior inferior regions of the left ventricle, respectively.

Both LBB and RBB divided into smaller branches and finally into terminal conducting system in the ventricles called Purkinje cells, whose firing rate 15–40 beats/min.

From the Purkinje cells, the muscle cells of both ventricles are stimulated, which produces the QRS complex in the ECG. The QRS complex represents electrical excitation of the ventricular muscles cells.

Impulse Formation and Conduction

In this process, three types of heart cells are involved:
1. *Pacemaker cells:* SA node, which initiates electrical impulses, at first.
2. *Specialized conducting cells:* Conduct electrical impulse, e.g. SA node, atrial internodal pathways, AV node, bundle of His, LBB, left anterior and posterior fascicles, Purkinje fibers.
3. *Muscle cells:* Have the functions of electrical conduction and mechanical contraction which produces the normal heart beat.

SEQUENCE OF HEART ACTIVATION

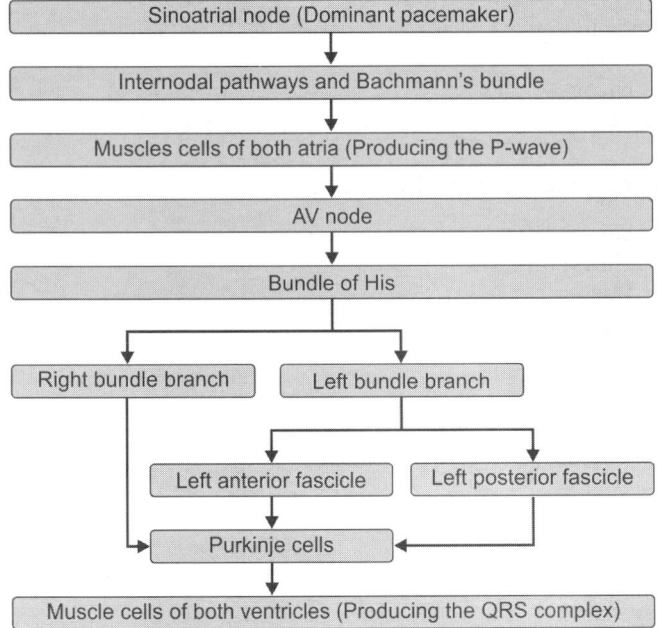

Note: Sinus rhythm: The normal heart rhythm with electrical activation beginning in the SA node, is called sinus rhythm if any disturbance of this sequence occurs, there is rhythm disturbance, called arrhythmia or abnormality of conduction, called heart block.

PROPERTIES OF CARDIAC CELLS

The inherent properties are:
- *Autorhythmicity:* Ability to spontaneously initiate and it maintain a rhythmic beat completely independent of neurologic input.
- *Conductivity:* Ability to conduct impulses to next cells.
- *Excitability:* Ability to respond to a stimulus inherent in both pacemaker and no-pacemaker cells.
- *Contractility:* Ability to contract after depolarization.
- Refractory period.

NERVE SUPPLY OF THE HEART

The heart is supplied by both:
- Parasympathetic nerve
- Sympathetic nerve

in cardiac plexus

Parasympathetic

Inhibitory nerve fibers supply the SA node, atrial muscle and AV junction of the heart by means of the vagus nerves.

Acetylcholine is a chemical messenger (neurotransmitter) that is released when parasympathetic nerves are stimulated. It binds to parasympathetic receptors Nicotinic and muscarinic receptors.

Nicotinic receptors are located in skeletal muscle. Muscarinic receptors are located in smooth muscle.

Parasympathetic Stimulation

- Slows the rate of discharge of the SA node
- Slows conduction through the AV node
- Decreases the strength of atrial contraction
- Can cause a small decrease in the force of ventricular contraction.

Sympathetic: Adrenergic receptors sites are alpha receptors, beta and dopaminergic receptors. Dopaminergic receptor sites are located in the coronary arteries, renal, mesenteric and visceral blood vessels stimulation of dopaminergic receptor sites results in dilatation.

Sympathetic (accelerator) nerves supply specific areas of the hearts electrical system, atrial muscle and ventricular myocardium.

When this nerves are stimulated norepinephrine is released. Then it results:

- Increased force of contraction
- Increased heart rate
- Increased BP.

3

Electrocardiographic Leads

DEFINITION

A lead is a graphic illustration of the electrical potential difference between two points on the skin surface that is being transmitted by the heart during the cardiac cycle.

Standard ECG (Fig. 3.1) consists of 12 different leads to provide a complete picture of the heart's electrical activity.

TYPES OF LEADS

Types: The conventional ECG records 12 leads. These 12 leads consists of the following:
- *The frontal plane leads*—are orientated in the frontal or coronal of the body, and consists of six limb or extremity leads:
    – Standard or bipolar limb leads (Table 3.1)
        - Lead I
        - Lead II
        - Lead III
    – Augmented unipolar limb leads (Table 3.2)
        - Lead aVR
        - Lead aVL
        - Lead aVF.

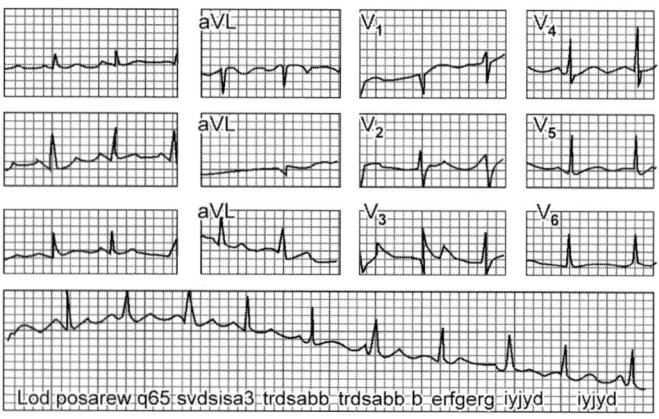

Fig. 3.1 A normal ECG

Table 3.1 | Standard limb leads

Lead	Positive electrode	Negative electrode	Heart surface viewed
Lead I	Left arm	Right arm	Lateral
Lead II	Left leg	Right arm	Inferior
Lead III	Left leg	Left arm	Inferior

Table 3.2 | Augmented leads

Lead	Positive electrode	Heart surface viewed
aVR	Right arm	None
aVL	Left arm	Lateral
aVF	Left leg	Inferior

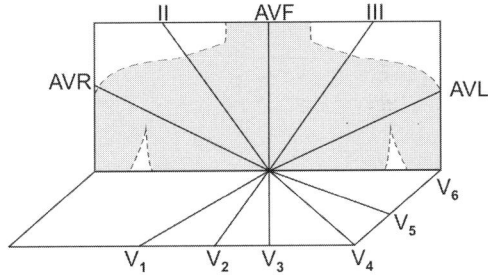

Fig. 3.2 Basic orientation of the frontal and horizontal plane leads

- *The horizontal plane leads*—are orientated in the transverse or horizontal plane of the body and formed by unipolar chest or precordial leads:
  Lead V_1 to Lead V_6 (V_1, V_2 V_3 V_4 V_5 V_6) (Fig. 3.2).

ELECTRODE PLACEMENT OF THE STANDARD LEADS

The standard leads are derived from electrodes placed on the right arm, left arm, left leg. The right leg electrode as a grounding electrode.

Lead I: Lead records difference of potential or electrical activity by connecting the negative electrode on the right arm (RA) and the positive electrode on the left arm (LA) (Fig. 3.3).

Lead II: Records electrical activity by connecting the negative electrodes on the right arm (RA) and the positive electrode on the left leg (LL) (Fig. 3.4).

Lead III: Difference of potential between the negative electrode of the left arm (LA) and the positive electrode on the left leg (LL) (Fig. 3.5).

The lead axis of these 3 leads form a equilateral triangle with the heart of the center (Fig. 3.6). This is Einthoven's triangle'.

12 ECG for Medical Diagnosis

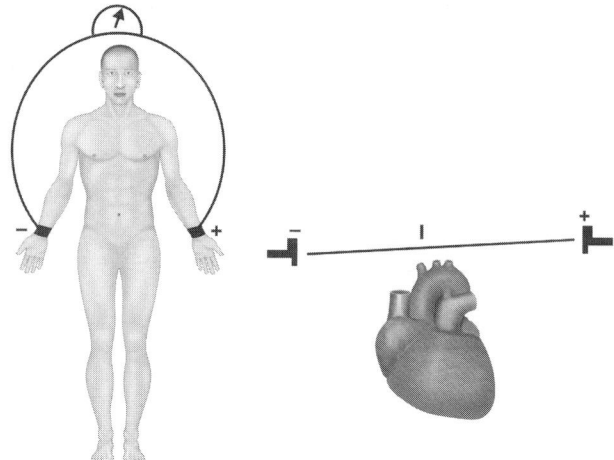

Fig. 3.3 Electrode placement of standard lead I

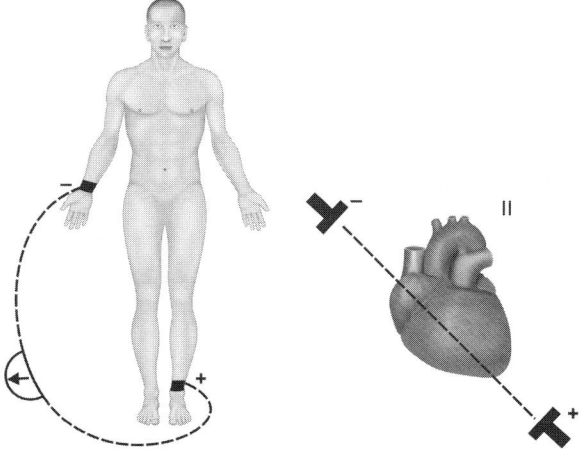

Fig. 3.4 Electrode placement of standard lead II

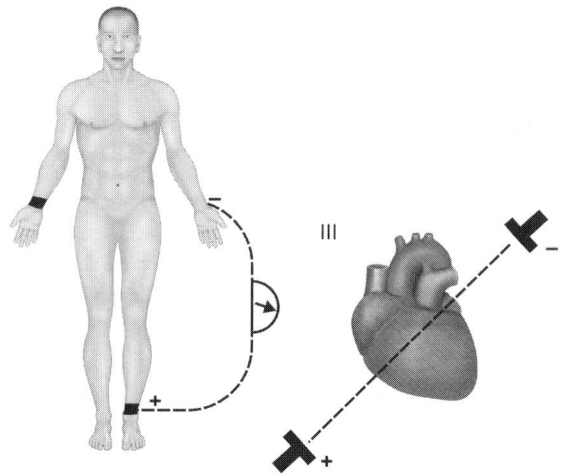

Fig. 3.5 Electrode placement of standard lead III

Electrocardiographic Leads

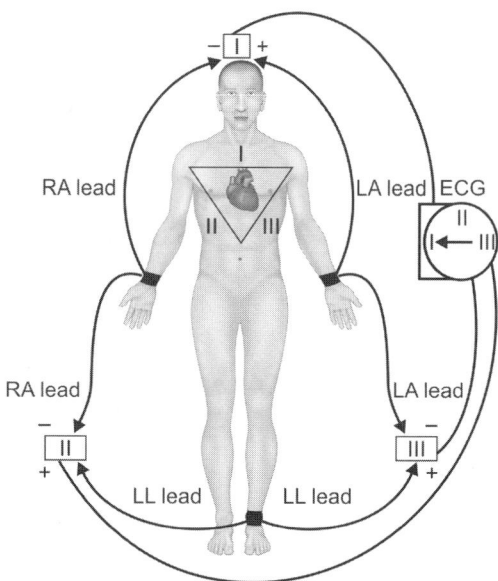

Fig. 3.6 Connection for limb leads

Triaxial Reference System (Fig. 3.7)

The Einthoven's triangle may be converted into a Triaxial system' by bringing the sides of the triangle to the common center.

Solid lines represent positive half of each lead whereas the broken lines, negative half. In assigning degrees to the triaxial reference system, the axis are 60° apart.

View of the Heart

- Lead I — A reflection of the lateral wall of the heart
- Lead II
- Lead III — Reflection of the inferior wall of the heart.

Augmented Unipolar Limb Leads (Figs 3.8A and B)

- Only one pole, positive, is attached to each limb, the negative is connected to a central terminal.
- Lead aVR—is the augmented unipolar right arm lead and is orientated to the heart from the right shoulder.
- Lead aVL—is the augmented unipolar left arm lead and is orientated to the heart from the left shoulder.
- Lead aVF—is the augmented unipolar left leg lead.

View of the Heart

- *aVR:* Provide cavity of the heart. Thus, all the deflexions—the p, QRS, T deflexions are normally negative in this lead.

14 ECG for Medical Diagnosis

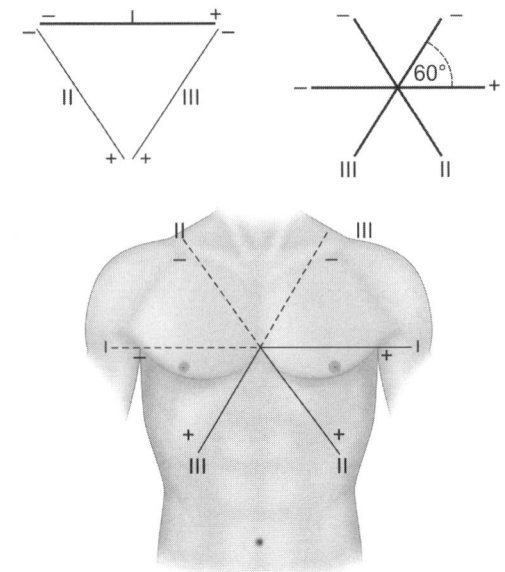

Fig. 3.7 Triaxial reference system

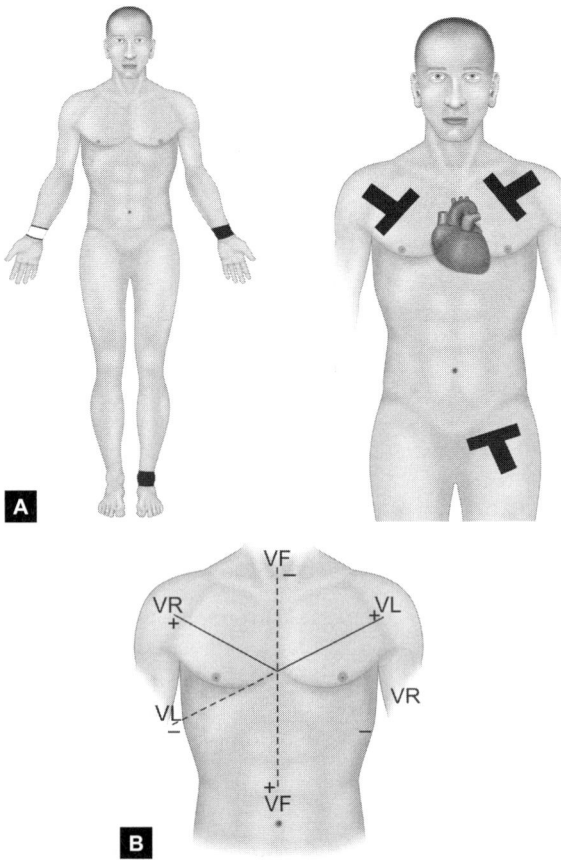

Figs 3.8A and B Unipolar limb leads

- *aVL:* A reflection of the anterolateral or lateral or superior surface of the left ventricle.
- *aVF:* A reflection of the inferior surface of the left ventricle.

Hexaxial Reference System (Fig. 3.9)

Lead I, lead II, lead III, aVR, aVL, aVF form a hexaxial system. The solid line represents the positive ends of the six limb leads. The broken line represents the negative ends.

An increase in the R wave with decrease in the S wave is normally seen from V_1-V_6.

View of the Heart

- Lead V_1-V_6 : Indicate anterior surface of the heart.
- Lead V_1-V_4 : Indicate anteroseptal wall.
- Lead V_5-V_6 : Indicate anterolateral wall.

REPRESENTATION OF THE SURFACE OF THE HEART BY ELECTRODE

- Lead I and Lead aVL : High or superior left lateral wall
- Lead II, Lead III, Lead aVF : Inferior surface of the heart
- Lead aVR : Cavity of the heart
- Lead V_1 : Cavity of the heart
- Lead V_1-V_6 : Anterior wall of the heart
- Lead V_1-V_4 : Anteroseptal wall
- Lead V_5-V_6 : Anterolateral or apical or lateral wall
- Lead I, aVL, V_5 to V_6 : Left-orientated leads
- Lead II, Lead III, aVF, L1, aVL, V_5-V_6 : Inferolateral wall

Note: There is no lead which is orientated directly to the posterior wall of the heart. The part of the circle used most frequently in clinical ECG contains:

- Positive lead I + 0°
- Positive lead aVL - 30°

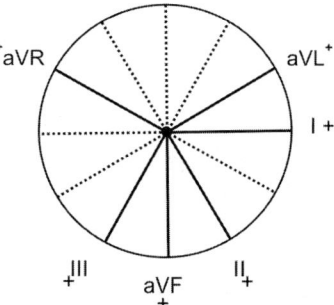

Fig. 3.9 Hexaxial reference system

- Positive lead aVR − 150°
- Positive lead II + 60°
- Positive lead III + 120°
- Positive lead aVF + 90°

Chest or Precordial Leads Placement (Fig. 3.10)

These leads are V_1, V_2, V_3, V_4 V_5, V_6, which are derived from six electrodes placed on the chest in designated areas (Fig. 3.11). The chest electrodes sites are as follows:
- V_1 : 4th intercostals space, right sternal border—heart surface septum
- V_2 : 4th intercostals space, left sternal border—heart surface septum
- V_3 : Midway between V_2 and V_4—Heart surface anterior
- V_4 : 5th intercostals space, left midclavicular line-Heart surface anterior
- V_5 : At the same horizontal level as lead V_4 but on the left anterior axillary line—heart surface lateral
- V_6 : At the same horizontal level as lead V_5 but on the left mid axillary line—heart surface lateral

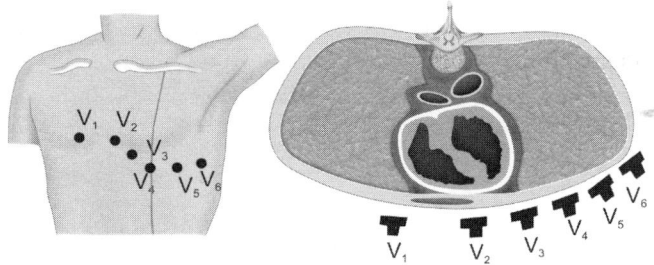

Fig. 3.10 Electrode placement of the chest leads

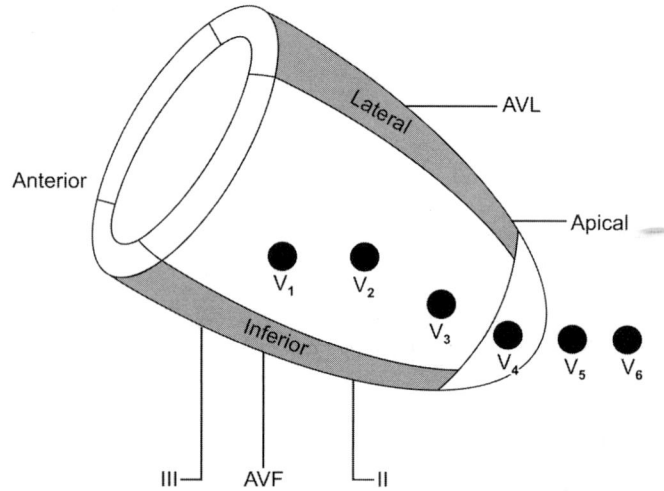

Fig. 3.11 Representation of the six limb leads

Electrodes V_1 and V_2 overlie the right ventricles. V_4, V_5, V_6 overlie of the ventricles and V_3 overlies the interventricular septum.

Now, right-sided chest leads are:
- V_1R : 4th intercostal space to left of sternum
- V_2R : 4th intercostal space to right of sternum
- V_3R : Point mid-way between V_2R and V_4R
- V_4R : 5th intercostal space in midclavicular line, and so on.

These leads are particularly useful for the assessment of the right ventricle.

R-WAVE PROGRESSION

Introduction

Each chest or precordial lead records in a unipolar fashion. Each records the hearts electrical forces in reference to a central terminal.

The left ventricle is larger of the two ventricles and lies to the left and behind the right ventricle. The chest electrodes record depolarization of the ventricles (QRS complexes) that become progressively more positive from the gradual increase in the positive QRS deflections from lead V_1-V_6 is known as R-wave progression.

'Poor R-wave progression' signifies that the QRS deflection is predominantly negative in lead V_1-V_4 and positive in V_5-V_6.

Causes of R-wave Progression (Fig. 3.12)

- Anterior or anteroseptal MI
- Left bundle branch block (LBBB)
- Chronic obstructive pulmonary disease (COPD)
- Left ventricular hypertrophy (though R is tall in most case)
- Dextrocardia
- Cardiomyopathy
- Left-sided pneumothorax
- Left-sided pleural effusion (massive)
- Chest electrode placed incorrectly
- Deformity of the chest wall
- Marked clockwise rotation
- Normal variation.

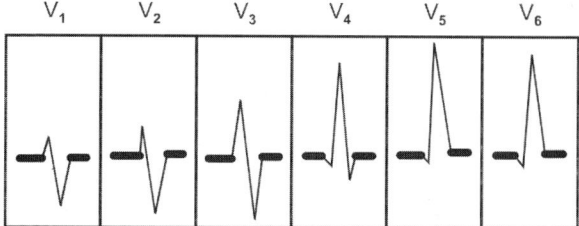

Fig. 3.12 Normal R-wave progression in chest leads

4

Essential Basic Electrocardiogram Principles

THE BASIC ACTION: DEPOLARIZATION AND REPOLARIZATION

In a healthy resting cardiac cell, certain molecules dissociates into positive and negative ions. The positively charged ions are on the outer surface and the negatively charged ions on the inner surface of the cell membrane. The positive charges are equal in number to the negative charges. When this occurs, the cell is in a state of electrical balance, named polarized or resting state (Fig. 4.1).

When two electrical charges of equal and opposite direction, i.e. one positive ion and one negative ion, are juxtaposed on either side of a membrane, they constitute a 'dipole' (Fig. 4.2).

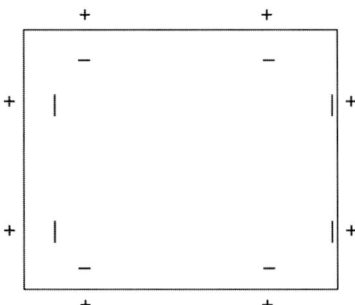

Fig. 4.1 A polarized or resting cell

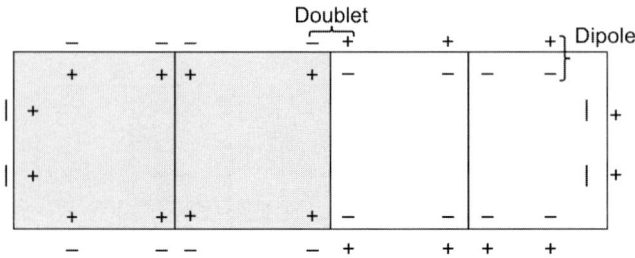

Fig. 4.2 Doublet and dipole

When two charged ions of equal and opposite direction are situated next to each other on the surface of an excitable tissue, they constitute a 'Doublet'.

When the cell is stimulated or injured, the negative ions migrate to the outer surface of the cell and the positive charges pass into the cell, i.e. the polarity is reversed. This process is 'depolarization' (Fig. 4.3).

With recovery, positive charges return to the outer surface and negative charges migrate into the cell. This process is 'Repolarization', i.e. the polarity or electrical balance of the cell is reestablished.

So each heart beat is comprised of two electrical processes depolarization and repolarization.

At first, cardiac cells remain in resting state. Then cells are activated to contract during depolarization. Depolarization is followed by repolarization, return to the resting electrical state but repolarization or 'recharging' is necessary before depolarization can recur. If cells are not allowed to repolarize fully (return in resting state) the cells will be 'refractory' to the next electrical impulse. In other words, the depolarized cells are unable to the stimulated to contract again until they are repolarized (Fig. 4.4).

What is Depolarization?

Depolarization: It means initial spread of the stimulus through the muscle causing activation or contraction.

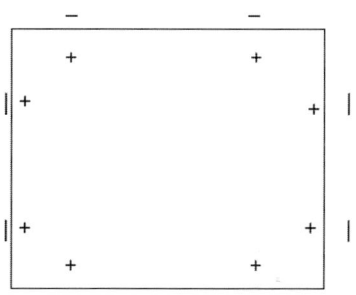

Fig. 4.3 A depolarized or activated cell

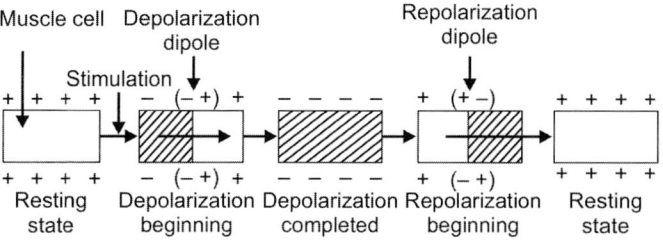

Fig. 4.4 Depolarization and repolarization in a single muscle cell

What is Repolarization?

Repolarization: It means return of the stimulated muscle to the resting state (recovery from activation or contraction).

RECORDING DEPOLARIZATION AND REPOLARIZATION

ECG Deflections

The ECG records the electrical processes of depolarization and repolarization for each heart beat. Upon electrical stimulation, depolarization is represented by a dipole (pair of electrical charges) consisting of a positive (+) charge followed by a negative (-) charge. As repolarization, with a negative (-) charge followed by a positive (+) charge.

When an electromagnetic force (current vector, activation front, depolarization front) flows, or is directed, towards the positive electrode of a lead, the electrocardiograph will record an 'upward' or positive deflection (Figs 4.5A and B).

When this force flows away from the positive electrode of a lead and thus towards the negative electrode, then it will be recorded as a 'downward or negative deflection' (Figs 4.6A and B).

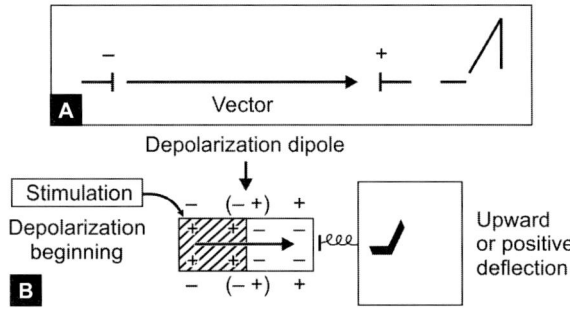

Figs 4.5A and B (A) Positive deflection; (B) Upward (positive) deflection

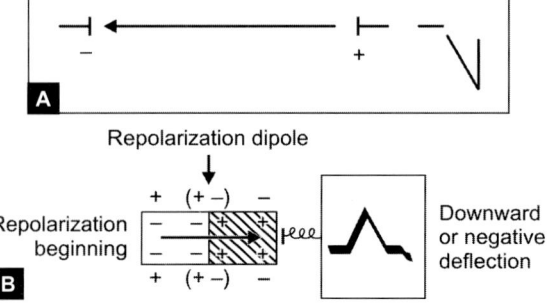

Figs 4.6A and B (A) Negative deflection; (B) Downward (negative) deflection

Essential Basic Electrocardiogram Principles

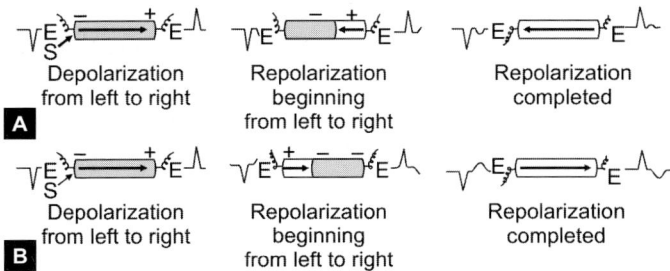

Figs 4.7A and B (A) Depolarization from left to right and repolarization in the opposite direction; (B) Depolarization form left to right and repolarization in the same direction

So, an electrode that faces the positive side of the depolarization dipole records 'positive deflection'.

And same electrode that faces the negative side of the repotarization dipole, records 'negative' deflexion.

Depolarization (electrical stimulation) cannot occur until repolarization (return to the resting state) is completed (Figs 4.7A and B).

Both electrical processes occur in the atria and ventricles and are recorded in the ECG.

5

Normal Electrocardiogram

BASIC SHAPE OF THE NORMAL ELECTROCARDIOGRAM (FIG. 5.1)

- P, Q, R, S, T, U deflection are all called 'waves'
- Q, R, S waves together make up a 'complex'
- The interval between the S-wave and T-wave is called the ST 'segment'.

The ECG consists of:
- Waves, complex
    - P-wave
    - QRS complex—Q, R, S-wave
    - T-wave
    - U-wave.
- Intervals
    - P-R interval
    - R-R interval
    - Q-T interval
    - P-P interval
    - QRS interval and ventricular activation time (VAT).
- Segments
    - S-T segment
    - P-R segment.

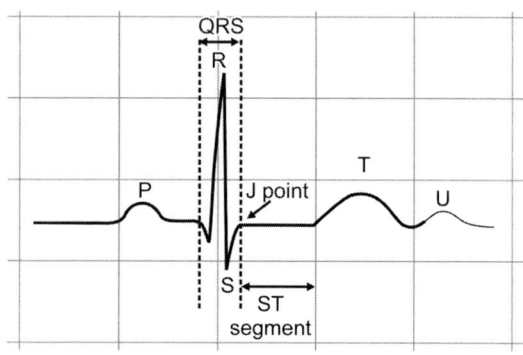

Fig. 5.1 Normal electrocardiogram deflection

Junctions

J-junction.

Waves and Complexes (Fig. 5.2)

Atrial Activation

P-wave: Depolarization of right and left atria.

Ventricular Activation

- *Q-wave*: Initial negative deflection resulting from ventricular depolarization.
- *R-wave*: First positive deflection produced by ventricular depolarization.
- *S-wave*: First negative deflection of ventricular depolarization.
- *QRS complex*: Depolarization of right and left ventricles. Ventricular repolarization.
- *T-wave*: Repolarization of right and left ventricles.
- *U-wave*: Not always seen, when present, it follows T-wave and represents late repolarization.

Points

- The ventricles contain the majority of the heart muscle or mass and this is the reason, the complex is much larger than the P-wave.

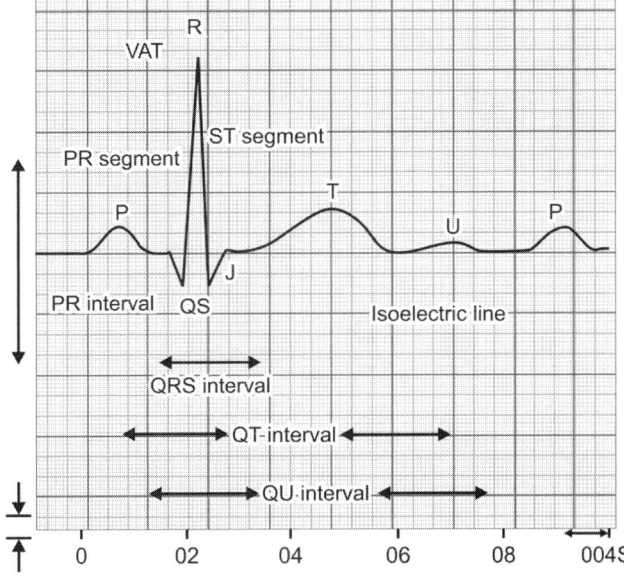

Fig. 5.2 Electrocardiographic complexes, interval and segments

- The deflection representing of the atria is small and is buried in the much large QRS complex (Fig. 5.3).

Intervals

- *P-R interval*: Interval between the onset of the P-wave and the onset of the QRS complex.
- *P-R interval*: Interval between two consecutive R-wave.
- *Q-T interval*: Interval between the onset of the Q-wave and the end of T-wave, and represents the duration of electrical systole.
- *P-P interval*: Interval between two consecutive P-wave.
- *QRS interval or duration*: Represents the ventricular depolarization time. It is measured from the onset of the Q-wave (or R wave) to the termination of the S-wave.
- *Ventricular activation time (VAT)*: Interval measured from the beginning of the Q-wave to the peak of the R-wave (Fig. 5.4).

Segments

- *ST segment*: Portion of the tracing from the j-point to the onset of the T-wave.
- *PR segment*: Portion of the tracing from the end of the P-wave to the onset of the QRS complex.

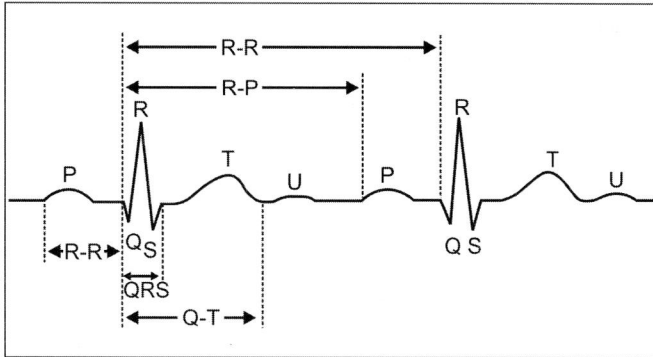

Fig. 5.3 Electrocardiogram complexes

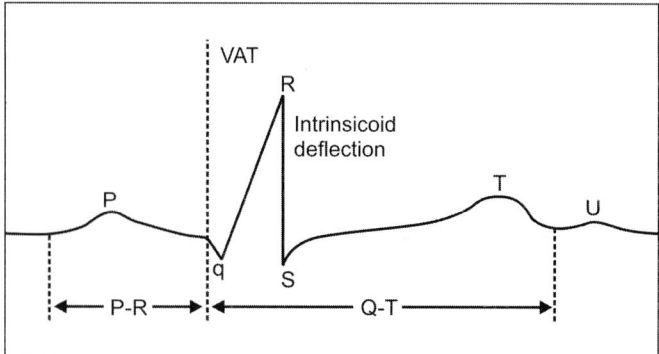

Fig. 5.4 Ventricular activation time

J-point (RST Junction)

The point at which the QRS complex ends and the ST segment begins.

Note:
- Vertricles contain majority of the heart muscles (Left ventricle contains more than the right). So, QRS is larger than P-wave.
- Atrial repolarization is small and is buried in QRS, so it is not seen in ECG (No wave is seen due to atrial repolarization in ECG).

VARIOUS FORMS OF THE QRS COMPLEX (FIG. 5.5)

The QRS complex reflects ventricular activation or depolarization. This complex can have various configuration. A capital or large letter (Q, R, S) denotes a large deflection. A small letter (Q, R, S) denotes a small deflection.

- *rS complex*: Small initial r wave followed by large S-wave.
- *RS complex*: A complex with an R- and S-wave of equal amplitudes.
- *Rs complex*: A large R-wave followed by small S-wave.
- *R-wave complex*: A single wave complex which is positive.
- *qRS complex*: Small initial downward deflection followed by a tall upward deflection which is followed by a large terminal downward deflection.
- *Qr complex*: Deep and wide initial negative deflection followed by a small terminal positive.
- *QS complex*: A complex with complete negative.
- *rSr' complex*: An rS complex followed by small terminal positive.
- *rSR' complex:* An rS complex followed by tall terminal positive.
- *RR' complex:* When deflexion is completely positive and notched.

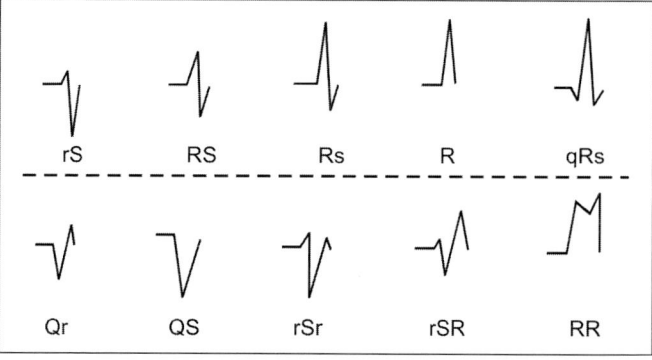

Fig. 5.5 Various forms of the ORS deflexions and their nomenclature

ELECTROCARDIOGRAM PAPER (FIG. 5.6)

The ECG paper is divided into small and large squares.
One small square = 1 mm = 0.04 sec
One large square = 5 mm sq = 0.04 × 5 = 0.2 sec
So, 0.2 sec = 5 mm

$$1 \text{ second} = \frac{5}{0.2} = \frac{10 \times 5}{2} = 25 \text{ mm}$$

The ECG is recorded at a paper speed of 25 mm/sec. So, 5 large squares 25 mm represent one second.

The squares from a grid which facilitates the measurement of:
- Time parameters (horizontal measurement).
- Deflection amplitudes (vertical measurement).

The vertical direction in the ECG measures voltage. Each small box equals 0.1 mV, 1 mm of height, when the ECG is standardized to the conventional 10 mm of height (1 mV) and this 'calibration' signal should be included with every record.

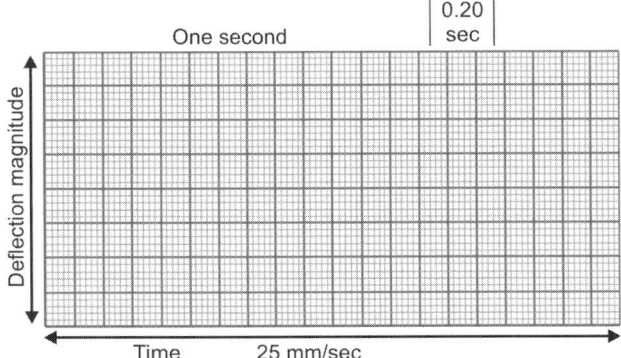

Fig. 5.6 The electrocardigram paper

CALIBRATION (FIG. 5.7)

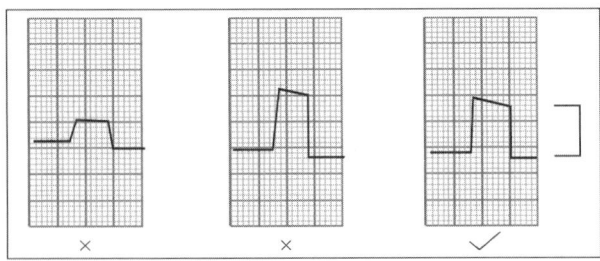

Fig. 5.7 Diagram of calibration

NORMAL ELECTROCARDIOGRAM MEASUREMENTS

Amplitude and Duration

- *P-wave*: Amplitude—not exceed 2-2.5 mm in height
  Duration—0.08-0.12 sec
  Duration—no longer than 0.10 sec
- *QRS complex:*
  - *P-R interval*: Duration—0.12-0.20 s
  - *R-R interval (Fig. 5.8)*:
    R-R interval of 0.2 sec = heart rate of 300/minute
    R-R interval of 0.4 sec = heart rate of 150/minute
    R-R interval of 0.6 sec = heart rate of 100/minute

Q-T interval: Varies inversely with heart rate (HR)
  if HR 40,   Q-T = 0.49-0.50 sec
  if HR 50,   Q-T = 0.45-0.47 sec
  if HR 60,   Q-T = 0.42-0.43 sec
  if HR 70,   Q-T = 0.35-0.36 sec
  if HR 90,   Q-T = 0.35-0.36 sec
  if HR 100,   Q-T = 0.33-0.34 sec

Ventricular activation time (VAT) (R-wave peak time): 0.03-0.05 sec.

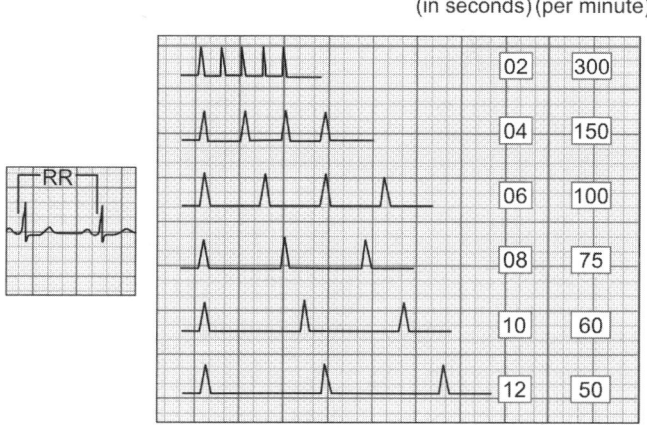

Fig. 5.8 RR interval

MAKING A RECORDING (FIG. 5.9)

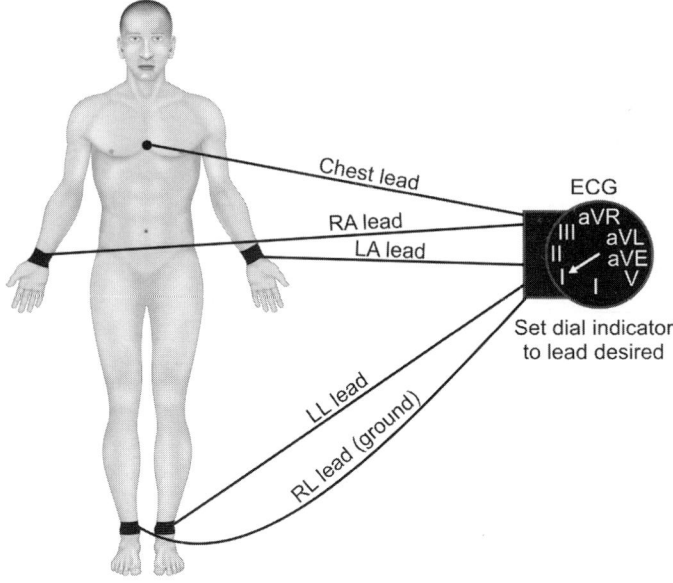

Fig. 5.9 Recording of leads

When Making a Recording

- The patient must lie down and relax (to prevent muscle tremor)
- Connect up the limb electrodes, making certain that they are applied to the correct limb
- Calibrate the record with the 1 mV signal
- Record the six standard leads—3-4 complexes are sufficient for each
- Record the six V leads.

HEART RATE DETERMINATION (FIGS 5.10 TO 5.12)

Heart rate can be readily determined from the ECG. It determines the atrial and the ventricular heart rate.

- *Method-1*: If cardiac rhythm is regular.
  - 1500 method:
    0.04 sec = 1 small sq
    0.02 sec = 5 small sq
    1 s = 25 small sq
    1 minute = 25 × 60 = 1500 small sq

$$\text{Heart rate (HR)} = \frac{1500}{\text{No of small sq between R-R or P-P interval}} \text{ per minute}$$

$$\left[\begin{array}{l} \text{Example: R-R or P-P interval} = 20 \text{ small sq} \\ \text{Then, HR} = \frac{1500}{20} = 75 \text{ beats/minute} \end{array} \right]$$

Normal Electrocardiogram

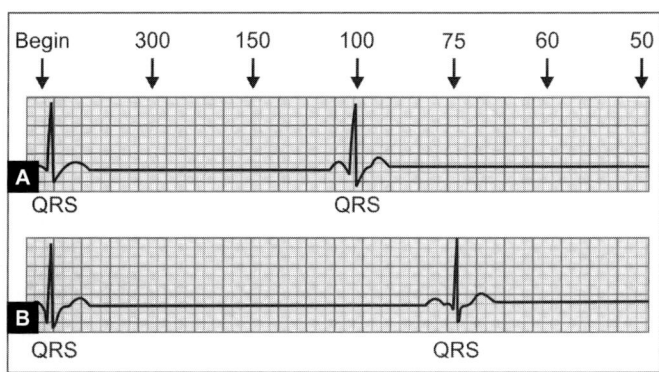

Figs 5.10A and B Determination of heart rate, counting from initial R-wave to next R-wave: (A) three large squares, heart rate is 100 beats/minute; (B) four large squares, heart rats is 75 beats/minute

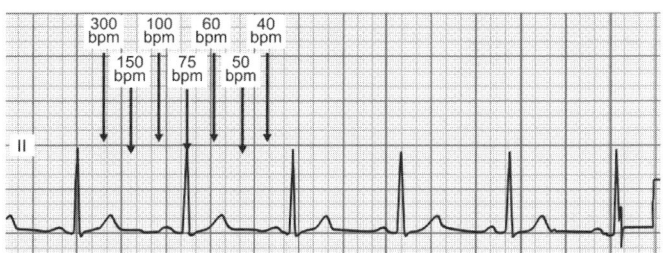

Fig. 5.11 Lead II beats/ minute

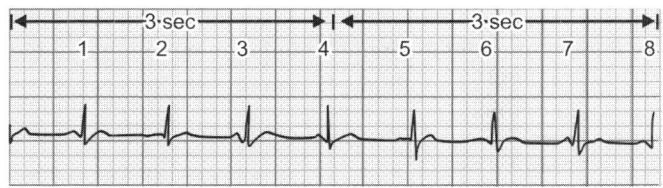

Fig. 5.12 The 8 QRS complexes within a 6 sec interval

- *300 method*:
  1 sec = 25 small sq = 5 large sq
  1 minute = 5 × 60 = 300 large sq

  $$HR = \frac{300}{\text{No of small sq between R-R or P-P interval}} \text{ per minute}$$

  if R-R or P-P interval is:
  1 large sq,   HR is 300 beats/minute
  2 large sq,   HR is 150 beats/minute
  3 large sq,   HR is 100 beats/minute
  4 large sq,   HR is 75 bears/minute
  5 large sq,   HR is 60 beats/minute
  6 large sq,   HR is 50 beats/minute

- *Atrial rate*: Count the number of squares between p-p interval.

- *Ventricular rate*: Count the number of squares between R-R interval.
- *Method-II*: If cardiac rhythm is irregular.
  - *Times 10:*
    HR = Number of cardiac cycle in 6 sec (between 30 large sq) 10 per minute.
    Example, No of cardiac cycle (R or p) in second is 8. Then, HR = 8 × 10 = 80 beats/minute.
  - *Time 20:*
    HR = Number of cardiac cycle in 3 sec (between 15 large sq) × 20 per minute.

STANDARDIZATION OF ELECTROCARDIOGRAM

1. Normally, 1 mv current - 10 mm height (10 small square)
2. Half strength - 5 mm
3. Double strength - 20 mm
4. Recording speed - 25 mm/sec
   (i.e. 1500 mm/minute)

ECG Conventions and Intervals

- *Depolarization towards the electrode*: Positive deflection (above the iso electric line)
- *Depolarization away from the electrode*: Negative deflection (below the isoelectric line)
- Sensitivity = 10 mm = 1 mv
- Paper speed = 25 mm/sec
- Each large square (5 mm) = 0.2 sec
- Each small square (1 mm) = 0.04 sec
- Normal standardization = 10 mm
- Rhythm = interval between two RR.

Cause of Low Voltage ECG Tracing

- Incorrect standardization (i.e. if <10 mm)
- Thick chest wall
- Obesity
- Pericardial effusion
- Chronic constrictive pericarditis
- Myxoedema
- Emphysema
- Hypothermia
- Dilated cardiomyopathy (DCM).

Criteria of Low Voltage Tracing

- In standard limb leads: QRS <5 mm (mainly the R-wave)
- In chest leads—QRS <10 mm (mainly the R-wave).

Note:
- If ryhthm disturbance—
  - Long rhythm strip (L_{11}) should be taken
- If strong arrhythmia—
  - Holter monitor ECG.

Heart Rhythm

- If RR interval is equal—
  - Regular rhythm
- If RR interval is irregular—
  - Irregular rhythm.

Cause of Irregular Rhythm

- *Physiological*: Sinus arrhythmia
- *Pathological*
  - Atrial fibrillation
  - Atrial flutter
  - Ectopic beat
  - SA block
  - Sinus arrest
  - Atrial tachycardia with block
  - 2° HB
  - Ventricular fibrillation.

Characters of Sinus Rhythm

- P-wave is of sinus origin
- P and QRS are regular (p-p and R-R constant and identical)
- Constant P configuration in a given lead
- PR and QRS interval—within normal limit
- *Rate*: 60–100 bpm.

6

Axis and Vectors

AXIS

The axis of the heart is a term used to describe the mean direction and magnitude of all electrical impulses generated by the heart during cardiac cycle in relation to the frontal plane of the body.
- Mean axis : Major direction of the depolarization forces in the atria
- Mean QRS axis : Major direction of depolarization forces in the ventricles (Fig. 6.1)
- Mean T axis : Major direction of the repolarization
- Mean ST axis : Forces in the ventricles

The mean QRS axis is the major direction which expressed as degrees on the hexaxial reference system.

This direction can be altered by many causes:
- Hypertrophy of the ventricles
- Conduction blocks in the ventricles
- Myocardial infarction
- Chronic obstructive pulmonary disease (COPD)—chronic bronchitis, emphysema
- Pre-excitation syndromes.

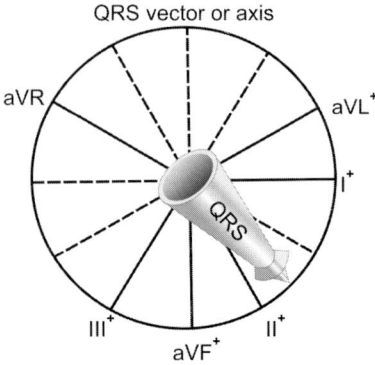

Fig. 6.1 Normal mean QRS axis or vector

VECTOR

It designates all of the electromotive forces of the cardiac cycle. It is a graphic method of representing the direction and magnitude of the hearts electrical forces using arrows instead of wave forms (Fig. 6.2).

A vector has:
1. Magnitude – Amount of electrical force.
2. Direction – Which way the force travels.
3. Polarity   – Positive and negative ends.

Graphically,
- A vector shows   – An arrow
- Magnitude shows   – The length of the arrow
- Direction shows   – Position of the arrow
- Polarity   – Tip of the arrow shows positive end
                        Tail of the arrow shows negative end
- Mean P-wave vector   Depolarization
- Mean ORS vector   Forces
- ST vector   Repolarization forces
- T vector

When, in the 12 lead ECG, P, QRS, ST wave—represent by vectors. On hexaxial reference system, these vectors are projected and represent P, QRS, ST, T-axis.

Instantaneous vector: It represents the net electrical forces generated by the heart at a given instant.

QRS AXIS

When the ventricles are depolarized, multiple small instantaneous vectors are present. The mean QRS vector or mean QRS axis is the average of these small instantaneous vectors. This vector (QRS) represents the main direction of depolarization in the ventricles (Figs 6.3A and B).

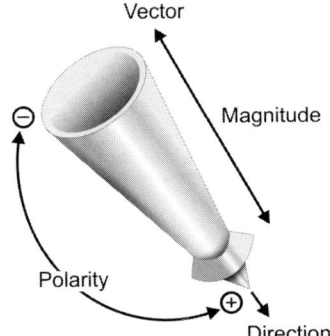

Fig. 6.2 Vector drawn as an arrow representing magnitude direction and polarity

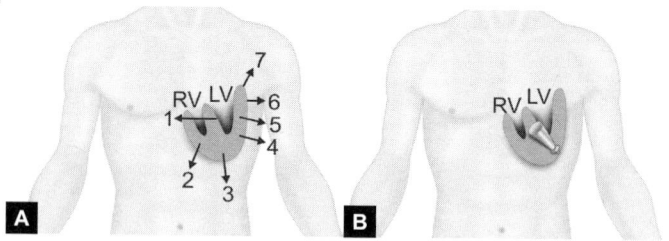

Figs 6.3A and B (A) Instantaneous vectors of ventricular depolarization in sequence (1 through 7) during ventricular activation; (B) Normal mean QRS axis of vector

Normally, left ventricle is much larger than the right and is responsible for most of the heart's electrical forces, so the mean QRS axis (major direction), normally, points towards the left side of the patient's body, as well as downward and posteriorly. When viewed from the front of the body (frontal plane), the mean QRS axis points to the left and downward.

RELATION OF ECG LEADS TO AXIS LEADS (FIG. 6.4)

- In hexaxial system, ECG lead is called 'axis lead'.
- As an example, ECG lead I → Axis lead I.
- Each axis lead has a positive (+) and a negative (−) end.
- In this system, specific leads represent certain areas of the heart.

For example,
- Lead II
- Lead III   : Represent inferior surface of the heart
- Lead aVF   : These are inferior leads
- Lead I   : High lateral or lateral surface of the heart
- Lead aVL   : These are lateral leads.

Positive ends of the limb leads are projected as axis leads.

AXIS LEADS AND CORRESPONDING DEGREES (FIG. 6.5)

- The hexaxial reference system is enclosed in a circle (360°) divided by six axis leads.
- The upper 180° = Negative
- The lower 180° = Positive

Positive ends of the standard limb leads (axis lead).
- Axis lead I = 0°
- Axis Lead II = + 60°
- Axis Lead III = + 120°

They are separated by 60° intervals in a clockwise direction

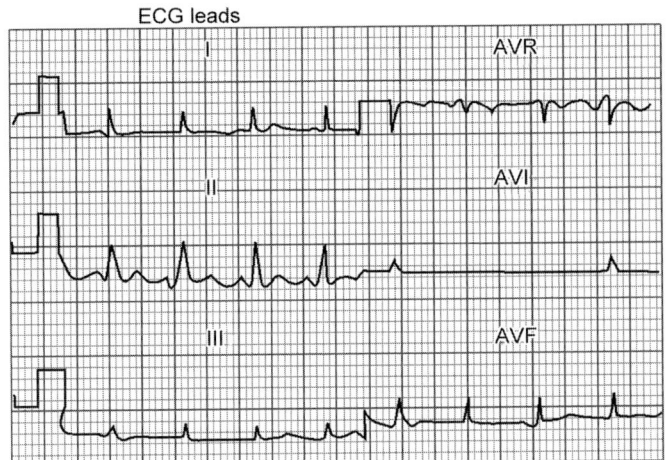

Fig. 6.4 Relation of ECG leads to axis leads

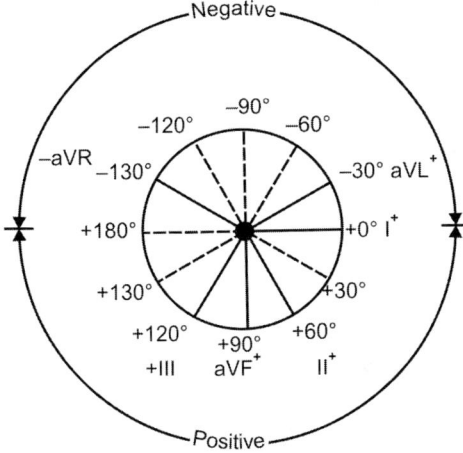

Fig. 6.5 The hexaxial reference system enclose in a 360° circle

Positive ends of the unipolar limb leads:
- Axis lead aVF = + 90°
- Axis lead aVL = −30°   They are separated by 120° intervals
- Axis lead aVR = −150°

DETERMINATION OF QRS VECTOR (FIGS 6.6A AND B)

- In the ECG lead, majority of the QRS deflection is positive (above the baseline), then vector will point toward the positive (+) end of that axis lead that is parallel.
- If QRS deflection is Negative (below the base line), vector, toward the negative (−) end of that axis lead that is parallel.

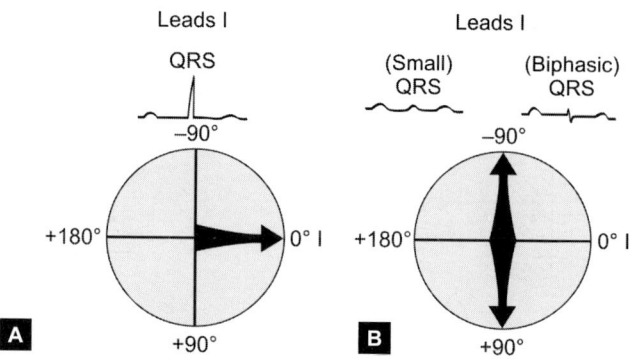

Figs 6.6A and B (A) The large positive QRS deflection in ECG lead; (B) Small or biphasic ORS deflection in lead

- If QRS deflection is small or no QRS deflection or same amount of positive as negative QRS deflection (biphasic) then vector will be perpendicular to that axis lead.
- For example, ECG lead I is positive, Vector points to the positive side of axis lead I, ECG lead I is small or biphasic vector points perpendicular to axis lead I.

DETERMINATION OF MEAN QRS AXIS (FIGS 6.7A TO C)

The ORS axis can be determined by several methods:

Method 1

- Find the lead with smallest or equiphasic deflection
- Determine the lead at right angles to the first lead
- See the net deflection in the second lead

Example 1
- Lead with smallest deflection is aVL
- Lead at right angles to aVL is LII
- Major deflection in LII is positive
- Axis is + 60°

Example 2
- Lead will smallest deflection is aVR
- Lead at right angle to aVR is LII
- Major deflection in LIII is negative
- Axis is – 60°

Method 2 (Fig. 6.8)

- Find the deflection in lead L_1 and aVF, which are perpendicular to each other.
- Plot the net deflection in these leads onto their respective axes, on a scale of 0 to 10

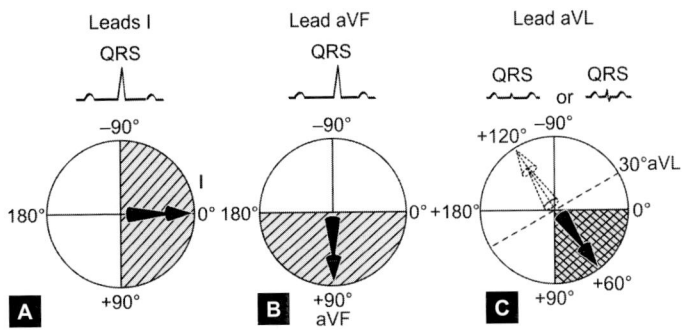

Figs 6.7A to C Determination of mean QRS axis

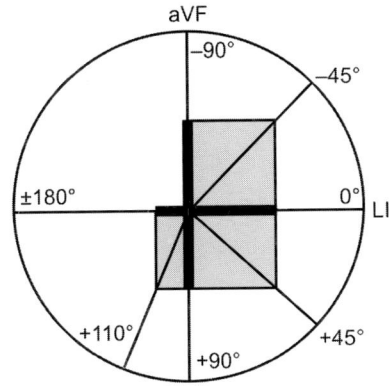

Fig. 6.8 Determination of the electrical axis

- Drop perpendicular lines from this points and plot a point where these lines intersect.
- Join the center of the circle to the intersection point and extend it to the circumference.
- The point on the circumference where this line intersects is the ORS axis.

Example 1
- Net deflection in L_1 is +5
- Net deflection in aVF is 0
- Axis is 0°

Example 2
- Net deflection in L_1 is + 5
- Net deflection in aVF is –5
- Axis is –45°

Example 3
- Net deflection in L_1 is + 6
- Net deflection in aVF is + 3
- Axis is + 30°

Method 3

- For rapid and easy estimation of ORS axis, just scan the direction of the dominant deflection in lead L_1 and aVF whether positive or negative.
- The mean QRS axis represents the main direction of depolarization in the ventricles. As an example,
  - ECG lead I is positive, so axis lead I is 0°
  - ECG lead aVF is positive, axis lead aVF is + 90°
- When these two vectors are averaged, the mean QRS axis points in between 0° and +90°
- But to localize more accurately the mean QRS axis, fine the ECG lead with the smallest or biphasic QRS deflection.
- So, here ECG lead aVL is small or biphasic: So the mean QRS axis lies perpendicular to axis lead aVL. The axis points towards + 60° or –120°
- So the mean QRS axis of + 60° is correct one, because it lies between 0° and + 90°

AXIS DEVIATION

Definition

A shifting of the heart's electrical axis beyond the normal range of 0°–90° on the hexaxial reference figure (Fig. 6.9).

Types (Figs 6.10 to 6.12)

1. Left axis deviation (LAD)
2. Right axis deviation (RAD)
3. Indeterminate or extreme right axis deviation.

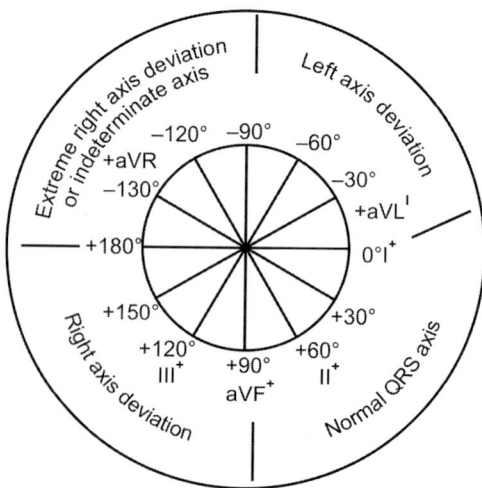

Fig. 6.9 QRS axis deviation

Axis and Vectors

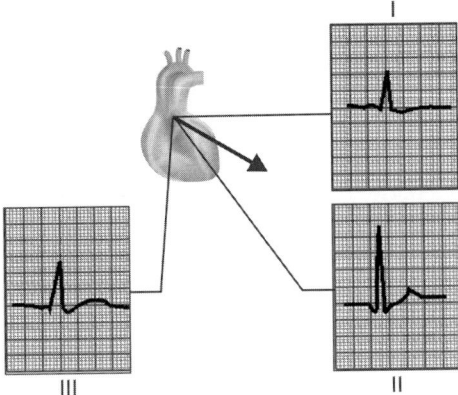

Fig. 6.10 Normal axis

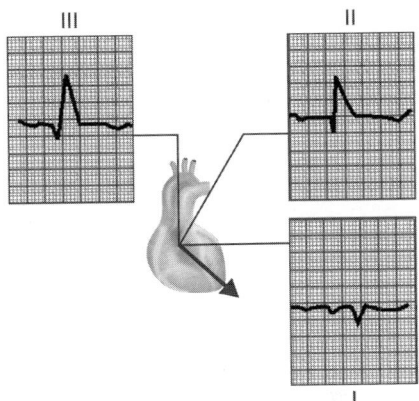

Fig. 6.11 Right axis deviation

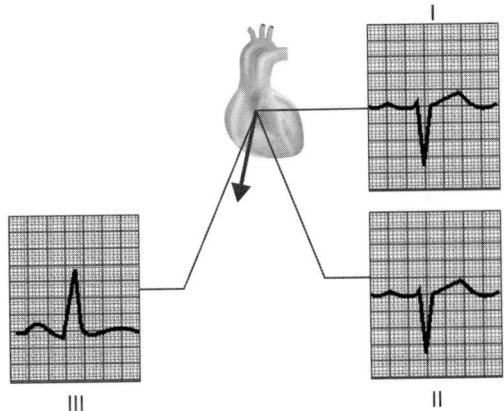

Fig. 6.12 Left axis deviation

Note:

- The range of normal QRS axis : Between + 90° and 30°
- Left axis deviation (LAD) : Between – 30° and –90°
- Right axis deviation (RAD) : Between + 90° and + 180°
- Extreme RAD or indeterminate : Between + 180° and – 90°

RAPID ESTIMATION OF MEAN QRS AXIS (FIG. 6.13)

By scanning, the main QRS deflections in ECG leads I and II, the mean QRS axis may be rapidly estimated.

	Main QRS deflection		QRS axis quadrant
	Lead I	Lead II/aVF	
Normal QRS axis	Positive	Positive	0 to + 90°
Left axis deviation	Positive	Negative	0 to –90°
Right axis deviation	Negative	Positive	+90° to +180°
Extreme right axis deviation	Negative	Negative	- 90° to - 180°

Causes of Left Axis Deviation (LAD) (Axis between –30° and 90°)

- Left anterior hemiblock (LAHB)
- Inferior myocardial infarction (MI)
- Pre-excitation syndromes (Wolff-Parkinson-White syndrome, WPW)
- Normal variant
- Old age, obesity, pregnancy or ascites
- Left ventricular hypertrophy (LVH) with LAHB

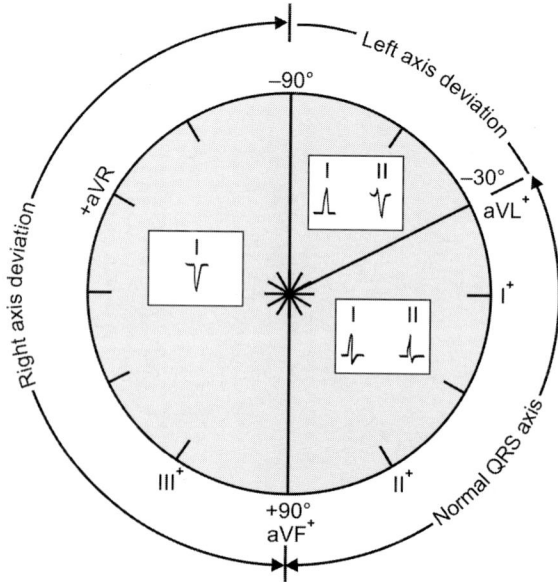

Fig. 6.13 Rapid estimation of mean QRS axis only ECG leads I and II

- Chronic obstructive pulmonary disease (COPD), emphysema
- Cardiomyopathy
- LBBB
- Pacing from the apex of the right or left ventricle (endocardial pacing).

Causes of Right Axis Deviation (RAD) (Axis between +90° and +180°):

- Normal variant
- Younger age—infants and children
- Right ventricular hypertrophy (RVH), TOF
- Anterolateral MI
- Cor pulmonale, pulmonary embolism
- Left posterior hemiblock (LPHB)
- WPW syndrome (Type A)
- RBBB (Right bundle-branch block due to ostium primum disease)
- Dextrocardia
- Epicardial pacing.

Note: A simple way to check for reversed limb electrodes is to observe the QRS voltage. If the limb electrodes are placed correctly the QRS voltage in lead I + lead II = ORS voltage in lead II.

Causes of Extreme RAD (North-west Axis or Indeterminate QRS Axis or no Mans Land)

- Congenital heart disease
- Left ventricular aneurysm.

7
Abnormalities of Wave Intervals and Segments

NORMAL P-WAVE

The P-wave is produced by atrial depolarization, it is the sum of right and left atrial activation, the right atrium being activated first since the pacemaker is located in it.

The normal P-wave meets the following:

Criteria

- *Location*: Precedes QRS complex
- *Amplitude*: 2–2.5 mm in height
- *Duration*: 0.08–0.12 sec
- *Configuration:* Rounded and upright or pyramidal shape
- *Deflexion:* Normally P-wave is positive (upright) deflexion in all leads except aVR in which negative (inverted) and V_1- in which biphasic (positive and negative).

P-wave, best seen in lead II, V_1

- *P-wave in V_1:* Usually biphasic having initial positivity and terminal negativity
- *Positive deflexion:* Less than 1.5 mm amplitude
- *Negative terminal deflexion:* Less than 1 mm in depth and 0.03 sec in duration.

ABNORMAL P-WAVE (CLINICAL SIGNIFICANCE) (FIGS 7.1A TO D)

Configuration	Leads best seen	Lead V_1	Found in
Peaked- >2.5 mm in height (P-pulmonale) or Tall-P	II, III, aVL	Initial positivity	Right atrial enlargement Pulmonary stenosis Tricuspid stenosis Pulmonary hypertension
Broad, notched or bifid, >0.12 sec in duration (P-mitrale)	I, II, aVL $V_4 – V_6$	Terminal negativity	Left atrial enlargement Mitral stenosis
Both peaked and broad	Any of above leads	Biphasic (peaked and broad)	Right and left atrial enlargement

Contd...

Contd...

Configuration	Leads best seen	Lead V_1	Found in
Inverted P-wave	Lead I		Dextrocardia Mechanical error (Incorrectly placed lead) Reverse electrode Nodal rhythm and retrograde conducting Low atrial and high nodal ectopics beat
	II, III, aVF		Retrograde activation of the sinoatrial (SA) node
Absent P-wave	All leads		Atrial fibrillation Atrial flutter Ventricular ectopics Ventricular tachycardia Supraventricular tachycardia (SVT) Atrioventricular (AV) nodal rhythm Hyperkalemias Idioventricular rhythm
Small P-wave	All leads		Atrial tachycardia Atrial ectopic Nodal rhythm (high nodal) Nodal ectopic (high nodal)
Variable P-wave			Wandering pacemaker
Multiple P-wave (Consecutive 2 or more			AV block (either partial or complete heart block (CHB) SVT and AV block

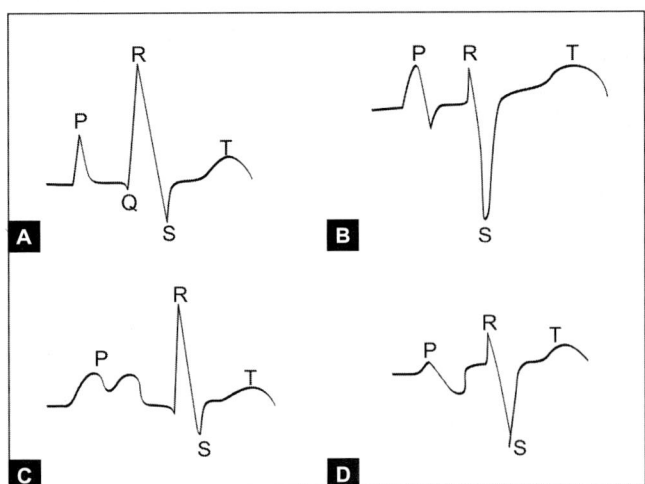

Figs 7.1A to D (A) Tall, peaked P in L_{11}, aVF; (B) Initial positive deflection in V_1; (C) Broad, notched P in L_1, aVF; (D) Terminal negative deflection in V_1

Various Causes of Atrial Enlargement

	Left atrial enlargement	Right atrial enlargement
Intracardiac shunt	VSD	ASD
AV valve disease	MS	TS
	MR	TR
Outflow obstruction	AS	PS
Hypertension	Systemic hypertension	Pulmonary hypertension
Myocardial disease	Cardiomyopathy	Cor pulmonale

NORMAL AND PATHOLOGICAL Q-WAVE

Normal Q-wave

- First negative (downward) deflexion QRS complex
- Normally found in I, aVL, V_4, V_5, V_6
- Not exceed 2 mm in depth or 0.03 sec in duration.

Pathological Q-wave (Fig. 7.2)

- *Duration:* 0.04 sec (1 small sq) or more
- *Depth:* More than 2 mm
- Associated with substantial loss of height of R-wave
- Q-wave at least $\frac{1}{4}$th of R-wave
- Must be present in multiple leads.

Note:
- A normal Q-wave may be present in lead III, but this Q-wave usually abolish during deep inspiration
- Deep but narrow Q-wave in I, aVL, V_5, V_6 for left ventricular volume overload
- Lead Q showing the site of myocardial infarction.

Causes of Pathological Q-wave

- Myocardial infarction (the most common cause)
- Ventricular hypertrophy (Lt or Rt)
- Cardiomyopathy
- Left bundle branch block (LBBB)

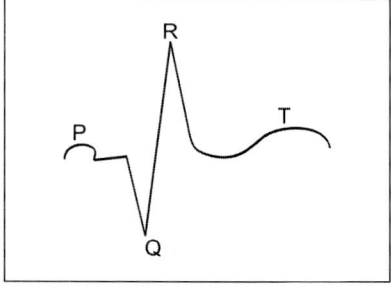

Fig. 7.2 Pathological Q-wave

- Emphysema
- Q only in L_{III} is associated for pulmonary embolism (S_1, Q_{III}, T_{III} pattern).

Note:
- Q-wave in V_1, V_2, V_3 may be seen LVH and may be mistaken as old myocardial infarction
- Abnormal Q-wave in L_3 may be found in pulmonary embolism
- Abnormal Q-wave in L_3 and aVF may be found Wolff-Parkinson-White (WPW) syndrome (confuses with old inferior myocardial infarction).

Area of Infarction from Q-wave Location

Location of Q-wave	Area of intraction
L_1, aVL	High lateral
L_{II}, L_{III}, aVF	Inferior
L_1, aVL, $V_1 - V_6$	Extensive anterior
$V_1 - V_6$	Anterior
$V_1 - V_{3-4}$	Anteroseptal or septal
$V_4 - V_6$	Anterolateral
L_1, aVL, $V_4 - V_6$	Lateral

NORMAL AND ABNORMAL R-WAVE

Normal R-wave (Fig. 7.3)

- First positive (upwards) deflection of QRS complex
- Normal height (amplitude)
  - *Lead aVL:* <13 mm
  - *Lead aVF:* <20 mm
  - *Chest leads ($V_1 - V_6$):* Gradual progression of R-wave from $V_1 - V_6$ but maximum in V_5 (<27 mm).

Abnormal R-wave (Fig. 7.4)

Tall R-wave

- *In aVL:* >13 mm
- *In aVF:* >20 mm   Found in left ventricular hypertrophy

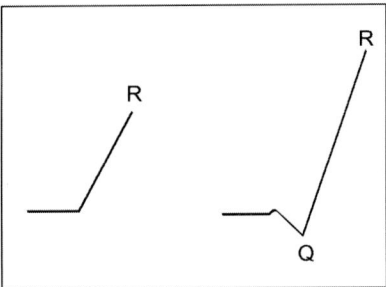

Fig. 7.3 Normal R-wave

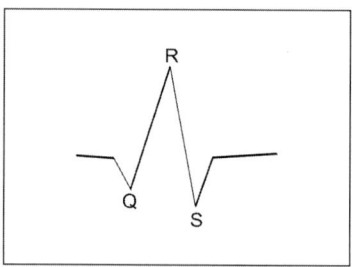

Fig. 7.4 Abnormal R-wave

- In $V_5 - V_6$: > 27 mm
- In V_1: R is greater than S (R > S): Found in-
  - Normal variant
  - Right bundle branch block (RBBB) and dominance
  - WPW syndrome (Type A)
  - Post-MI
  - Dextrocardia.

S-wave

- The negative deflexion, follows the R-wave
- It is dominant in V_1 to V_3
- It is progressively diminished from V_1 to V_6.

Causes of Nonprogressing of R-wave

- Old anterior wall infarction
- Pulmonary emphysema
- Diffuse myocardial disease
- Left ventricular hypertrophy (LVH)
- LBBB.

NORMAL AND ABNORMAL QRS COMPLEX

Normal QRS Complex (Fig. 7.5)

- Components of Q, R and S-wave
- *Duration:* Not greater than 0.10 sec

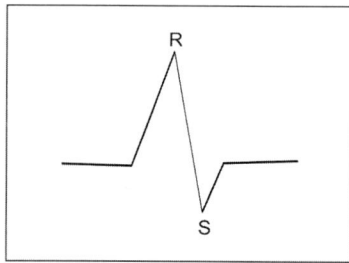

Fig. 7.5 QRS complete

- In a right ventricular lead (V_1), the S-wave is greater than the R-wave
- In a left ventricular lead (V_5 or V_6) the height of the R-wave is less than 25 mm
- Left ventricular leads may show Q-waves due to septal depolarization, but these are less than 1 mm across and less than 2 mm deep.

Abnormalities of QRS Complex

QRS may be

- High voltage
- Low voltage
- Wide
- Change in shape
- Variable.

Causes of High Voltage QRS

- Incorrect calibration
- Thin chest wall
- Ventricular hypertrophy (Right or left or both)
- WPW syndrome
- True posterior myocardial infarction (in V_1 and V_2).

Causes of Low Voltage QRS (<5 mm in L1, L2, L3 and <10 mm in Chest Leads)

- Incorrect calibration
- Thick chest wall (obesity)
- Emphysema
- Hypothyroidism
- Pericardial effusion
- Chronic constrictive pericarditis
- Hypothermia
- Cardiomyopathy
- Diffuse coronary artery disease.

Causes of Wide QRS (>0.12 sec, 3 Small Squares)

- Ventricular ectopics
- Ventricular tachycardia
- Idioventricular rhythm
- Ventricular hypertrophy
- BBB (LBBB or RBBB)
- WPW syndrome
- Hyperkalemia
- Pacemaker (looks like LBBB and spike)
- Drugs
  - Quinidine
  - Procainamide

- Phenothiazine
- Tricyclic antidepressants.

Causes of Changes Shape of QRS

- Right or left bundle block (slurred or M-pattern)
- Ventricular tachycardia
- Ventricular fibrillation
- Hyperkalemia
- WPW syndrome.

Causes of Variable QRS

- Multifocal ventricular ectopics
- Torsades de-pointes
- Ventricular fibrillation.

NORMAL AND ABNORMAL T-WAVE

Normal T-wave

- Follows the S-wave and the ST segment
- *Amplitude:* 5 mm or less in limb lead, 10 mm or less in chest leads
- *Configuration:* Rounded and smooth
- *Deflexion:* Normally upright in leads I, II, V_3 to V_6 and inverted in leads III, aVR, V_1 to V_{3-4} (Infancy). May occasionally persist in adulthood. Persistent inverted T-wave in V_1 common in young adulthood
- T taller in lead V_6 than in lead V_1 and taller L_1 than in lead L_3.

Note:
- T-wave relatively taller in athletes.
- T-wave amplitude diminish with age.
- PJP (persistent juvenile pattern)—T-wave inversion V_1-V_4 in infancy and childhood if it enters into adulthood—called PJP.

Abnormal T-wave

Causes

- *Tall, peaked, pointed, tented T-wave*
  - Hyperacute myocardial infarction (MI)
  - Hyperkalemia
  - Acute true posterior MI (Tall, T in V_1 to V_2).
- *Inverted T-wave*
  - Myocardial ischemia (IHD) and infarction
  - Strain pattern and ventricular hypertrophy
  - Bundle branch block (BBB)
  - WPW syndrome
  - Normal in aVR, V_1, V_2, lead III
  - Ventricular ectopics

- Non-Q-wave MI (Subendocardial MI)
- Cardiomyopathy
- Acute pericarditis, myocarditis
- Drugs—digitalis, quinidine (Figs 7.6A and B)
- Metabolic—hypothermic, hypokalemic (Fig. 7.7)
- Physiological states
    - Heavy meals
    - Smoking anxiety, tachycardia
    - Hyperventilation
- Extracardiac cause
    - *Systemic*: Hemorrhage, shock
    - *Cerebral*: Vascular accident
    - *Abdominal*: Pancreatitis, cholecystitis
    - *Respiratory*: Pulmonary embolism
    - *Endocrine*: Hypothyroidism.

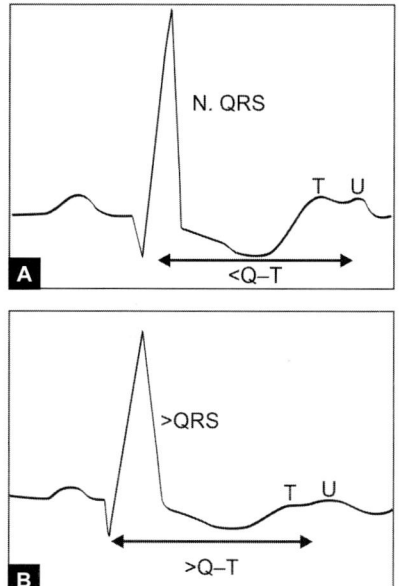

Figs 7.6A and B (A) Effects of digitalis on the P-QRS-T; (B) Effects of quinidine on the P-QRS-T

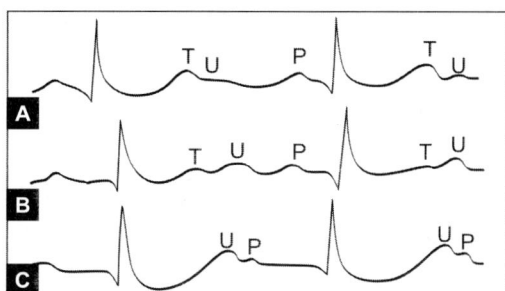

Fig. 7.7 Effects of progressively increasing hypokalemia

- *If giant T-wave inversion in V_2 to V_4 (large, broad, bizarre, inverted)*
  - Recent syncopal attack
  - Adams attack
  - Paroxysmal VF or flutter
  - If asymmetrical T-wave inversion
    - Digoxin toxicity
    - Ventricular strain
  - If giant symmetrical T-wave inversion in chest leads—Acute subendocardial ischemia (Non-Q-wave MI) (Fig. 7.8).
- *Heavily notched T-waves*
  - Pericarditis in adult
  - Normal in children.
- *Tall symmetrical T-wave (in precordial leads)*
  - Hyperkalemia
  - Acute subendocardial ischemia, injury or infarction
  - Recovering inferior wall myocardial infarction
  - Hyperacute phase of anterior MI
  - True posterior wall MI
  - Prinzmetal's angina
  - Coronary insufficiency.

Note:
T-wave Inversion (Figs 7.9 to 7.11)
- *In leads L_1, aVL, V_5, V_6*
  - Lateral wall ischemia/infarction
  - LVH
  - LBBB
  - Digitalis effect or toxicity.

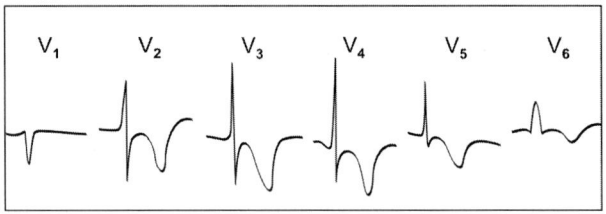

Fig. 7.8 Acute non-Q-wave anterior wall myocardial infarction convex ST-segment symmetrical T-wave

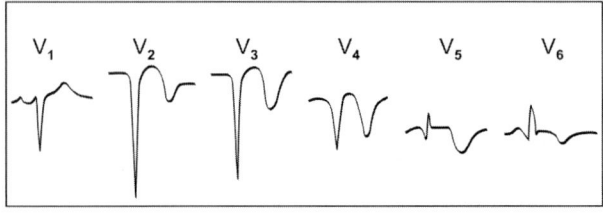

Fig. 7.9 Acute extensive anterior wall myocardial infarction fully evolved phase QS in V_1, qR in V_5 to V_6

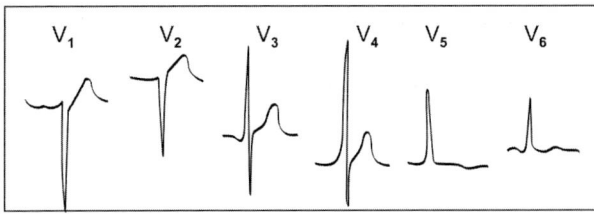

Fig. 7.10 Coronary insufficiency: T-wave in V_1 is taller than in V_6

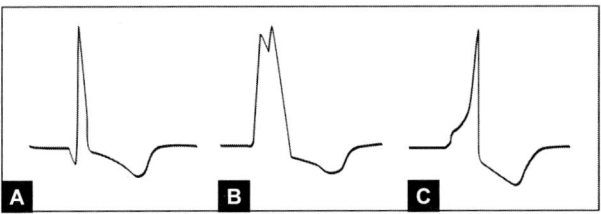

Figs 7.11A to C Causes of secondary T-wave inversion. (A) Ventricular hypertrophy; (B) Bundle branch block; (C) WPW syndrome

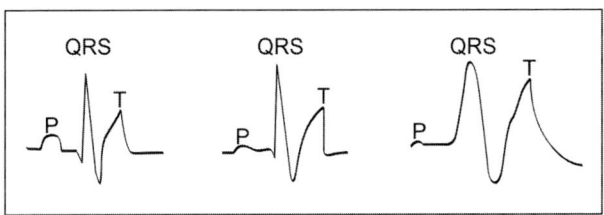

Fig. 7.12 ECG findings of hyperkalemia according to serum K⁺

- In leads V_1, V_2, V_3
  - Anteroseptal ischemia/infarction
  - RVH
  - RBBB
  - WPW syndrome, Type A.
- In leads L_{II} L_{III}, aVF
  - Inferior wall ischemia/infarction
  - Mitral valve prolapse syndrome.

Electrocardiogram Finding of Hyperkalemia Depend Upon Serum Potassium (Fig. 7.12)

- If serum K > 6.8 mEq/L
  - Tall, tented T
  - Short Q-T interval.
- If serum K > 8.4 mEq/L
  - Low or absent P-waves
  - Tall tented T
  - Short Q-T interval
- If serum K > 9.1 mEq/L
  - Wide, bizarre QRS
  - AV block and arrhythmias

Relationship between Locations of Electrocardiogram Changes and Coronary Artery Spasm

Coronary artery spasm of	Locations of ECG changes
Right coronary artery	L_{II}, L_{III}, aVF
Left anterior descending (LAD) artery	V_1, V_2, V_3, V_4
Left circumflex (LCX) artery	L_1, aVL, V_5, V_6

JUVENILE T-WAVE PATTERN

- It is a condition in which T is inverted in V_1 to V_3 (rarely V_4 to V_6)
- In this case, T inversion is neither symmetrical nor deep. It is common in children and young adults, more in female <40 years.
- Frequently, it is associated with sinus arrhythmia and high left ventricular voltage.

Diagnostic Pearls

Juvenile T-wave pattern (JTWP) should be differentiated from other clinical conditions that produce inverted T-wave in the chest leads, including anterior myocardial, pulmonary embolism and myocarditis. It should be noted that JTWP does not produce symmetric or deep T-wave inversion.

NORMAL AND ABNORMAL U-WAVE

Normal U-wave (Fig. 7.13)

- Positive deflection immediately after T-wave
- Small, rounded
- *Amplitude*: Usually 1–2 mm in athletes
- Best seen in V_2–V_4.

Abnormal U-wave (Fig. 7.14)

Inverted in Lead I, Lead II, V_6

- Coronary heart disease
- Hypertensive heart disease
  - LV systolic overload
  - LV diastolic overload.

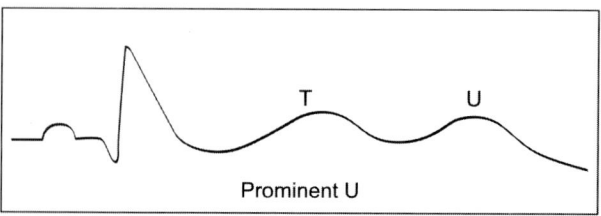

Fig. 7.13 Normal U-wave

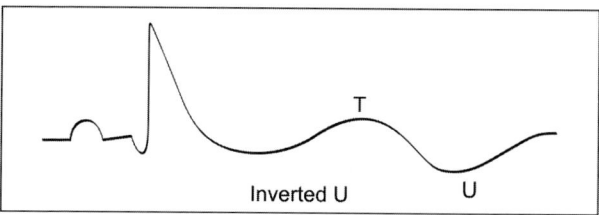

Fig. 7.14 Abnormal U-wave

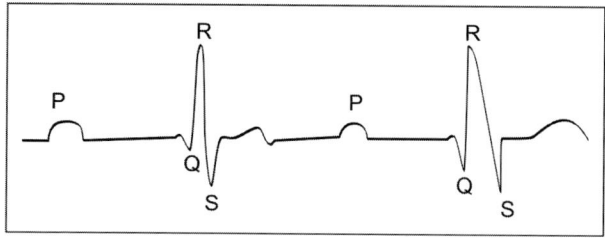

Fig. 7.15 Prolonged PR interval

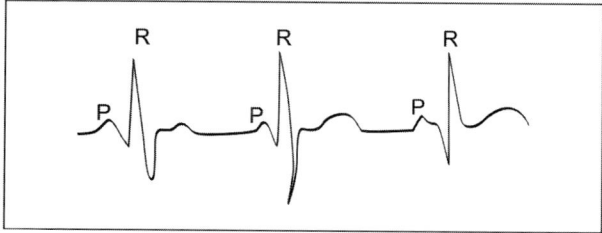

Fig. 7.16 Short PR interval

Prominent U-wave in V_3–V_5

- Hypokalemia
- Cardiovascular drugs, e.g. digitalis quinidine
- Psychotropic drugs, e.g. phenothiazines, tricyclics.

NORMAL AND ABNORMAL P-INTERVAL

Location: Extends from beginning of P-wave to beginning of QRS complex.

Duration: 0.12–0.20 sec.

Abnormal PR Interval

- *Prolong PR interval:* >0.20 sec (Fig. 7.15)
  First degree heart block (1° HB) PR >0.2 sec
  Causes
    - Rheumatic carditis, myocarditis
    - Coronary artery disease
    - Hypokalemia
    - Digitalis toxicity
    - Atrial hypertrophy.
- *Short PR interval:* <0.12 sec (Fig. 7.16)
  A dissociated beat—Atrial ectopic beat

WPW syndrome
LGL (Lown-ganong-Levine) syndrome
AV nodal rhythm.

Causes
- WPW syndrome
- LGL syndrome
- Nodal rhythm
- Nodal ectopic (high nodal).

- *Variable PR interval (Fig. 7.17)*
  - Wenckebach's phenomenon (Mobitz type-I)
  - Partial heart block (Mob type II)
  - 2 : 1 AV block
  - Complete AV block (CHB)
  - Wandering pacemaker-variable configuration of P.

Causes of PR Segment Depression (Fig. 7.18)

- *Primary causes*
  - Acute pericarditis
  - Atrial infarction
  - Chest wall trauma.
- *Secondary causes*
  - Sinus tachycardia
  - Atrial enlargement.

QT INTERVAL: NORMAL AND ABNORMAL

Normal QT Interval

- It is the distance from the beginning of the QRS to the end of the T-wave, it represents the total time required for both depolarization and repolarization of the ventricles.

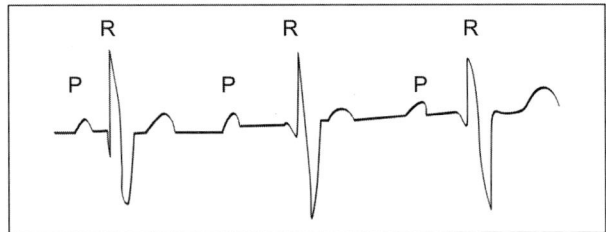

Fig. 7.17 Variable PR interval

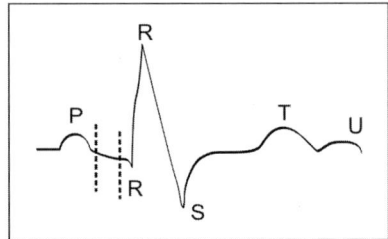

Fig. 7.18 Depressed PR segment

- *Normal QT interval:* 0.35–0.43 sec or 0.39 ± 0.04 sec.
- Its duration varies with heart rate, becoming shorter as the HR increases and longer as the HR decreases.
- In general, the QT interval at heart rate between 60–90/min does not exceed in duration half the preceding RR interval.
- It is better seen in aVL (because there is no U-wave).

Abnormalities of QT Interval

QT interval may be—
- Short (Fig. 7.19)
- Long (Fig. 7.20).

Causes of Short QT Interval

- Tachycardia
- Digoxin effect
- Hyperthermia
- Hypercalcemia
- Hyperkalemia.

Causes of Long QT Interval

- Bradycardia AV block
- *Drugs:*
    - Quinidine
    - Procainamide
    - Amiodarone
    - Tricyclic antidepressant

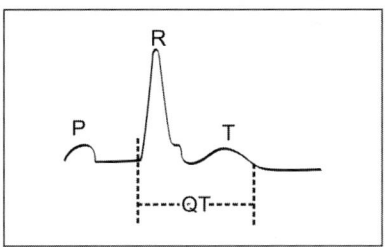

Fig. 7.19 Short QT interval

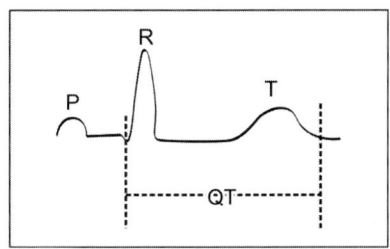

Fig. 7.20 Long QT interval

- Acute myocardial infarction
- *Acute myocarditis:* Viral rheumatic fever
- Hypertrophic cardiomyopathy
- Cerebral injury
  - Head injury
  - Intracerebral hemorrhage
- Hypothermia
- Hypocalcemia, hypomagnesemia
- During sleep
- Hereditary syndrome
  - *Jervell lange:* Nielsen syndrome
  - *Romano:* Ward syndrome
- *Congenital*
  - QT prolongation
  - Mitral valve prolapse syndrome.

Note: It may be associated and ventricular arrhythmia. Rarely can it cause 'torsades de pointes' tachycardia and sudden death.

Interpretation

The QT interval must be corrected for the heart rate. The corrected QT interval is known as the QTc interval. The QTc interval is determined using the formula:

$$QTc = \frac{QT}{\sqrt{RR}}$$

Here, QT is the measured QT interval. $\sqrt{RR}$ is square-root of R-R interval

When, RR interval = 25 mm or 1 sec (25 × 0.04 sec = 1 sec)
Then $\sqrt{RR}$ is 1
Then QTc = QT
Then Heart rate occurs 60 bpm.

NORMAL AND ABNORMAL ST SEGMENT

Normal ST Segment

- Between the QRS complex and T-wave
- Amplitude (*Height*: Usually in isoelectric line but height up to 1 mm in standard leads and 2 mm in right chest leads ($V_1 - V_3$).

Abnormal ST Segment

ST Segment Depression

- Horizontal ST depression with a sharp-angled ST-T junction, e.g. earliest sign of coronary insufficiency (acute myocardial ischemia) (Fig. 7.21).
- Upward-sloping ST segment depression, e.g. pathological, impaired coronary blood flow, physiological (Fig. 7.22).

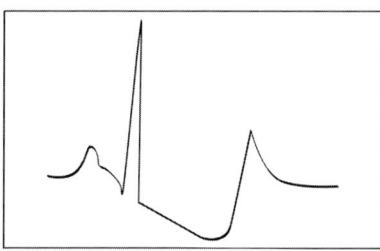

Fig. 7.21 Horizontal ST depression with a sharp-angled ST–T junction, e.g. earliest sign of coronary insufficiency (acute myocardial ischemia)

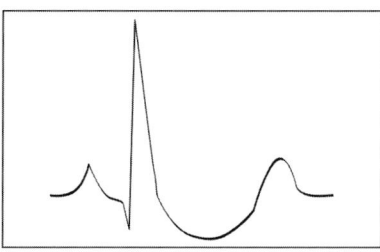

Fig. 7.22 Upward-sloping ST-segment depression, e.g. pathological, impaired coronary blood flow, physiological

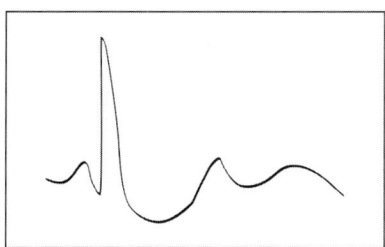

Fig. 7.23 Junctional ST depression, e.g. pathology, physiological

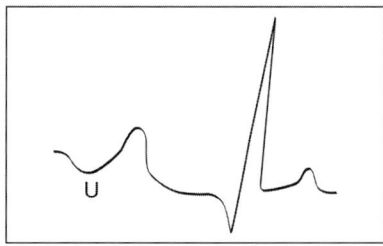

Fig. 7.24 Plane ST depression, e.g. angina pectoris

- Junctional ST depression, e.g. pathology, physiological (Fig. 7.23).
- Plane ST depression, e.g. angina pectoris (Fig. 7.24).
- Downward sloping ST depression, e.g. severe impaired coronary blood flow, digoxin toxicity (Fig. 7.25).
- Sagging ST depression (Fig. 7.26)

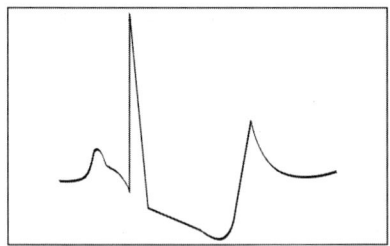

Fig. 7.25 Downward sloping ST depression, e.g. severe impaired coronary blood flow, digoxin toxicity

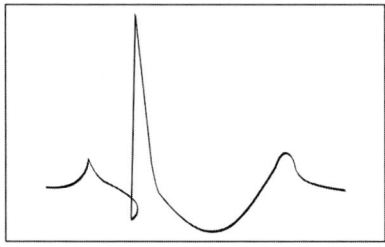

Fig. 7.26 Sagging ST depression

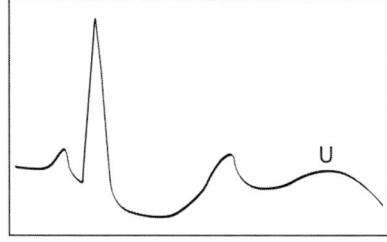

Fig. 7.27 Sagging ST depression with U-wave

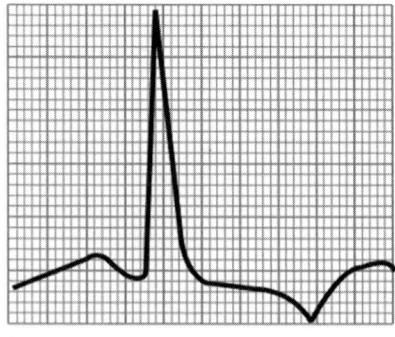

Fig. 7.28

- Sagging ST depression with U-wave (Fig. 7.27)
- Strain pattern ST depression with convexity upwards with asymmetric T-wave inversion, e.g. ventricular hypertrophy (Fig. 7.28)

Basic mechanism: ST-depression most marked in leads V_5-V_6. Injury to the subendocardial region of the left ventricle. The ST segment vector will be directed towards the cavity of the left ventricle and away from the lead V_5 and V_6. This will result in ST segment depression in V_5 or V_6.

ST Segment Elevation (Fig. 7.29)

More marked in mid-precordial leads (V_2 or V_4), but frequently manifested in V_2 - V_6 and lead I, III, aVF. ST-segment elevation—amplitude about 4 mm, but it can be high as 40 mm.

- ST segment elevation with convexity upwards with T-inversion (coving pattern ST-elevation), e.g. acute MI.
- ST elevation with concavity upward, e.g. pericarditis (Fig. 7.30).
- ST elevation with tall T-wave, e.g. V_2-V_5, Prinzmetal's angina (Fig. 7.31).

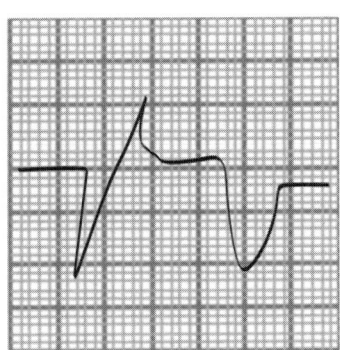

Fig. 7.29

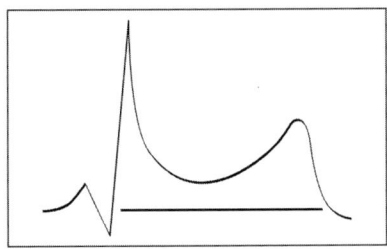

Fig. 7.30

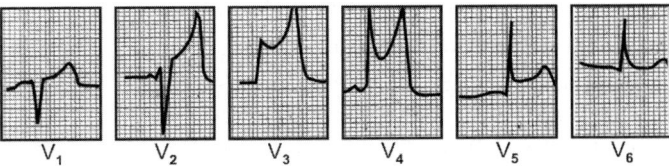

Fig. 7.31

Causes of ST Segment Elevation (>2 mm)

- Acute MI (ST elevation and convexity upwards), Dressler's syndrome
- Coronary vasospasm e.g. Prinzmetal's angina, rest angina, variant angina, vasospastic angina
- Organic stenosis of the coronary arteries
- Left ventricular aneurysm or LV tumor
- Impaired left ventricular function (ventricular aneurysm)
- Pericarditis (ST elevation and concavity upwards)
- Early repolarization syndrome (high take off)
- Normal variant in Asians and Africa
- *Noncardiac*: Acute pancreatitis, cholecystitis, diaphragmatic pleurisy.

Note:
- Higher ST elevation—more severe coronary artery disease
- ST segment depression in one attack and elevation in another attack may be seen in same lead
- ST depression during exercise and ST elevation in post-exercise.

Causes of ST Depression

- Physiological
    - Anxiety
    - Tachycardia
    - Hyperventilation
- Extracardiac
    - *Systemic:* Hemorrhage, shock
    - *Cerebral:* Vascular accident
    - *Abdominal:* Pancreatitis cholecystitis
    - *Respiratory:* Pulmonary embolism
- *Specific cause:*
    - Primary
        - Digitalis quinidine
        - Hypokalemia hypothermia
        - Cardiomyopathy, myocarditis
        - Infarction, coronary insufficiency
    - Secondary
        - Ventricular hypertrophy
        - BBB
        - WPW syndrome.

Electrocardiogram Features of Myocardial Infarction (Besides ST Elevation)

- Symmetrical T inversion
- Appearance of Q-wave
- Loss of R-wave height
- Regional location of changes

- Reciprocal ST depression in other leads
- Arrhythmias and conduction defects
- Serial evolution of ECG changes.

Specific Features of Dresslers Syndrome (Postinfarction Syndrome)

- ST elevation without reciprocal depression
- Precordial pain increasing on inspiration
- Fever and tachycardia
- Raised erythrocyte sedimentation rate (ESR) but normal cardiac enzymes
- Appearance of pleuropericardial rub
- Responsiveness to steroid therapy.

EARLY REPOLARIZATION (HIGH TAKE OFF) SYNDROME

- It is a benign, normal findings in young healthy person more in black males
- It is seen in chest leads commonly V_4 to V_6 (rarely other chest lead)
- ST elevation is usually associated with j-point elevation
- It is not associated with inversion of T-wave or abnormal Q-wave.

Note:
- Early repolarization syndrome confuses with acute pericarditis and acute MI
- To differentiate from these, detail history, serial ECG tracing (that shows no change) and comparison and old ECG are helpful.

Electrocardiogram Criteria of Early Repolarization Syndrome (Fig. 7.32)

- Tall R in V_4 to V_6
- Deep and narrow initial Q-waves
- Concave upward ST elevation
- Initial slur on ST segment the J-wave
- Tall and upright symmetrical T

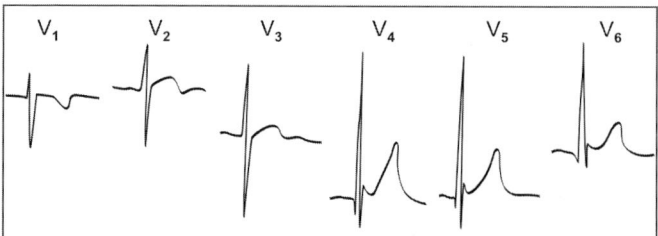

Fig. 7.32 ECG features of early repolarization syndrome

Clinical Features

- Young black male
- Healthy and athletic built
- He is active and free from symptoms
- Clinical evaluation is entirely normal
- ST returns to baseline after exercise.

RHYTHM OF THE HEART

At first, calculate the RR interval. If the RR interval is equal, it is called regular rhythm. If the RR interval is irregular, then it is called irregular rhythm.

Causes of Irregular Rhythm

- *Physiological:* Sinus arrhythmia
- *Pathological*
    - Atrial fibrillation
    - Atrial flutter
    - Ectopic beat
- Atrial tachycardia with block
    - SA block or sinus arrest
    - $2°$ heart block
    - Ventricular fibrillation.

Sinus Rhythm

Characters

- P-wave is of sinus origin
- Wave and QRS complexes are regular
- Constant P-wave configuration in a given lead
- PR interval and QRS interval should be within normal limit
- Rate should be between 60 and 100 beats/minute.

Arrhythmia

Arrhythmia is the abnormality in initiation or propagation of cardiac impulse.

NORMAL VARIANTS IN ELECTROCARDIOGRAM

These are commonly found in young adults and children:
- Early repolarization syndromes (in young black males)
- Left ventricular hypertrophy (in children and young adults)
- Short PR interval
- Sinus arrhythmia with or without wandering pacemaker
- Right axis deviation
- Low voltage in obese people
- $1°$ heart block
- Wenckebach's phenomenon
- Juvenile T-wave pattern in children and young adults.

8

Hypertrophy

ATRIAL HYPERTROPHY

Myocardial hypertrophy denotes increase in the thickness of the walls of the atria or ventricles. The right atrium lies anterior to the left atrium. Atrial activation begins in the sinoatrial (SA) node, which is located in the superior and posterior part of the right atrium, atrial depolarization proceeds first through the right atrium, then through the left atrium. Thus, right atrial activation is responsible for the initial part of the P-wave and left atrial activation is responsible for the terminal portion of the P-wave. Depolarization of both atria is represented in the electrocardiography (ECG) by the P-wave. The normal P-wave is less than 0.12 sec in duration and less than 2.5 mm in height (Figs 8.1 and 8.2).

RIGHT ATRIAL HYPERTROPHY (FIG. 8.3)

(P-pulmonale, P-congenitale)

Definition: Right atrial hypertrophy (RAH) is characterized by an increased right atrial electrical force manifested by tall P-waves in Lead II, III, and aVF that are associated with tall P-wave in Lead $V_1 - V_2$.

The ECG Criteria

- Tall, peaked P-wave (> 2.5 mm) in leads II, II, aVF (Tall P is called P-pulmonales).

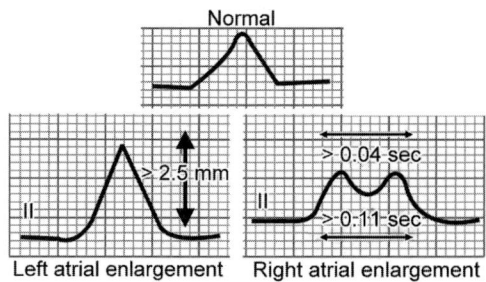

Fig. 8.1 Atrial enlargement

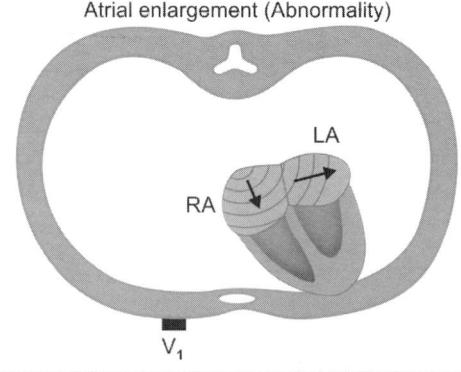

Fig. 8.2 Atrial enlargement
Abbreviations: RA, right atrial; LA, left atrial

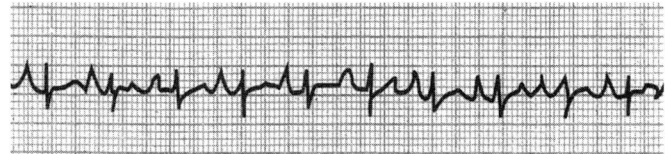

Fig. 8.3 Right atrial hypertrophy

- Large initial positive deflection of the P-wave (proximal part) more than 1.5 mm in lead V_1), Biphasic
- Duration of P-wave normal (<0.12 sec)
- Right ward P-wave (between + 75° + 90°).

LEFT ATRIAL HYPERTROPHY (FIG. 8.4)

(P-Mitrale)

Definition: Left atrial hypertrophy (LAH) is characterized by an increased left atrial electrical force manifested by broad (often notched) P-waves in limb leads that are associated with deep and broad P-waves of the negative component in Lead $V_1 - V_2$.

The ECG Criteria

- Broad, notched P-wave greater than 0.12 sec in duration in lead I, II, aVL (Like M), called P-mitrale

Hypertrophy

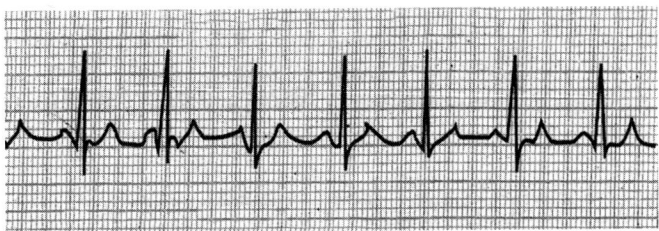

Fig. 8.4 Left atrial hypertrophy

- Large terminal negative P-wave deflection duration >0.4 sec, depth >1 mm in V_1 representing the depolarization forces traveling posteriorly in the large left atrium.
- Leftward P-wave axis (between+ 30° and – 30°).

Others

What does P-pulmonale indicate?
It indicates right atrial hypertrophy or enlargement. It is commonly seen in severe pulmonary disease.

What does P-mitrale indicate?
It indicates left atrial hypertrophy or enlargement.

Cause of P-pulmonale

- Chronic obstructive pulmonary disease (COPD) and chronic cor pulmonale (the most common) or right ventricular failure
- Pulmonary stenosis
- Pulmonary hypertension
- Atrial septal defect (ASD)
- Tricuspid stenosis or regurgitation
- Transient P-pulmonale occurs in acute pulmonary embolism and acute severe asthma.

Causes of P-mitrale

- Mitral stenosis (the most common)
- Mitral regurgitation
- Secondary to ventricular hypertrophy due to any cause
- ASD.

BOTH RIGHT AND LEFT ATRIAL HYPERTROPHY (P-TRICUSPIDALE) (FIGS 8.5 AND 8.6)

ECG Criteria

Left atrial enlargement reflected by:
- Wide and notched P-wave in all limb leads and V_4 to V_6 the duration of the notch in V_5 and V_6 measures >0.04 sec.
- Widening of the terminal P-wave deflection—in V_1 (1.5 mm depth × 0.04 sec duration).

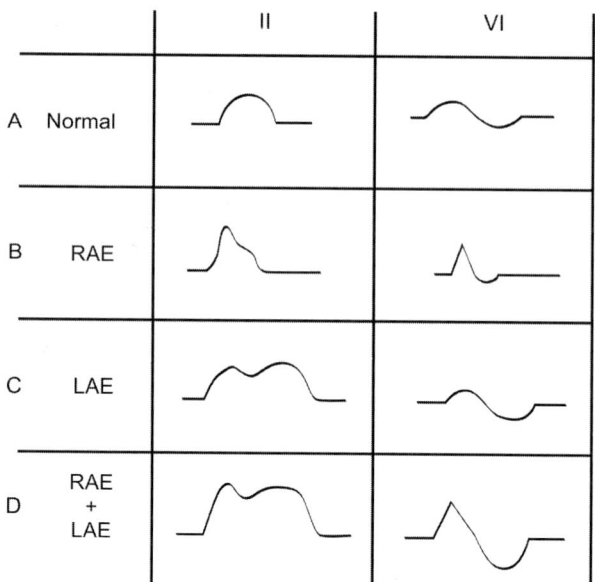

Fig. 8.5 Both atrial hypertrophies
Abbreviations: RAE, right atrial enlargement; LAE, left atrial enlargement

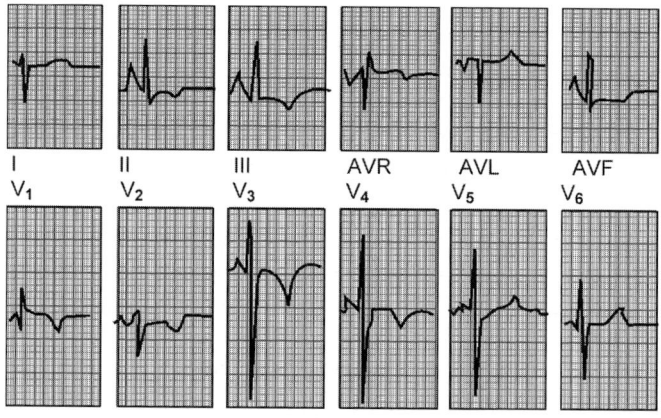

Fig. 8.6 Both right and left atrial hypertrophies

Right atrial enlargement reflected by:
Large amplitude of the initial P-wave in limb leads >2.5 mm and tall, peaked P-wave in V_2, V_3.

Causes

- Mitral stenosis associated with pulmonary hypertension (MS and PH)
- Mitral stenosis associated with tricuspid incompetence
- Mitral stenosis associated with tricuspid stenosis
- Atrial septal defect (ASD)
- *Lutembacher's syndrome*: Atrial septal defect with acquired mitral stenosis.

Various Causes of Atrial Enlargement

	Left atrial enlargement	Right atrial enlargement
Intracardiac shut	Ventricular septal defect (VSD)	Atrial septal defect (ASD)
A-V valve disease	Mitral stenosis (MS) Mitral regurgitation (MR)	Tricuspid stenosis (TS)
Outflow obstruction	Aortic stenosis (AS)	Pulmonary stenosis (PS)
Hypertension	Systemic hypertension	Pulmonary hypertension
Myocardial disease	Cardiomyopathy	Cor pulmonale

VENTRICULAR HYPERTROPHY

The right ventricle lies anterior to the left ventricle. Because, the left ventricle possesses 3–4 times the mass of the right ventricle, depolarization of the left ventricle produces the majority of the QRS deflection. Depolarization of both ventricle is represented in ECG by QRS complex which is >0.10 sec in duration. LV is three times thicker than the right ventricle the electrical potential of the LV is about 10 times greater than that of the right ventricle.

LEFT VENTRICULAR HYPERTROPHY (FIG. 8.7)

Definition: Left ventricular hypertrophy (LVH) is characterized by an increased left ventricular electrical force manifested by Tall R-waves in Leads V_5 - V_6 and a deep S-wave in V_1 that is associated with a secondary T-wave change (strain pattern) in Lead V_5 - V_6.

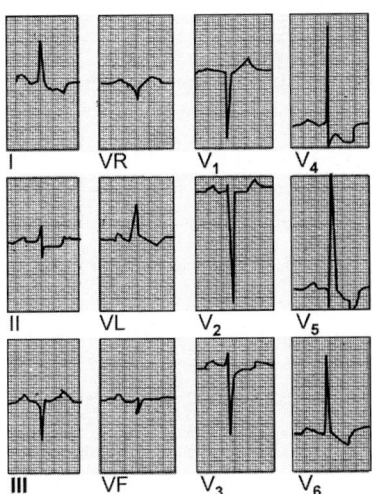

Fig. 8.7 Left ventricular hypertrophy

ECG Criteria

- Increased voltage of QRS complexes (Voltage criteria)
  - R-wave in V_5 or V_6 + S-wave in V_1 > 35 mm, or (SV_1 + RV_6 > 35 mm)
  - R-wave in V_5 or V_6 > 26 mm, or
  - R-wave in aVL > 11 mm, or
  - R-wave in 1 + S-wave in III > 25 mm, or
  - R-wave in a VF > 20 mm
  - R in L_1 > 15 mm
  - S in V_1 or V_2 > 25 mm
  - R in $V_6 \geq$ R in V_5
  - Total voltage of QRS in all 12 leads > 175 mm
- Repolarization changes
  - Minimum S-T depression with convexity upwards and T-inversion opposite in direction to the R-wave in I, aVL V_5, V_6 (Strain pattern)
- Left atrial enlargement
- *Left axis deviation (LAD)*: Tall R in I, aVL and deep S in II or III
- Delayed onset of intrinsicoid deflection or ventricular activation time (VAT) or R-peak time, greater than 0.05 sec in V_5, V_6.

Causes of LVH

As follows:
- Systemic hypertension
- Aortic stenosis
- Hypertrophic cardiomyopathy
- Coarctation of aorta
- Ventricular septal defect (VSD)
- Mitral regurgitation (MR)
- Aortic regurgitation (AR)
- Patent ductus arteriosus (PDA)
- Coronary artery disease (long standing).

Diagnosis of LVH clinically?
- Apex beat is heaving in nature
- Apex beat is not shifted as the hypertrophy is concentric type—at the expense of the cavity.

How to confirm the diagnosis of LVH?
By echocardiography (M-mode).

ECG criteria of LVH with strain
- Findings of LVH
- ST^- and T^- in L_1, aVL, $V_4 - V_6$.

Differential diagnosis of LVH and strain
- Hypertrophic cardiomyopathy
- Subendocardial MI (T inversion-symmetrically).

Romhilt-Estes Scoring System for LVH

	Points
	3

- R or S wave in any Limb $\geq$ 2 mv
  - Or, S in V_1 or V_2
  - Or, R in V_5 or $V_6 \geq$ 3 mv
- Left ventricular strain
  - ST segment and T in opposite direction to QRS
  - Without digitalis — 3
  - With digitalis — 1
- Left atrial enlargement
  - Terminal negativity of the P in V_1 is $\geq$ 0.10 mv in depth and $\geq$ 0.04 S in duration — 3
- Left axis deviation $\geq$ –30° — 2
- QRS duration $\geq$ 0.09 S — 1
- Intrinsicoid detection in V_5 or $V_6 \geq$ 0.05 S — 1

Sokolow-Lyon Criteria for LVH

- S-wave in V_1 + R-wave in V_5 or $V_6 \geq$ 3.50 mv or
- R-wave in V_5 or V_6 > 2.6 mv.

Cornell Voltage Criteria for LVH

- *Females*: R in aVL + S in V_3 > 2.00 mv
- *Males*: R in aVL + S in V_3 > 2.80 mv

Cause of Systolic and Diastolic Overload on LVH

Systolic	Diastolic
Aortic stenosis, i.e. valvular Supravalvular or, subvalvular	Mitral regurgitation (MR) or incompetence
Coarctation of aorta (CoA)	Aortic regurgitation (AR) or incompetence
Systemic hypertension	Moderate to large left to right shunt (PDA, VSD, etc.)
Hypertrophic cardiomyopathy	Beriberi or high cardiac output syndromes

Right Ventricular Hypertrophy (Fig. 8.8)

Definition: Right ventricular hypertrophy (RVH) is characterized by an increased anterior and rightward force manifested by a tall R-wave in V_1 that associated with right axis deviation (RAD) of the QRS.

ECG Criteria

- Right axis deviation (RAD)—between + 90° and + 180° deep S in lead I Tall R in aVF or III.

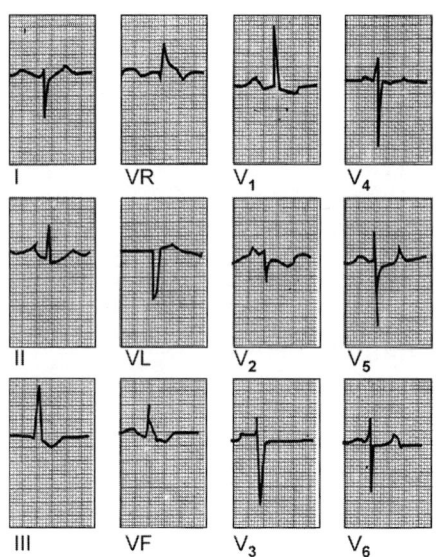

Fig. 8.8 Right ventricular hypertrophy

- Increased voltage of QRS-
  - R> S in V_1 or, V_2, or
  - R/S ratio in V_1 or V_2 greater than I, or
  - R-wave in V_1 + S-wave in V_5 or $V_6 \geq 10.5$ mm, or
  - R-wave in V_1 > 7 mm or
  - Prominent S-wave in V_5 or V_6 (S-wave ≥ 7 mm)
- Repolarization changes—ST depression and T inversion (strain pattern) in V_1, V_2
- *Mild increase in duration of QRS*: 0.10 sec or more
- Delayed onset of intrinsicoid deflection or VAT> 0.02 sec in V_1, V_2
- Incomplete right bundle branch block (RBBB) pattern (rSR in V_1)
- Small Q wave in V_1.

ECG Criteria for RVH in Age

- R in VI > 20 mm in all age
- S in V6 > 14 mm in 0–17 day
  - S in V6 > 10 mm in 1–6 month
  - S in V6 > 7 mm in 6–12 month
  - S in V6 > 5 mm in above 1 year
- 3. R: S in V_1
  - > 6.5 mm in 0–3 month
  - > 4 mm in 3–6 month
  - > 2.4 mm in 6 month to 3 years
  - > 1.6 mm in 3 yrs to 5 years
  - > 0.8 mm in 6 yrs to 15 years.

Hypertrophy

Causes of RVH

As follows:
- Chronic cor pulmonale
- MS and pulmonary hypertension
- Pulmonary hypertension (PH)
- Pulmonary stenosis (PS)
- Eisenmenger's syndrome
- Tetralogy of Fallot (TOF)
- ASD
- VSD
- Tricuspid regurgitation (TR).

Cause of tall R in V_1
- Normal variant
- RVH
- True posterior MI
- Wolff-Parkinson-White (WPW) syndrome (Type A)
- RBBB
- Dextrocardia.

Diagnosis of RVH clinically?

As follows:
- Left parasternal heave
- Epigastric pulsation

⎱ by palpation of precordium

RVH with strain
- Features of RVH
- ST depression and T-inversion (in V_1 and V_2).

Butler-Leggett Formula for RVH

Direction	Anterior (A)	Right ward (R)	Posterior left ward (PL)
Amplitude	Tallest R or R' in V_1 or V_2	Deepest S in 1 or V_6	S in V_1
RVH formula	A+ R– PL ≥ 0.70 mv		

Sokolow-Lyon Criteria for RVH

As follows:
R in Lead V_1 + S in V_5 or V_6 ≥ 1.10 mv

OVERLOAD CONCEPT OF LEFT VENTRICULAR HYPERTROPHY

Types

Left ventricular hypertrophy may occur as a result of two basic hemodynamic abnormalities (Figs 8.9A to C):
1. Systolic overload (pressure overload).
2. Diastolic overload (volume overload).

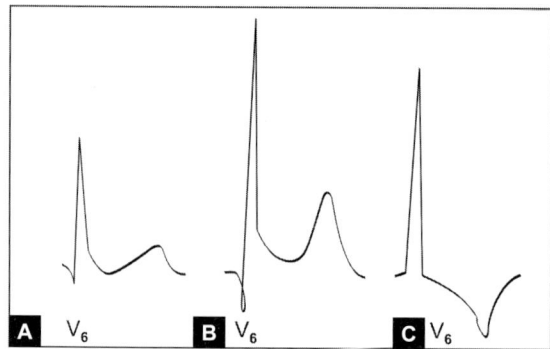

Figs 8.9A to C Normal QRS diastolic and systolic overload

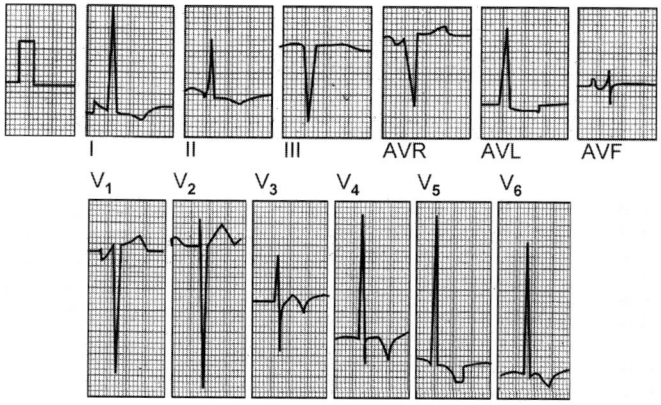

Fig. 8.10 Left ventricular systolic overload

Systolic overload: It is the expression of resistance to left ventricular systolic outflow and hence left ventricular systolic contraction (Fig. 8.10).

Cause

- Aortic stenosis (AS)
- Systemic hypertension
- Hypertrophic cardiomyopathy (HCM)
- Coarctation of the aorta (CoA).

Diastolic overload: It is due to overfilling of the left ventricle in diastole so that the left ventricular compromise occurs during diastole (Fig. 8.11).

Causes

- Mitral incompetence (MR)
- Aortic incompetence (AR)
- Ventricular septal defect (VSD)
- Patent ductus arteriosus (PDA).

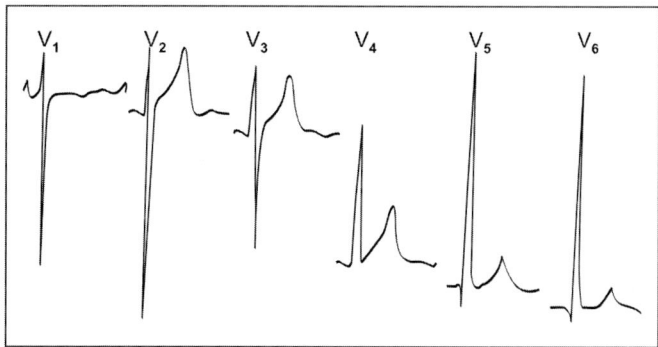

Fig. 8.11 Left ventricular diastolic overload

SYSTOLIC OVERLOAD (PRESSURE OVERLOAD) OF LEFT VENTRICULAR HYPERTROPHY

ECG Criteria

- Deep S-wave and T upright in $V_1 - V_4$
- Tall R-wave and T inversion in $V_5 - V_6$
- Minimal depression of ST segment with convexity upwards.

DIASTOLIC OVERLOAD (VOLUME OVERLOAD) OF LEFT VENTRICULAR HYPERTROPHY

ECG Criteria

- Long narrow Q-wave in I, aVL, V_5, V_6
- Long narrow Q-wave with tall R-wave with T-upright in V_5, V_6
- Minimal elevation of ST segment with concavity upwards.

ECG Criteria in Systolic Overload of LVH

As follows:
- Attenuation of small q in $V_5 - V_6$
- VAT (Ventricular activation time)—Increased due to hypertrophied ventricle
- ST strain pattern ie depression with slight convexity upwards in $V_5 - V_6$
- T in version in $V_5 - V_6$, I, aVL and upright in V_1, V_2 and aVR.

ECG Criteria in Diastolic Overload of LVH

As follows:
- Initial q is increased in amplitude in $V_5 - V_6$
- It remains usually normal
- Minimally elevated ST in $V_5 - V_6$ with concavity up wards and slight elevation of J point
- Tall symmetric upright T in $V_5 - V_6$. It is inverted in aVR.

BIVENTRICULAR HYPERTROPHY (FIG. 8.12)

(LVH and RVH)

Definition: Biventricular hypertrophy (BVH) is characterized by increased electrical forces of both ventricles as a result of the ventricular enlargement of both ventricles.

ECG Criteria

- ECG presentation of LVH with right axis deviation (RAD)
- ECG presentation of LVH with a degree of clockwise electrical rotation: a shift of the transition zone to the left.
- ECG presentation of LVH with tall R and V_1
  This is seen in ventricular septal defect (VSD) with pulmonary hypertension (Eisenmenger syndrome) with:
  - Tall R in left precordial leads
  - Tall R in right precordial leads
  - Large equiphasic QRS complexes in midprecordial leads (Katz-Wachtel phenomenon) (Fig. 8.13).
- Left atrial hypertrophy (LAH) with any one of the following three:
  1. R/s ratio in V_5 or $V_6 \leq 1$ mm
  2. S-wave in V_5 or $V_6 \geq 7$ mm
  3. Right axis deviation to the right of $+ 90°$
- Other findings:
  - LVH + RAD
  - LVH + R>S in V_1.

Causes of Biventricular Hypertrophy

As follows:
- Eisenmenger's syndrome (VSD or ASD or PDA with reversal of shunt)
- Hypertrophic cardiomyopathy (HCM)
- Multiple valvular disease (AS + PS).

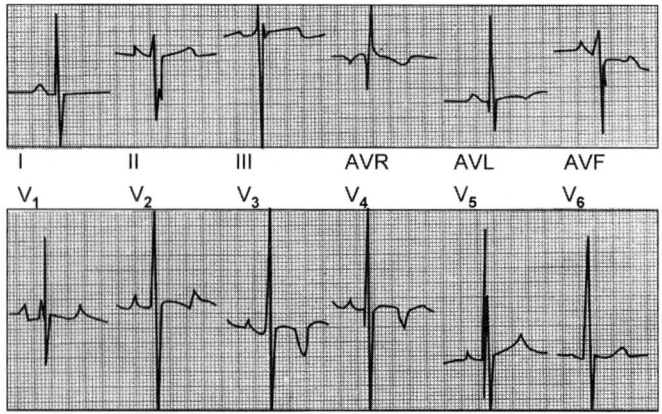

Fig. 8.12 Biventricular hypertrophy

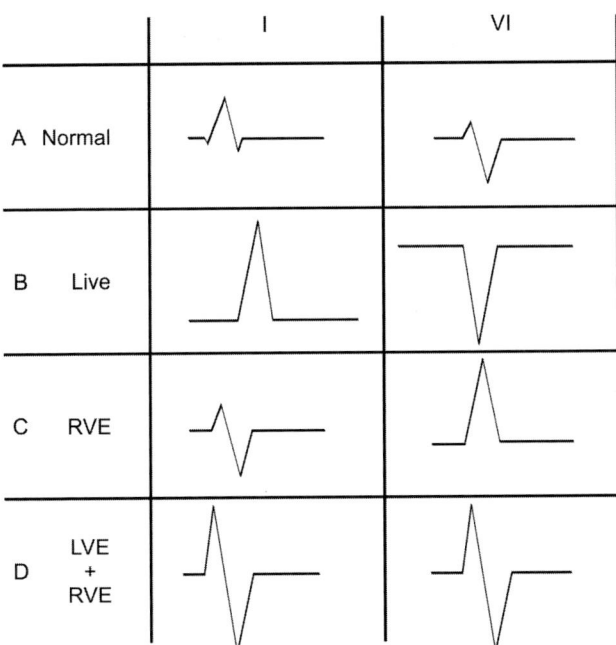

Fig. 8.13 QRS complex typical of ventricular enlargement in leads I and V_1.

Abbreviations: LVE, left-ventricular enlargement; RVE, right-ventricular enlargement

Common Diagnostic Criteria

- Left ventricular hypertrophy (LVH) or LBBB in precordial Leads with RAD in limb leads (most common)
- Tall R in all precordial leads with RAD
- *Katz-Wachtel phenomenon*: Large amplitude of positive and negative components of the QRS complexes in Lead V_2-V_4—usually RS complex
- P-pulmonale or P-congenitale in limb leads and LVH in precordial leads.

Note: RAD may be due to pulmonary embolism or left posterior hemiblock (LPHB)

RAD develops acutely in pulmonary embolism with various tachyarrhythmias, whereas LPHB almost always coexists with RBBB, Leading to Bifascicular Block.

9

Arrhythmias: Disorders of the Cardiac Rhythms

ARRHYTHMIAS

Definition: An arrhythmia is a disturbance in the electrical activity of the heart in a form of either disorder of impulse formation or disorder of impulse conduction or combined which may be paroxysmal or continuous.

Classification of Arrhythmias

- Primary disorders of rhythm
  - Disturbances of impulse formation
    - Sinus rhythms
      - Sinus premature beats
      - Sinus tachycardia
      - Sinus bradycardia
      - Sinus arrhythmia (respiratory and nonrespiratory)
      - Sinus arrest (pause or standstill) or vagotonic block
    - Atrial rhythms
      - Atrial premature beats
      - Paroxysmal atrial tachycardia
      - Multifocal chaotic atrial tachycardia
      - Wandering atrial pacemaker
      - Atrial flutter
      - Atrial fibrillation
    - AV nodal (junctional) rhythms
      - AV nodal ectopics or premature complexes
      - AV nodal tachycardia (paroxysmal and non-paroxysmal)
      - Extrasystolic AV nodal (idionodal) tachycardia
    - Ventricular rhythms
      - Ventricular premature complexes or ectopics
      - Idioventricular rhythm
      - Accelerated idioventricular rhythm
      - Ventricular tachycardia
      - Torsade de pointes
      - Ventricular flutter
      - Ventricular fibrillation
      - Chaotic rhythm

- Ventricular parasystole
- Ventricular asystole
  - Conduction defects
    - SA blocks
      - First degree
      - Second degree
      - Third degree
    - Intra-atrial blocks
    - AV blocks
      - First degree
      - Second degree (Mobitz type 1 and 11)
      - Complete AV block
      - Dual AV conduction
      - Supernormal AV conduction
    - Intraventricular blocks
      - Right bundle branch block (complete or incomplete)
      - Left bundle branch block (complete or incomplete)
      - Bilateral bundle branch block
      - Intermittent bundle branch block (right or left)
      - Peri-infarction block
    - Exit block
  - Miscellaneous disturbances (disturbance of both impulse formation and conduction)
    - aV dissociation (complete or incomplete)
    - Pre-excitation syndromes
    - Reciprocal beats, rhythm and tachycardia
    - Parasystole (atrial, AV nodal and ventricular)
    - Electrical alternans
    - Slow atrial rhythm
    - Left atrial rhythm
    - Coronary sinus rhythm
    - Concealed conduction
    - Phasic aberrant intraventricular conduction
  - Artificial pacemaker induced arrhythmias.
- Secondary disorders
  - Escapes rhythms
  - AV dissociation
  - Aberrant ventricular conduction.

Clinical Classification

- Tachyarrhythmia
  - Narrow QRS tachycardia
    - Regular
      - Sinus tachycardia
      - AV nodal reentrant tachycardia (SVT)
      - Atrial tachycardia
      - Atrial flutter and fixed AV-conduction
      - W-P-W syndrome
    - Irregular

- Atrial fibrillation (AF)
- Atrial flutter with variable AV conduction
- Multifocal atrial tachycardia (MAT)
  - Wide QRS tachycarida:
    - Regular
      - VT
      - SVT with BBB or with aberrant conduction
      - Atrial flutter and WPW conduction
      - Pre-excited tachycardia
    - Irregular
      - AF and WPW anterograde conduction
      - AF and intraventricular conduction defect.
- Brady arrhythmias:
  - Failure of impulse formation:
    - Sinus bradycardia
    - Sinus pauses, sinus arrest, SA block
    - SSS (sick-sinus-syndrome)
    - Carotid sinus hypersensitivity syndrome
    - Neuro-cardiogenic syncope.
  - AV conduction abnormalities
    - AV block: 1°, 2° CHB
    - AV dissociation.

Anatomy and Physiology of Conduction System (Fig. 9.1)

Normally the cardiac stimulus starts in pacemaker cells of the sinus node (SN) also called the sinoatrial (SA) node located high in the right atrium (RA) near the opening of the superior vena cave (SVC). From there the stimulus spreads downward and to the left, through the right and left atria and reaches the atrioventricular (AV) node, located near the top of the interventricular septum (IVS).

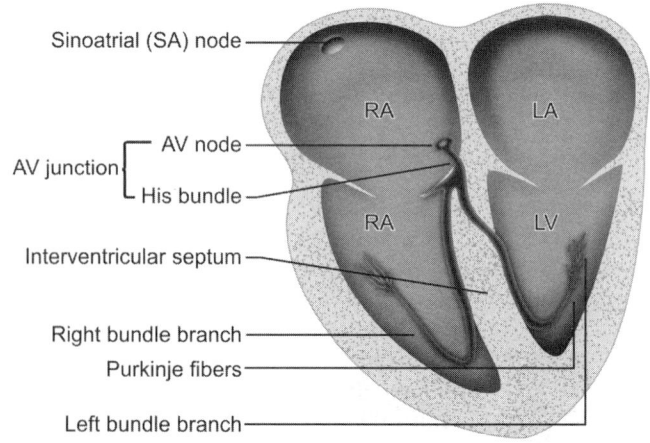

Fig. 9.1 Conduction system

After a delay, the stimulus spreads through the AV junction (AV node and bundle of His). The bundle of His then subdivided into right and left bundle branches.

The right bundle branch (RBB) runs down the interventricular septum and into the right ventricle. From there the small Purkinje fibers rapidly distribute the stimulus outward into the main muscle mass of the right ventricle.

Simultaneously, the left main bundle branch (LBB) carries the stimulus down the interventricular septum to the muscle mass of the left ventricle, also by way of the Purkinje fibers.

Disturbances in this process may produce abnormalities of heart rhythm, termed cardiac arrhythmias.

Discharge Rates of Potential Pacemakers of the Heart

Pacemaker   Discharge rate/minute
- SA node   – 75–80 approx
- AV node   – 50–60 approx
- Bundle of His   – 40–50 approx
- Purkinje cells   – 15–40 approx

Description of Abnormal Cardiac Rhythm

For description of a cardiac rhythm, three things are essential:
- Anatomical site
- Discharge sequence
- Conduction sequence.

Anatomical site: The rhythm may arise either from SA node, atria AV node, and bundle of his, bundle branches or ventricles.

Discharge sequence: Every rhythm has a discharge sequence, such as, normal sinus rhythm or an escape rhythm or idionodal or idioventricular rhythm. Bradycardia, tachycardia, extrasystoles, flutter, fibrillation also indicate the discharge sequence of a rhythm.

Conduction sequence: Conduction sequence must be described while interpreting a rhythm strip, i.e. 2:1 AV block, 3:2 SA or AV block, complete heart block (CHB) atrial flutter with 3:1 block, etc.

Genesis of Abnormal Cardiac Rhythm

Two main categories:
1. *Abnormalities of automaticity*: The abnormal automaticity arises from a single disordered cell or an ectopic focus of few cells.
2. *Abnormalities of conduction*: The abnormalities in conduction arise due to abnormal interaction between the cells.

Mechanisms of arrhythmias: Three mechanisms:
1. Accelerated automatcity.
2. Triggered activity:

- Due to early after depolarization called reflection
- Due to delayed after depolarization
3. Re-entry-Excitation, circus movement, reciprocal beats.

Tachyarrhythmias Due to Re-entry

SA node SA node tachycardia	Atrial Atrial flutter Atrial fibrillation	Nodal AV nodal re-entrant Tachycardia Atrio-ventricular tachycardia (AVRT) Pre-excitation syndrome tachycardia	Ventricular tachycardia Ventricular fibrillation

NORMAL SINUS RHYTHM (FIG. 9.2)

ECG Criteria

- Normal P, QRS complex
- P-P, R-R interval constant and equal
- Rate of 60–100 beats/minute
- P-R interval normal (0.12–0.20 sec)
- No ectopic activity.

Characteristics of Sinus Rhythm

- Rate   : 60–100 bpm
- Rhythm   : Regular
- P-wave   : Positive in lead
- PR interval   : 0.12–0.20 sec
- QRS duration : 0.10 sec or less

SINUS TACHYCARDIA (Fig. 9.3)

ECG Criteria

- P, QRS complex normal (P-wave of sinus origin)
- Rhythm (R-R interval) regular

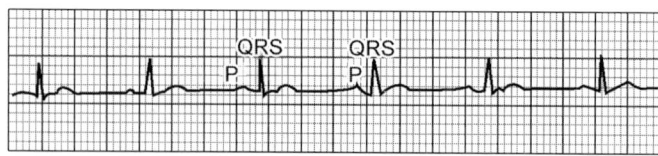

Fig. 9.2 Normal sinus rhythm at a rate of 60–100 beats/minute

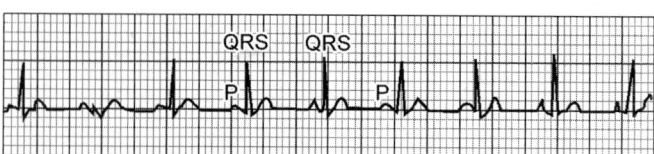

Fig. 9.3 Sinus tachycardia at a rate of 104 beats/minute

- Heart rate >100 beats/minute (not more than 150/minute)
- Constant and normal P-R interval (0.12–0.20 s).

Question: What is sinus Tachycardia?
Answer: Sinus tachycardia is the sinus rhythm with a heart rate greater than 100 bpm.

Causes of Sinus Tachycardia

Physiological

- Anxiety in neonates
- Emotion during REM sleep
- Exercise
- Pregnancy.

Pathological

- Anemia
- Fever
- Thyrotoxicosis
- Shock
- Heart failure (HF)
- Sick sinus syndrome (SSS)
- Chronic constrictive pericarditis
- Acute anterior MI
- Drugs
    - Salbutamol
    - Atropin
    - Adrenaline
    - Thyroid medications
    - Nicotine, alcohol
    - Caffeine
    - Amylnitrate
    - Nifedipine.

Causes of Narrow Complex Tachycardia

- Sinus tachycardia
- Atrial tachycardia
- Atrial flutter
- Atrial fibrillation
- AV re-entry tachycardia (SVT).

Causes of Broad Complex Tachycardia

- Ventricular tachycardia
- SVT and aberrant conduction
- WPW syndrome.

Treatment

Tablet propranolol 100 mg 1–2 tds orally.

Characteristics

- Rate   : 101–180 bpm
- Rhythm   : Regular
- P-wave   : Positive in Lead II
- PR interval : 0.12–0.20 s and constant
- QRS duration : 0.10 s or less

SINUS BRADYCARDIA (FIG. 9.4)

ECG Criteria

- P, QRS complex normal, P-wave of sinus origin
- R-R interval regular
- Heart rate is less than 60/minute
- Constant and normal P-R interval (0.12–0.20 sec).

Question: What is sinus bradycardia?
Answer: Sinus bradycardia is the sinus rhythm and heart rate less than 60 bpm.

Note: Sinus bradycardia may be associated with sinus arrhythmia.

Causes of Sinus Bradycardia

- Physiological (due to increased vagal tone)
  - Athlete
  - Sleep
  - Vagotonic persons—induced by carotid sinus compression
- Pathological
  - Acute inferior MI
  - Sick sinus syndrome
  - Raised intracranial pressure (due to inhibitory effect on sympathetic outflow)
  - Drugs   - Digoxin
            - β-blocker
            - Verapamil (CCB)
  - Hypothyroidism
  - Obstruction jaundice
  - Hypothermia
  - Electrolyte imbalance, i.e. hyperkalemia, hypermagnesemia

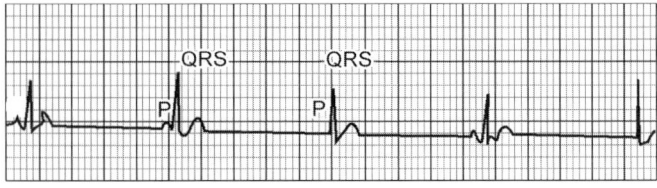

Fig. 9.4 Sinus bradycardia at a rate of 54 beats/minute

- Uremia
- Poisoning—organophosphorus
- Hyperactive carotid sinus.

Causes of Bradycardia

- Sinus bradycardia due to any cause
- Sick sinus syndrome
- 2° HB (Mobitz type II)
- Complete heart block
- Nodal rhythm
- Idioventricular rhythm
- Drugs   – β-blocker
            – Digoxin

Treatment

- If pulse <60 beats/minute and BP normal: no treatment
- If BP low: Inj-Atropine 0.5 mg IV stat and repeat.

Characteristics of Sinus Bradycardia

- Rate   : Less than 60 bpm
- Rhythm   : Regular
- P-wave   : Positive (upright) in Lead II
- PR interval   : 0.12–20 sec and constant
- QRS duration : 0.10 sec or less

SINUS ARRHYTHMIA (FIG. 9.5)

Definition: Sinus arrhythmia is an irregular cardiac rhythm originating from the sinus node in which heart rate increases in inspiration and decreases in expiration.

Types: Three major types:
1. *Respiratory sinus arrhythmia*: In this form, the sinus rate increases with inspiration and slows with expiration. This is due to reflex stimulation of vagal receptors in the lungs it is benign condition. In ECG, the R-R interval shortens during inspiration and lengthens during expiration. It is common in children and young adults.
2. *Nonrespiratory sinus arrhythmia*: This form has no relation ship to respiration.

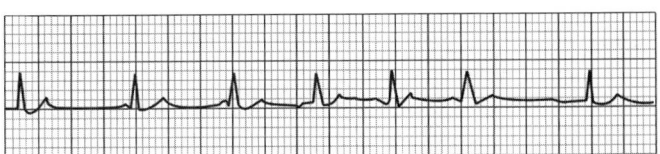

Fig. 9.5 Sinus arrhythmia

This is observed during certain conditions where vagal tone fluctuates such as in persons with a cardiac disease or myocardial infarction.

This is often called idiopathic. In ECG, there are alternate periods of lengthening and shortening of R-R intervals.

3. *Ventriculophasic sinus arrhythymia*: This arrhythmia occurs due to the influence of autonomic nervous system in response to changes. In ventricular stroke volume example complete heart block (CHB).

Diagnostic Clues

- Maximum R-R interval – minimum R-R interval in the same lead exceeds 0.12 sec.
- Maximum R-R interval – minimum R-R interval ÷ minimum R-R interval exceeds 10% in the same lead.

ECG Criteria

- P, QRS-T complex: Normal. P-wave of sinus origin
- *Heart rate*: Increases during inspiration and decreases during expiration which is characterized by gradually lengthening of P-P intervals or R-R intervals during expiration and shortening of R-R intervals during inspiration.
- *Constant and normal P-R interval*: Constant P-wave configuration.

Note:

- Physiologically—common in young adult.
- Accentuated by vagotonic procedure
  - Digitalis administration
  - Carotid sinus massage
- Abolished by vagolytic procedures
  - Exercise
  - Atropine
  - Amylnitrite
- Nonrespiratory sinus arrhythmia in adult
  - Heart disease
  - After MI.

Mechanism

It is the manifestation of autonomic activity which varies and respiration

- In inspiration, parasympathetic activity diminishes, so heart rate increases. It reverses during expiration.
- Sinus arrhythmia is a benign condition common in children and young adults
- It is absent in autonomic neuropathy.

Note: Sinus arrhythmia may be associated with:
- Sinus bradycardia
- Wandering pacemaker
- Sinus tachycardia.

Characteristics of Sinus Arrhythmia

- Rate : Usually 60–100 bpm may be slower on faster
- Rhythm : Irregular
  Phasic with respiration
  Heart rate increases gradually during inspiration (R-R shorten) and decreases with expiration (R-R lengthen)
- P-wave : Positive (upright) in Lead II
- PR interval : 0.12–0.20 sec and constant from beat to beat
- QRS duration : 0.10 sec or less

PACEMAKER SITES OF THE HEART (FIG. 9.6)

The SA node, in right atrium, is the pacemaker site where impulses are normally initiated.

Ectopic: Impulses originating outside of the SA node are termed ectopic.

If SA node fails, either a lower escape pacemaker site takes over or the heart stops beating. Potential ectopic pacemaker sites are located throughout the heart in the atria AV-junction and the ventricles.

Rate of SA node: 60–100 beats/minute in adults. So lower ectopic pacemaker site have slower intrinsic rate. When a higher pacemaker site fails to discharge, a lower site normally takes over. This is called 'escape rhythm'.

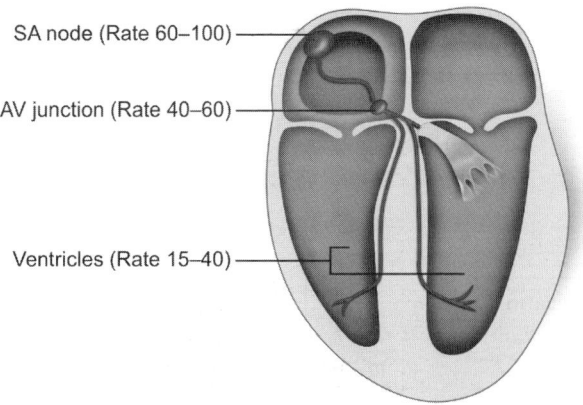

Fig. 9.6 Pacemaker sites

Rate of AV-junction: 40–60 beats/minute; if ectopic impulses originate in this area as an it is called 'junctional escape rhythm'.

Intrinsic rate of ventricles: 15–40 beats/minute, if ectopic impulses originate in the ventricles, called ventricular escape rhythm.

ECTOPIC BEAT (FIG. 9.7)

Definition: Ectopic beat or extrasystole is a premature extra beat that comes earlier than the normal beat. It arises from abnormal focus from atria AV node or ventricle.

ECG criteria: In ECG sequence is as follows:
 Normal beat → short pause → ectopic beat → long pause → strong beat.

Types of Ectopic (Extra Systole) (Figs 9.8A and B)

Three types:
1. *Atrial ectopic beat*: High atrial, low atrial
2. *Nodal ectopic beat*: High nodal (P inverted)
   Mid nodal (P is not seen buried in QRS)
   Low nodal (P after QRS)
3. Ventricular ectopic beat (VES).

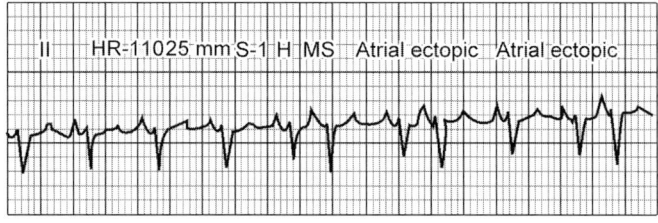

Fig. 9.7 Ectopic beat

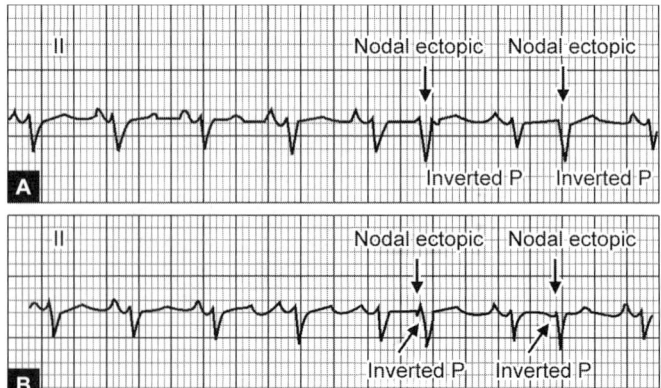

Figs 9.8A and B (A) Low nodal ectopic; (B) High nodal ectopic

ATRIAL EXTRASYSTOLES (AES) OR ATRIAL PREMATURE CONTRACTION (APC) OR ATRIAL PREMATURE OR ECTOPIC BEATS (FIG. 9.9)

This is an ectopic, supraventricular impulse that originates in the atria outside of the SA node.

ECG Criteria

- *P*: Small or inverted (abnormal shape)
- *PR interval*: Short (followed by wide pause)
- *PP interval*: Irregular.

Note: When atrial ectopic is associated with tachycardia, it is called chaotic or multifocal atrial tachycardia atrial ectopic may not be followed by QRS. It is called blocked or non-conducted atrial ectopic.

Causes of Atrial Ectopic (Fig. 9.10)

- Normal people
- Excess tea, coffee, smoking, alcohol, stress, anxiety
- *Organic heart disease*: Myocarditis, Ischemia, HF, cardiomyopath, valvular heart disease, digitalis intoxication
- *Electrolyte imbalance*: Hypokalemia
- COPD (Multifocal atrial tachycardia due to hypoxemia)
- Endogenous—   Febrile illness
   Thyrotoxicosis
   Emotional stress
- Systemic factors—   Infection.

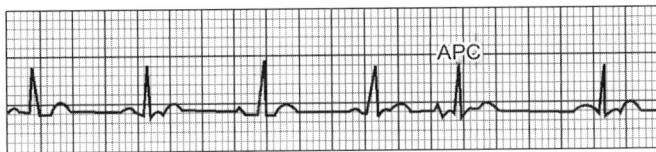

Fig. 9.9 Atrial premature contraction

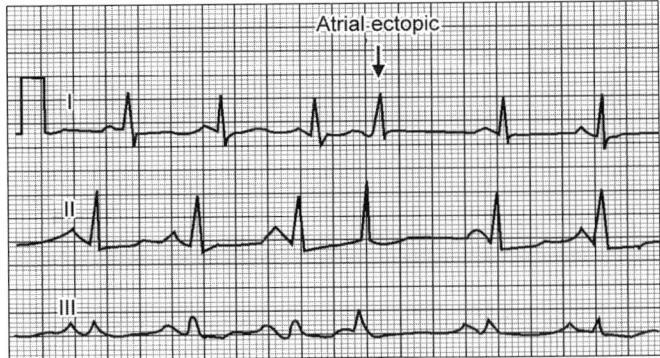

Fig. 9.10 Atrial ectopic

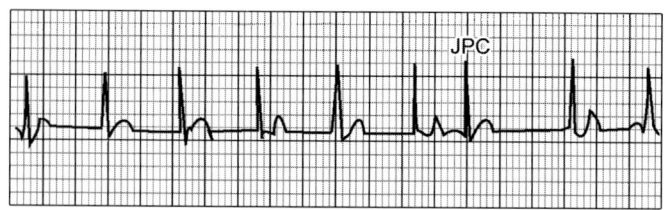

Fig. 9.11 Junctional premature contraction (JPC)

Types of Atrial Ectopic

Two types:
1. High atrial–P is upright in L_1 aVF.
2. Low atrial–P is inverted in L_{II}, L_{III}, aVF (confuse with high nodal ectopic).

JUNCTIONAL PREMATURE CONTRACTION (FIG. 9.11)

The junctional premature contraction (JPC) is an ectopic, supraventricular impulse that originates in the junction.

Types

- High nodal
- Mid nodal
- Low nodal.

ECG Criteria

- P-wave inverted in II, III, aVF
- *Inverted* P-wave immediately precedes the early QRS complex
- P-wave may occur just before or just after the QRS complex or may be buried in QRS complex.

NODAL RHYTHM (JUNCTIONAL RHYTHM)

Definition: When the impulse originate from AV node.

It is called nodal or junctional rhythm. If the rate is high, it is called junctional tachycardia. Usually it occurs due to depressed activity of SA node.

ECG Criteria

- Heart rate—40-60 bpm
- P-small, inverted (P-may not be seen, buried in QRS or after QRS)
- PR interval short.

Types: 3 types:
- High nodal rhythm—small inverted P before ORS
- Mid nodal rhythm—P is not seen (buried in ORS)
- Low nodal rhythm—P after ORS.

Causes of Nodal Rhythm (Fig. 9.12)

It may be transient or permanent.

As follows:
- Digitalis toxicity
- Ischemic heart disease (Commonly inferior MI)
- Rheumatic myocarditis
- Myocarditis.

WANDERING ATRIAL PACEMAKER (WANDERING PACEMAKER) (FIGS 9.13 AND 9.14)

In Wandering Pacemaker in the sinus node, the pacemaker shifts from one part of the sinus node to another so that the P-wave configuration changes from beat to beat and P-R interval is also variable.

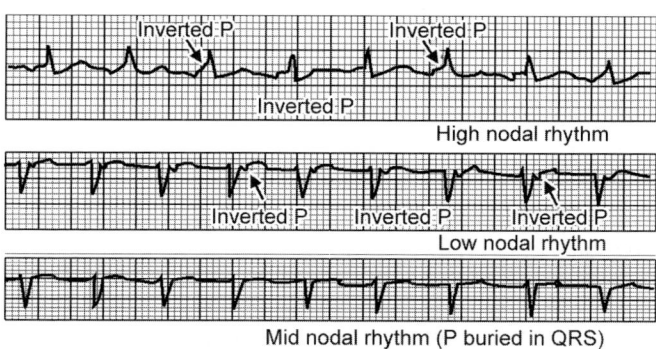

Fig. 9.12 Nodal rhythm

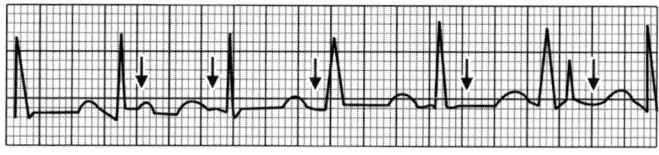

Fig. 9.13 Wandering atrial pacemaker between the SA node and the AV junction

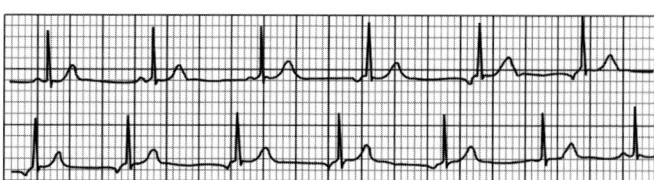

Fig. 9.14 Wandering atrial pacemaker

It is quite distinct from multifocal atrial tachycardia (MAT), another arrhythmia with multiple different P-wave. In Wandering atrial pacemaker the rate is normal or slow. In MAT, it is rapid.

This is a supraventricular rhythm where the pacemaker impulses originate from two or more different foci in the SA node, atria, or AV junction at a rate between 60 beats/minute and 100 beats/minute.

ECG Criteria

- P-wave configurations vary (some inverted, some small, some upright), P-wave of sinus origin
- P-R intervals vary, slightly irregular or regular P-P cycles
- Heart rate between 60 beats/minute and 100 beats/minute
- QRS normal.

Causes of Wandering Pacemaker

As follows:
- Normal individual (due to increase in vagal tone), athletes
- Rheumatic carditis
- Chronic lung disease (COPD)
- Digitalis toxicity
- Valvular disease (Mitral and tricuspid valve disease)
- Sick sinus syndrome.

Note:
- *Supraventricular arrhythmias*: The pacemaker impulses originate above the ventricles, i.e. SA node, the atria, the AV junction then bundle of His. It produces narrow QRS complexes.
- *Ventricular arrhythmias*: The pacemaker impulses originate in the ventricles. It produces wide QRS complex.
- Wandering pacemaker may be associated with sinus arrrhthmia.

Characteristics of Wandering Pacemaker

- *Rate*: Usually 60–100 bpm. But be slow if the rate is greater than 100 bpm, the rhythm is termed multifocal (chaotic) atrial tachycardia.
- *Rhythm*: May be irregular as the pacemaker site shifts from SA node to ectopic atrial locations and the AV junction.
  - *P-wave*: Size, shape and direction may change from beat to beat
  - *PR interval*: Variable
  - *QRS duration*: 0.10 sec or less unless an intraventricular conduction delay exists.

MULTIFOCAL ATRIAL TACHYCARDIA (FIG. 9.15)

It is an ectopic supraventricular tachycardia that originates from three or more atrial foci at a rate between 100 bpm and 250 bpm. Multifocal atrial tachycardia (MAT) can also occur without inducing tachycardia.

Definition: MAT is a rapid and irregular cardiac rhythm originating from two or more different sites of the atrium.

ECG Criteria

- Three or more different P-wave configuration and varying P-R intervals (due to different ectopic atrial foci)
- Varying P-P intervals (P-wave irregularly)
- Tachycardia, rate 100–250 beats/minute
- AV blocks of varying degree (Non-conducted ectopic P-wave).

If P-wave are not readily identifiable, MAT may be atrial fibrillation.

Note: MAT is found in patients with COPD and acute respiratory distress with resulting hypoxemia (decreased arterial PO_2).

Causes

- Pulmonary diseases
  - COPD
  - Cor-pulmonale
  - Acute respiratory distress or failure
  - Acute interstitial lung disease
  - Pulmonary embolism
  - Pneumonias
- Congestive heart failure
- Drugs—theophylline.

Treatment

- Correction of hypoxemia
- Correction of underlying causes.

Clinical Significance

It is easily confused with atrial fibrillation due to variable morphologies of the P-wave which may be confused with

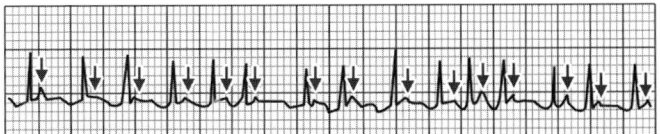

Fig. 9.15 Multifocal atrial tachycardia, greater than 3 different foci (arrows) discharge irregularly (90–180) beats/minute

fibrillatory (f) waves. Atrial fibrillation (AF) needs digitalis to slow the ventricular rate, if not differentiated from MAT, then unnecessary high doses of digitalis may be given. But MAT does not respond and results in digitalis toxicity. MAT may develop into atrial fibrillation.

ACCELERATED JUNCTIONAL RHYTHM (FIGS 9.16 AND 9.17)

(Nonparoxysmal Junctional Tachycardia)

Definition: Nonparoxysmal junctional tachycardia is moderately rapid and regular tachycardia with normal QRS complexes originating from any portion of the AV junctional tissues. The QRS complexes may be preceded by or followed by retrograde P-wave.

This is a supraventricular rhythm that originates from an enhanced focus in the AV junction at a rate faster than the normal intrinsic junctional rate of 40–60/minute.

ECG Criteria

- Inverted P-wave in II, III, aVF
- P-wave may occur just before or after the QRS or may be hidden in the QRS and not seen at all
- QRS normal and narrow
- *Heart rate*: 60–150 beats/minute
- Tachycardia is not paroxysmal in nature.

Causes

- Digoxin toxicity
- Acute inferior MI
- Effect of thrombolytic therapy.

Note: The QRS complexes are usually narrow and unchanged in configuration and occur at a rate of 60–150 bpm. If there is

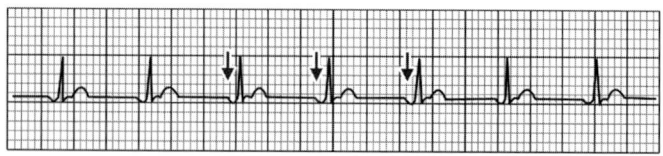

Fig. 9.16 Accelerated junctional rhythm, the inverted P (arrows) immediately preceding the narrow ORS complexes)

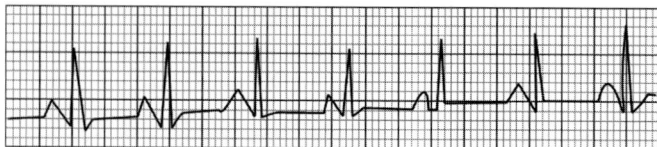

Fig. 9.17 Accelerated junction rhythm

retrograde conduction from the junctional pacemaker to the atria, inverted P-wave may be seen in Leads II, III, aVF.

Impulse formation in accelerated junctional rhythm is enhanced automatic focus in the AV junction that usurps SA node activity and fires at a rate between 60 bpm and 150 bpm. But paroxysmal junctional tachycardia involves a re-entry circuit as its mechanism of impulse formation.

It may begin abruptly and persist for longer periods of time than paroxysmal junctional tachycardia.

SUPRAVENTRICULAR TACHYCARDIA (SVT) OR PAROXYSMAL ATRIAL TACHYCARDIA (PAT) (FIG. 9.18)

Definition: SVT is a tachycardia which originates above the bifurcation of the bundle tissues proximal of the bundle re-entrant >100 bpm of His or incorporates to the bifurcation of His in a circuit and a rate.

ECG Criteria

- P-wave absent (hidden in QRS complex)
- Narrow QRS complex (<0.06 sec) and normal
- *R-R interval (rhythm):* Regular
- *Heart rate:* 150–250 beats/minute.

Note:
The PAT refers to a SVT derived from impulses that follows a re-entry circuit in the atria or in the AV junction area. The re-entry circuit causing PAT may be located in the:
- SA node (sinus node re-entrant tachycardia)
- Atria (intra-atrial re-entrant tachycardia)
- AV junction (AV junction re-entrant tachycardia).

Management of SVT

- Bedrest, reassurance
- *Diet*: Liquid
- O_2 *inhalalion:* SOS (if necessary)
- Maintain IV channel
- Continuous cardiac monitoring

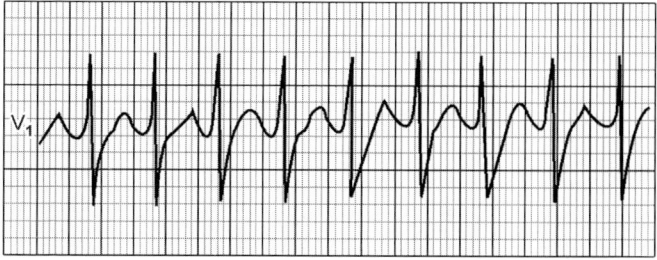

Fig. 9.18 Supraventricular tachycardia

- Valsalva maneuver it acts by increasing the vagal tone
- If fail, carotid sinus massage
- If fail, inj. diazepam (e.g. Sedil) 1 amp IV slowly diluted with distilled water
  If fail, IV adenosin—3 mg over 2 sec, if no response in 1-2 minutes, then 6 mg IV. If no response, then 12 mg (maximum dose)
- If fail Inj. verapamil 2.5-10 mg IV slowly, then table verapamil as a maintenance if QRS >0.12 sec or history of WPW syndrome or if the patient is on β-blocker, verapamil should be avoided.
- If fail, again Inj. verapamil
- If fail, DC (Direct current shock) (if patient is hemodynamically unstable, e.g. hypotension, pulmonary edema)
- Drugs—β-blocker disophyramide or digoxin
- If the attack is frequent prophylactic oral therapy with β-blocker, verapamil digoxin
- In Wolff-Parkinson-white syndrome—transvenous radio-frequency catheter ablation (RFA)
- In some cases—antitachycardial pacing (overdrive atrial pacing).

Causes of Supraventricular Tachycardia

- Physiological
  Anxiety, tension, drinking of coffee, tea, alcohol
- Pathological
  - Thyrotoxic crisis
  - Coronary artery disease
  - Wolff-Parkinson-white syndrome
  - Digitalis toxicity.

Differences between Sinus Tachycardia and SVT

Points	Sinus tachycardia	Supraventricular tachycardia
1. Onset	Gradual	Sudden
2. Pulse	<160 bpm	>160 bpm (140–220)
3. ECG	P, QRS T-normal	P-absent QRS-narrow
4. Symptoms	Palpitation	Sudden palpitation, dizziness, syncope, breathlessness, polyuria after attack (Due to ANP)
5. Carotid sinus massage or Valsalva maneuver	No or little response	May respond abruptly
6. Prognosis	Not serious	Hemodynamic instability is common

Complication of SVT

In SVT, because of rapid heart rate, there is short diastolic filling time. This results in reduction of stroke volume and precipitate heart failure.

Types of SVT

As follows:
- Sinus tachycardia
- AV nodal reentry tachycardia (AVNRT)
- Atrial tachycardia
- Atrial flutter
- Atrial fibrillation
- Multifocal atrial tachycardia
- Accelerated junctional tachycardia
- AV re-entrant tachycardia (AVRT).

Note:
- SVT is a misnomer, the types mentioned above are all SVT
- Sinus tachycardia neither starts abruptly nor stops abruptly
- If SVT is associated with WPW syndrome, verapamil should not be given intravenously
- Adenosine is safe in such case
- Look for carotid bruit before carotid sinus massage otherwise, thrombus may be dislodged and may cause cerebral embolism.

Adenosine

- Mode of action : It courses transient AV block
  Lasting for few seconds
  Half Life—8–10 sec
- Side effects : Chest pain
  Bronchospasm
  Dyspnea
  Choking sensation
  Transient flushing
  Hypotension
- Contraindication : Sick sinus syndrome (SSS)
  History of bronchial asthma $2°$ or $3°$ heart block

Supraventricular tachycardia (SVT) may be (Fig. 9.19):
- Regular
  - SVT
  - PSVT (Paroxysmal SVT)
  - Atrial flutter
- Irregular
  - Atrial fibrillation (AF)
  - Atrial flutter—sometimes
  - Multifocal atrial tachycardia (MAT).

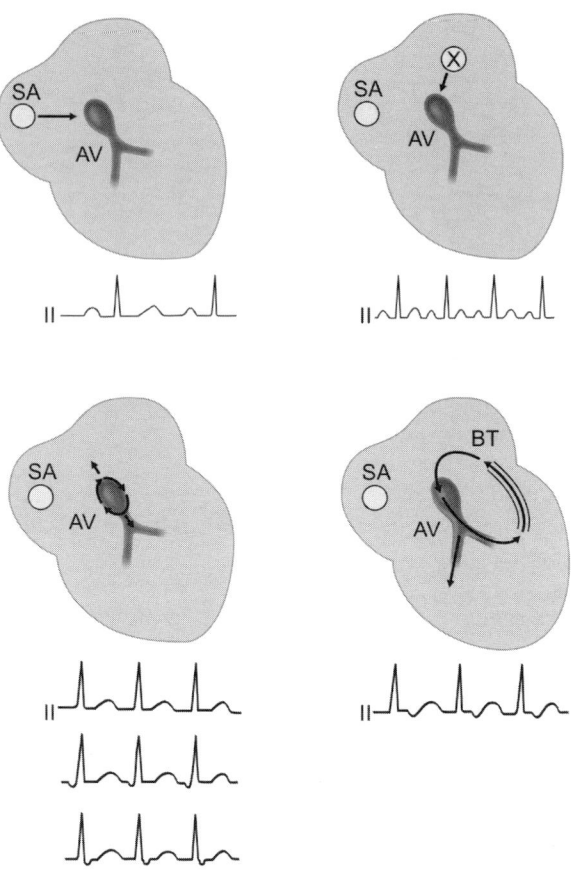

Fig. 9.19 Supraventricular tachycardia

PSVT: It is defined as conduction of supraventricular impulses at a rate of more than 100 bpm with narrow QRS, regular R-R interval and without an evidence of pre-excitation. If associated with wide QRS it is called paroxysmal SVT with aberrant conduction.

Classification of SVT (According to Duration)

- Paroxysmal SVT
  - Paroxysmal in onset and offset
  - Tends to be recurrent
  - Duration—seconds to hours
  - Found in
    - PSVT due to AV nodal reentry
    - PSVT due to WPW syndrome
    - PSVT due to paroxysmal AF
    - PSVT due to paroxysmal atrial flutter
- Persistant SVT
  - Lasts for days to weeks

- Contributing pathophysiologic factors
  - Decompensated COPD
  - Pulmonary embolism
  - Electrolyte imbalance
  - Drug toxicity
- Found in
  - Sinus tachycardia
  - Ectopic atrial tachycardia (Nonparoxysmal)
  - Multifocal atrial tachycardia
- Chronic SVT
  - Chronic atrial flutter
  - Chronic atrial fibrillation

Do not revert if untreated often fails to revert with treatment.

SVT: P-R and R-P relationship
- Short P-R/Long R-P relationship
  - Atrial tachycardia—Sinus node re-entrant tachycardia
  - Atypical AV nodal reentry—AVRT with slowly conducting pathway
- Long P-R/Short R-P interval
  - AV nodal re-entry—Atrioventricular re-entrant tachycardia (AVNRT).

ATRIAL TACHYCARDIA (FIG. 9.20)

Definition: Atrial tachycardia (AT) is the regular and rapid cardiac rhythm originating from any position of the atria.

Three Major Types of Paroxysmal SVT

- Atrial tachycardia (AT) and related rhythms
- Atrio ventricular nodal re-entrant tachycardia (AVNRT)
- AV re-entrant tachycardia (AVRT) involving a bypass tract of the type seen in the Wolf-Parkinson-White (WPW) syndrome.

Characteristics of AT

- Rate   : 100–250 bpm
- Rhythm   : Regular
- P-wave   : One positive P-wave precedes each QRS in Lead II P-wave differ in shape from sinus P-wave
- PR interval : May be shorter or longer than normal
- QRS duration : 0.10 sec or less unless an intraventricular conduction delay exists.

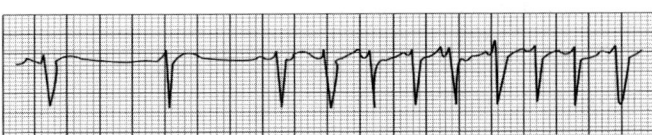

Fig. 9.20 Atrial tachycardia

ECG Criteria

- P-wave abnormal
- *Atrial rate*: 140–220 beats/minute
- 2 : 1, 3 : 1 or variable heart block
- QRS—normal may be broad and bizarre because of LBBB, RBBB or aberrant ventricular contraction (AVC)
- Rhythm-normal.

Note: Atrial tachycardia and AV block is common in digoxin toxicity.

AT is frequently initiated by atrial premature contraction (APC).

Causes of Atrial Tachycardia

- Digoxin toxicity
- Ischemic heart disease
- Rheumatic heart disease
- Cardio myopathy
- Sick sinus syndrome (SSS).

Mechanism

Atrial tachycardia is due to the ectopic focus that arise from any part of atrial muscle.

Treatment

As follows:
- If due to digoxin—it should be stopped
- It not due to digoxin
    - To control the HR—digoxin
        β-blocker
        Verapamil
        Amiodarone
    - If no response— Flecanide
        DC cardioversion
    - Atrial overdrive pacing in selected cases
    - Transvenous radio-frequency catheter ablation (in persistent and troublesome symptoms).

Note:
- Carotid sinus massage will not terminate the atrial tachycardia
- Atrial tachycardia is usually paroxymal, so it is called paroxysmal atrial tachycardia (PAT).

Characteristics of AV Nodal Re-entrant Tachycardia (AVNRT)

- Rate   : 150–250 bpm
- Rhythm   : Ventricular rhythm is usually very regular

- P-wave   : P-wave are often hidden in the QRS if the ventricles are stimulated first and then the atria, a negative (Inverted) P-wave will appear after the QRS in leads II, III, and aVF when the atria are depolarized after the ventricles, the P-wave typically distorts the end of the QRS complex.
- PR interval : P-wave are not seen before the QRS, therefore the PR interval is not measurable
- QRS duration : 0.10 s or less unless an intraventricular conduction delay exists.

Differences between Sinus and Atrial Tachycardia

	Sinus tachycardia	Atrial tachycardia
Heart rate	100–150 bpm	150–220 bpm
Regularity	Respiratory variation	Clock-like
Onset	Gradual warming up	Sudden
P-wave	Normal	Ectopic or inverted
ECG	Often normal	
Effect of vagal maneuvers	Slowing of rate	APCs or WPW syndrome Termination

Differences between Ectopic and Re-entrant Tachycardia

	Ectopic tachycardia	Re-entrant tachycardia
Heart rate	120–150 bpm	>150 bpm
Onset and offset	Gradual	Sudden
Past history	Not significant	Of previous episodes
Organic heart disease	May be present	Generally absent
P-wave	Ectopic, visible	Inverted, rarely visible
AV block	Can Co-exit	Never, 1:1 conduction
Effect of vagal maneuvers	Slowing	Termination

Differences between AVNRT and AVRT

AVNRT	AVRT (orthodromic conduction)
• Re-entry circuit is formed between fast and slow pathways within AV node (Micro reentry circuit)	• Re-entry circuit is constituted by the AV node and accessory pathway for reciprocation (Macro re-entry circuit)
• P-wave may not be visible	• Inverted visible P-wave generally follow narrow QRS
• QRS alternans can occur when rate is very fast	• No such alternans is seen
• Carotid sinus massage can slow the tachycardia	• There is either no effect or there may be slight slowing
• More common cause of PSVT	• Less common

NORMAL RANGES AND VARIATIONS IN THE ADULT ECG

Lead	P	Q	R	S	ST	T
I	Upright	Small (less than 0.04 s and less than 25% of R)	Dominant, Largest deflection of the QRS complex	Less than R, or none	Usually isoelectric; may vary from +1 to 0.5 mm	Upright
II	Upright	Small or none	Dominant	Less than R, or none	Usually isoelectric; may vary from +1 to −0.5 mm	Upright
III	Upright, flat, diphasic, or inverted, depending on frontal plane axis	Small or none, depending on frontal plane axis; or large (0.04–0.05 s or greater than 25% of R)	None to dominant, depending on frontal plane axis	None to dominant, depending on frontal plane axis	Usually isoelectric; may vary from +1 to −0.5 mm	Upright, flat diphasic, or inverted, depending on frontal plane axis
aVR	Inverted	Small, none, or large	Small or none, depending on frontal plane axis	Dominant (may be QS)	Usually isoelectric; may vary from +1 to −0.5 mm	Inverted
aVL	Upright, flat, diphasic or inverted, depending on frontal plane axis	Small, none, or large depending on frontal plane axis	Small, none, or dominant, depending on frontal plane axis	None to dominant, depending on frontal plane axis	Usually isoelectric; may vary from +1 to −0.5 mm	Upright, flat, diphasic, or inverted depending on frontal plane axis

Contd...

Contd...

Lead	P	Q	R	S	ST	T
aVF	Upright	Small or none	Small, none, or dominant, depending on frontal plane axis	None to dominant; depending on frontal plane axis	Usually isoelectric; may vary from +1 to −0.5 mm	Upright, flat, diphasic, or inverted depending on frontal plane axis
V_1	Inverted, flat, upright, or diphasic	None (may be QS)	Less than S, or none (QR); small r may be present	Dominant (may be QS)	0 to +3 mm	Upright, flat, diphasic, or inverted
V_2	Upright, less commonly diphasic or inverted	None (may be QS)	Less than S, or none (QS); small r may be present	Dominant (may be QS)	0 to +3 mm	Upright, less commonly flat diphasic, or inverted
V_3	Upright	Small or none	R less than, greater than, or equal to S	S greater than, less than, or equal to R	0 to +3 mm	Upright
V_4	Upright	Small or none	R > S	S less than R	Usually isoelectric; may vary from +1 to −0.5 mm	Upright
V_5	Upright	Small	Dominant (< 26 mm)	S less than SV		Upright
V_6	Upright	Small	Dominant (< 26 mm)	S less than SV		Upright

Atrial Arrhythmias

- Common
  - Atrial premature contraction (APC)
  - Atrial tachycardia (AT)
  - Atrial fibrillation (AF)
  - Atrial flutter
  - Atrial flutter—fibrillation.
- Less common
  - Slow atrial tachycardia
  - Multifocal atrial tachycardia (MAT)
  - Atrial escape rhythm
  - Left atrial rhythm
  - Right atrial rhythm.
- Rare
  - Atrial parasystol
  - Atrial dissociation
  - Atrial standstill.

AN APPROACH TO INTERPRETATION OF ECG

The QRS Rhythm

(i)

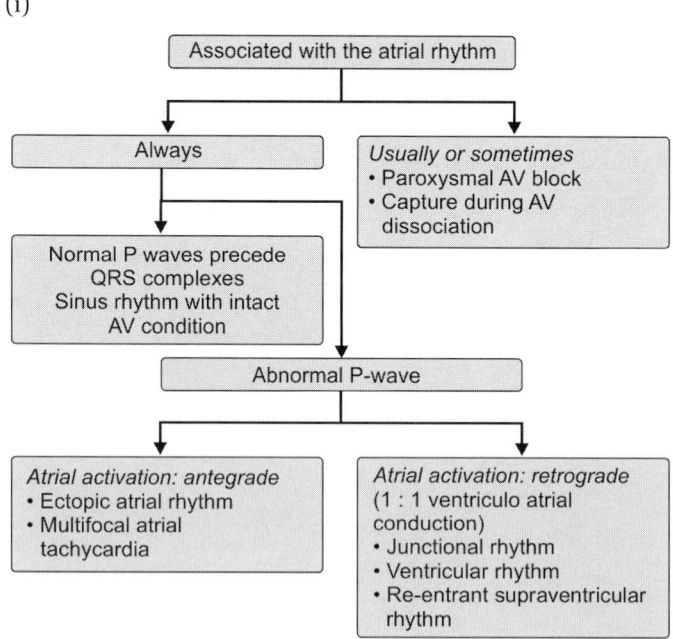

(ii)

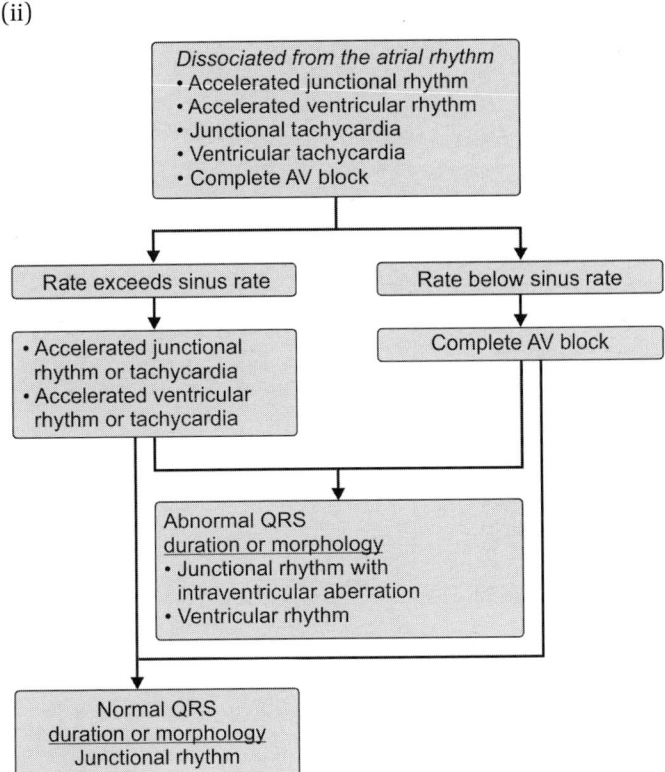

The Atrial Rhythm

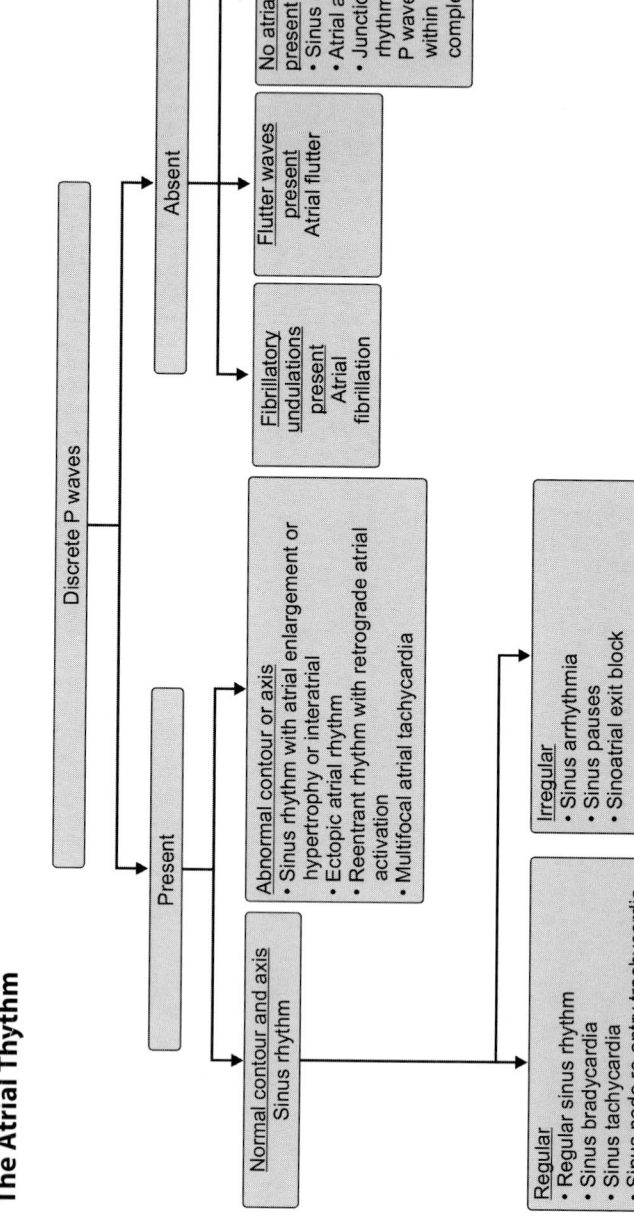

Atrial Premature Contraction (APC) with Aberrant Ventricular Conduction (AVC) (Fig. 9.21)

Definition: APC with AVC is the premature occurrence of ectopic P-wave associated with bizarre QRS complex as a result of AVC.

ECG Criteria

- APC with a bizarre QRS complex because the atrial impulse is conducted to the ventricles during their partial refractory period
- AVC occurs as a result of a short coupling interval, Ashmans phenomenon, or both.

Diagnostic pearls: APC with AVS closely mimics a ventricular premature contraction (VPC) especially when the premature P-wave is not easily visible an APC is not followed by a full compensatory pause, whereas a VPC is almost always followed by a full compensatory pause.

NONCONDUCTED (BLOCKED) ATRIAL PREMATURE CONTRACTION (FIG. 9.22)

Definition: Blocked APC is the premature occurrence of an ectopic P-wave not followed by a QRS complex.

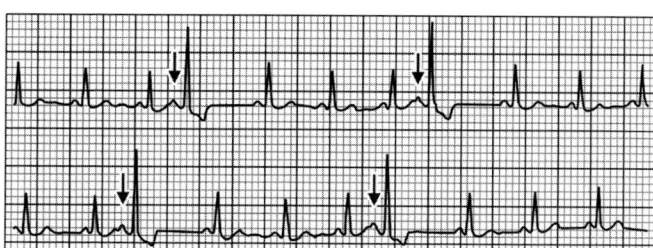

Fig. 9.21 Sinus rhythm and atrial premature contractions (indicated by arrows) with aberrant ventricular conduction due to a short coupling interval

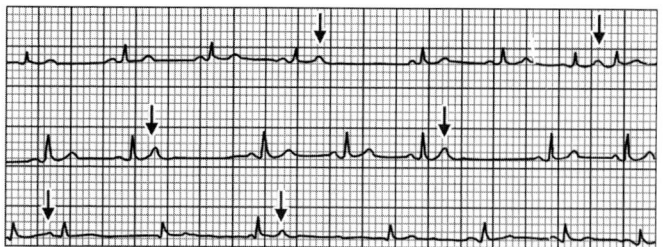

Fig. 9.22 Sinus rhythm with frequent atrial premature contractions (marked with arrows) and many atrial premature contractions are not followed by QRS complexes (blocked atrial premature contractions)

Diagnostic Criteria

- APC not followed by a QRS complex because the premature atrial impulse is conduction to the AV junction during its absolute refractory period.
- Blocked or nonconducted APC occurs as a result of a short coupling interval, Ashmans phenomenon, or preexisting AV block.

Diagnostic pearls: Blocked APC is the most common cause of a ventricular pause.

It resembles marked sinus arrhythmia, second degree or advanced AV block, sinus arrest and sinoatrial block.

ATRIAL TACHYCARDIA ASSOCIATED WITH ATRIOVENTRICULAR BLOCK (FIG. 9.23)

Definition: AT associated with AV block is a rapid and regular atrial rhythm origination from any position of atria associated with AV block.

Criteria

- ECG criteria same as atrial tachycardia.
- AT associated with AV block of varying degrees and any types.

Atrial tachycardia most commonly associated with 2 : 1 AV block and with Wenckebach AV block.

Diagnostic pearls: Paroxysmal atrial tachycardia (PAT) is often associated with Wenckbach AV block. Clinically, PAT with block is most commonly found in patients with digitalis toxication.

ATRIAL TACHYCARDIA WITH ABERRANT VENTRICULAR CONDUCTION (AVC) (FIG. 9.24)

Definition: AT with AVC is a regular and rapid atrial rhythm originating from any portion of the atria associated with bizarre QRS complexes as a result of AVC.

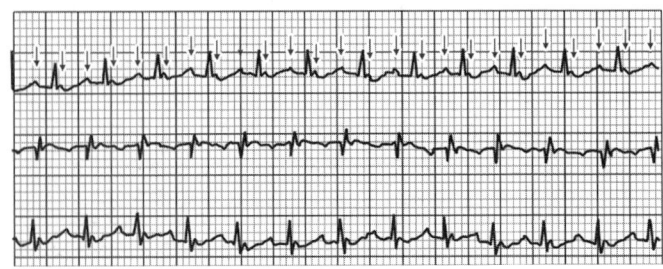

Fig. 9.23 Atrial tachycardia (indicated by arrows, rate of 187 bpm) with a 2.1 atrioventricular block

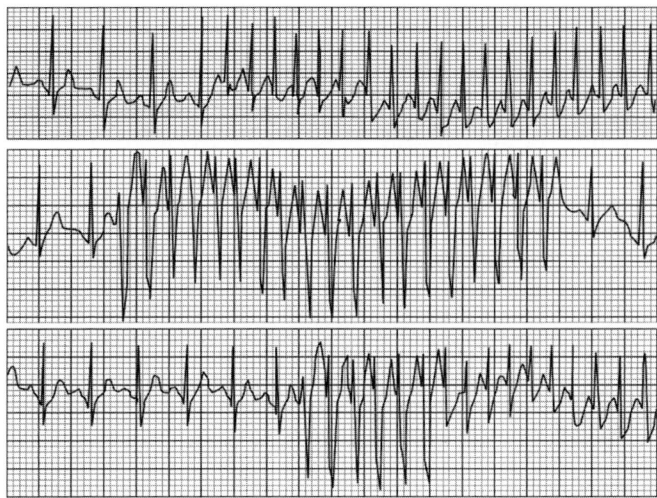

Fig. 9.24 Sinus rhythm and paroxysmal atrial tachycardia (rate of 210 beats per minute) with aberrant ventricular conduction of varying degrees

Criteria

- ECG criteria—same as atrial tachycardia.
- AT with AVC because of rapid rate when the rapidly occurring atrial impulses are conducted to the ventricles during their partial refractory period.
- AVC in AT is often initiated by Ashmans phenomenon.

Diagnostic pearls: AT with AVC closely mimics ventricular tachycardia (VT), the ectopic P-wave are often superimposed on the T-waves of preceding beats. In depth understanding of AVC and Ashmans phenomenon is extremely important to make the correct diagnosis of AT with AVC.

ATRIAL FLUTTER (FIG. 9.25)

Definition: It is a rapid regular atrial tachyarrhythmia, re-entrant type arrhythmia with typical atrial flutter, this wave originates in the right atriam generally traveling in a counter clock wise direction from top to bottom to top.

ECG Criteria

- P-wave replaced by flutter (ft) wave that have the configuration of a 'Saw tooth' or 'picket fence' pattern (best seen in II, III, aVF V_1)
- *Rhythm*: Regular, rapid
- *Atrial rate*: 250–350 beats/minute
- *Ventricular rate (R-R)*: Multiple of atrial rate, e.g. 2 : 1, 3 : 1, 4 : 1.

Note:
- Atrial rate 250–350 bpm. Ventricular rate—variable, may be 2 : 1, 3 : 1, 4 : 1, it is then called 'flutter with variable block'.

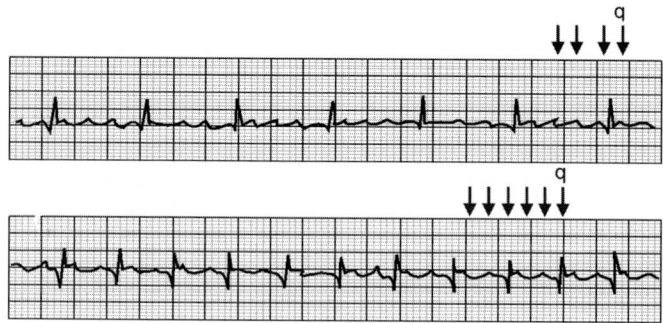

Fig. 9.25 Atrial flutter 4:1 Atrial flutter 2:1

- If atrial fibrillation and flutter may be present together, it is called flutter-fibrillation.

Causes of Atrial Flutter

As follows:
- May occur in normal individual
- Chronic rheumatic heart disease and valvular lesions
- Coronary artery disease (MI)
- Thyrotoxicosis
- Hypertension
- Congenital heart disease, e.g. transposition of great vessels
- Cardiomyopathy, TOF
- Pericarditis, myocarditis, ASD
- Thoracic surgery
- Electrolyte imbalance.

Classification

- Clinically
  - Paroxysmal atrial flutter
  - Persistent atrial flutter
  - Chronic atrial flutter
- Elctrocardiographically
  - *Type I*: Atrial rate 240–340 bpm (classical atrial fibrillation)
  - *Type II*: (Faster atrial rate) 340–450 bpm.

Differential Diagnosis of Atrial Flutter

When atrial flutter is associated with regular 2 : 1 AV block, it is difficult to differentiate from SVT or sinus tachycardia, because flutter waves are buried in QRS complex.

Diagnosis can be done by carotid sinus massage (CSM) or IV adenosine which temporarily increases the degree of AV block and reveals the flutter waves (F-wave).

Note:
- DC cardioversion is the easiest way to convert sinus rhythm.
- Atrial flutter is always associated with organic heart disease.

Characteristics of Atrial Flutter

- Rate : Atrial rate 250–450 bpm, typically 300 bpm ventricular rate variable-determined by AV blockade. The ventricular rate will usually not exceed 180 bpm due to the intrinsic conduction rate of the AV junction.
- Rhythm : Atrial regular ventricular regular or irregular depending on AV conduction or blockade.
- P-wave : No identifiable P-wave, saw-toothed flutter waves are present.
- PR interval : Not measurable
- QRS duration : 0.10 s or less but may be widened if flutter waves are buried in the QRS complex or an intraventricular conduction delay exists.

Management of Atrial Flutter

- Carotid sinus messages (CSM), slows ventricular rate
- Pharmacological treatment.

Aims

- Revert to a sinus rhythm
- To control the ventricular rate.

Drugs

- Digoxin
- CCB—Verapamil, Diltiazem
- When ventricular rate is poorly tolerated
  - Elective cardioversion (Dc shock) 10–50 joules
  - Atrial overdrive pacing
- Recurrent
  - Long-term use of drugs—Ia, Ib, Ic, III (Anti-arrhythmic drugs)
  - Digitalis
  - Beta-blocker
  - RF catheter ablation.

Difference between Atrial Flutter and Atrial Tachycardia

	Atrial tachycardia	Atrial flutter
Atrial rate	150–220 bpm	220–350 bpm
Ventricular rate	Same as atrial rate (1.1 AV conduction)	½ or ¼ of atrial rate (2 : 1 or 4 : 1 AV block)
P-wave	Ectopic or inverted	Saw-tooth like flutter waves
Effect of carotid sinus pressure	Termination in PAT slowing in ectopic tachycardia	Increased degree of AV block

Atrial Flutter With 2 : 1 AV Block

Definition: Atrial flutter with a 2 : 1 AV block is characterized by regular and rapid atrial waves with a saw-tooth appearance that originate from any portion of the atria, with a 2 : 1 AV conduction ratio (Fig. 9.25).

ECG Criteria

- Regular and rapid saw tooth appearance atrial waves with atrial rate ranging from 250–350 bpm
- Constant 2 : 1 AV conduction ratio
- Ventricular rate of 125–175 bpm
- Atrial rate may be slightly slower than 250 bpm in some cases.

Diagnostic Pearls

Atrial flutter with 2 : 1 AV block is the most common uncompleted from of atrial flutter, its rate is often reduced by quinidine or other antiarrhythmic agents conversely, atrial flutter rate is acclerated by digitalis. It is most common arrhymias in humans.

Atrial Flutter with A 4 : 1 AV Block

Definition: Atrial flutter with a 4 : 1 AV block is characterized by regular and rapid atrial waves with a saw tooth appearance and a 4 : 1 AV conduction ratio (Fig. 9.25).

ECG Criteria

- Regular and rapid atrial waves with a saw tooth appearance
- Atrial rate of 250–350 bpm
- Constant 4 : 1 AV conduction ratio.

Diagnostic Pearls

The 4 : 1 AV conduction ratio is a pathologic phenomenon due to prolonged refractory period. Recognizing atrial flutter waves is relatively easy because the ventricular rate is relatively slow (around 65–80 bpm) (Figs 9.26 and 9.27).

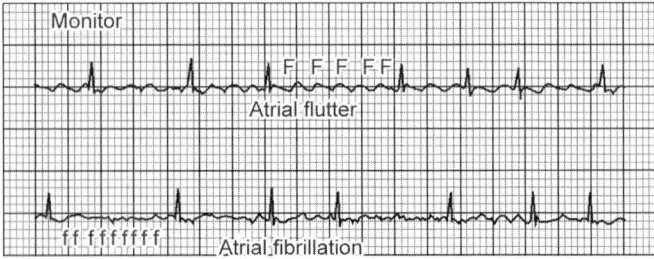

Fig. 9.26 Atrial flutter and fibrillation. Notice the "sawtooth" waves (F-waves) with atrial flutter and the irregular fibrillatory waves (F-waves) with atrial fibrillation

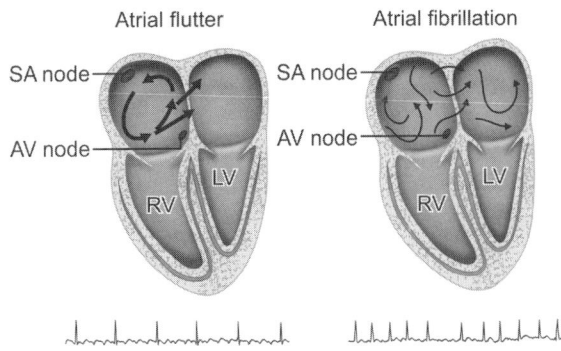

Fig. 9.27 Comparison of mechanisms of atrial flutter and atrial fibrillation (AF)

ATRIAL FIBRILLATION (FIG. 9.28)

Definition: Atrial fibrillation (AF) is an arrhythmia where atria beat rapidly, chaotically and ineffectively while the ventricles respond at irregular intervals, producing the characteristic irregularly irregular pulse. So AF is very rapid and chaotic atrial rhythm originating from any portion of the atria and having a rapid and irregular ventricular response.

ECG Criteria

- P-wave absent and replaced by fibrillation (f) waves, (best seen in II, V_1)
- *R-R interval:* Irregularly irregular
- *QRS complex:* Narrow
- *Atrial rate:* 350–600 beats/minute
- *Ventricular rate (R-R):* Up to 175 beats/minute.

Types of AF

- According to clinical expression:
  - *Paroxysmal AF:* Discreate self-limiting episodes, stops spontaneously with in 48 hours
    - *Short lasting:* <1 hour
    - *Long lasting:* >1 hour– <48 hours
  - *Persistent AF*: Prolonged episodes 2 days to week and usually requires cardioversion.
  - *Chronic or permanent AF*: Months to years, sinus rhythm cannot be restored even if cardioversion is attempted.
- According to rate
  - *Fast AF*: HR >100 bpm
  - *Slow AF*: HR <100 bpm
- According to amplitude:
  - *Fine AF*: Due to AMI, thyrotoxicosis
  - *Course AF*: Mitral stenosis.

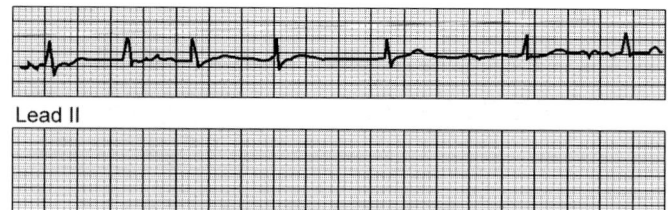

Fig. 9.28 Atrial fibrillation

Causes of Atrial Fibrillation

- Cardiac causes
  - Chronic rheumatic heart disease and valvular lesions commonly MS
  - Coronary artery disease (CAD)
  - Hypertension
  - Lone AF (Idiopathic 10% case)
  - Atrial septal defect (ASD)
  - Acute pericarditis
  - Chronic constrictive pericarditis
  - Myocarditis
  - Cardiomyopthy (CM→DCM, HCM)
  - Sick sinus syndrome (SSS)
  - Congenital heart disease—WPW syndrome
  - Cardio pulmonary surgery.
- Noncardiac cause
  - Acute chest infection (pneumonia, corpulmonale)
  - Thyrotoxicosis
  - Thoracic surgery
  - Pulmonary embolism
  - Electrolyte imbalance
    - Hypokalemia
    - Hyponatremia
  - Alcohol
  - Drugs—antiarrhythmic.

Causes of AF in Elderly Patient

- Acute myocardial infarction (AMI)
- Thyrotoxicosis
- Hypertension
- Lone AF
- Chronic rheumatic heart disease.

Causes of AF in Young Patient

- Chronic rheumatic heart disease with valvular lesions, commonly MS
- Atrial septal defect (ASD)
- Acute pericarditis

- Myocarditis
- Pneumonia.

Causes of Paroxysmal AF

- AMI
- Myocarditis
- Pneumonia (chest infection)
- Electrolyte imbalance
- Early stage of thyrotoxicosis
- End stage of mitral valve disease.

Clinical Presentation of AF

As follows:
- *Pulse*: Irregularly irregular (irregular in rhythm and volume)
- *Venous pulse*: Loss of JVP
- *BP*: May be hypertensive
- Examination of heart
    - Pulsus deficit
    - Mitral valvular or other cardiac/disease
    - Heart sound—Variable intensity of heart sound
    - Features of LVF and pulmonary edema
- Thyroid status
    - Warm and sweaty hands
    - Tremor
    - Tachycardia
    - Exopthalmus
    - Enlarged thyroid gland
- Features of complications
  Patient is AF with unconscious, what is the likely cause?
  Cerebral embolism (usually with right sided hemiplegia).

Complication of AF

As follows:
- Systemic and pulmonary embolism
- Heart failure
- MI
- Hypotension.

Lone AF

Lone AF means atrial fibrillation without any causes:
- *Lone AF*: Prognosis good
- *Chronic lone AF*: A higher risk
- 50% patients with paroxysmal AF and 20% with persistent or permanent AF have no cause and the heart is normal
- Lone AF usually occurs below 60 years of age
- It may be intermittent, later may become permanent
- *Prognosis*: Low risk of CVD (0.5% per year)
- Life span is normal

- Lone AF occurs by exogenous precipitating factors—such as:
  - Excessive cigarette
  - Alcohol
  - Coffee consumption
  - Recreational drugs—cocaine amphetamine
  - Stress or fatigue
  - Cessation of extreme exercise.

Aim of Treatment of AF

As follows:
- Control of ventricular rate (heart rate)
- Restoration of sinus rhythm
- Maintenance of sinus rhythm (prevention of recurrence)
- Prevention of embolism and primary causes.

Diagnostic Pearls

Uncomplicated (pure) AF always exhibits a rapid ventricular rate of 120–180 bpm. The atrial rate in AF is 400–650 bpm. In a practical sense, the atrial rate in AF is rather difficult or even impossible to determine.

Characteristics of AF

- Rate : Atrial rate usually 400–600 bpm ventricular rate variable
- Rhythm : Ventricular rhythm usually irregularly irregular
- P-wave : No identifiable P-wave, fibrillatory waves (f) present, erratic, wavy baseline.
- PR interval : Not measurable
- QRS duration : 0.10 sec or less but may be widened if an intraventricular conduction delay exists.

Difference between Atrial Fibrillation and Atrial Flutter

	Atrial fibrillation	Atrial flutter
Atrial rate	Over 350 bpm	220–350 bpm
Ventricular rate	Variable, no relation to atrial rate	Regular ½ to ¼th of atrial rate
Atrial activity	Fine fibrillatory (f) waves ragged base line	Visible flutter (F) waves saw-toothed base line
Ventricular activity	Variable R-R interval	Constant R-R interval

Atrial Fibrillation with Bundle Branch Block (BBB) (Fig. 9.29)

Definition: AF with BBB is a very rapid and chaotic atrial rhythm origination from any portion of the atria and having grossly irregular ventricular cycles that are associated with left bundle branch block (LBBB) or right bundle branch block (RBBB).

ECG Criteria

- Grossly irregular and rapid ventricular cycles with no discernible P-wave (Ventricular rate of 120–180 bpm)
- LBBB or RBBB in the presence of AF.

Note: When LBBB or RBBB is associated with underlying AF, ventricular tachycardia is closely simulated. Grossly irregular ventricular cycles exclude the diaggnosis of ventricular tachycardia.

Atrial Fibrillation with Aberrant Ventricular Conduction (AVC) (Fig. 9.30)

Definition: AF with AVC is a very rapid and chaotic atrial rhythm origination from any portion of the atria having grossly

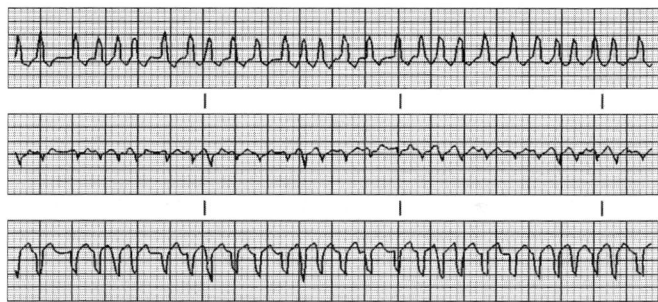

Fig. 9.29 Atrial fibrillation with rapid ventricular response (rate of 160–185 bpm) and left bundle branch block

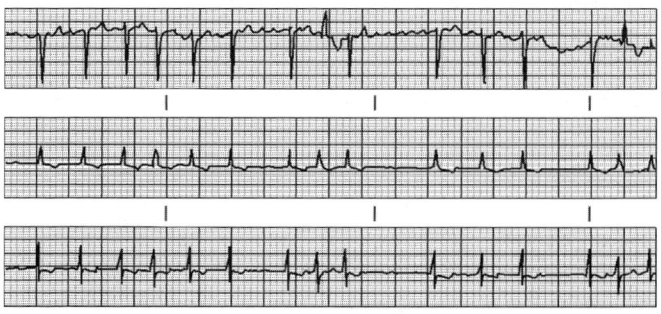

Fig. 9.30 Atrial flutter-fibrillation with occasional aberrant ventricular conduction

irregular ventricular cycles and occasional bizarre QRS because the atrial impulses are conducted to the ventricles during their partial refractory period.

ECG Criteria

- Grossly irregular and rapid ventricular cycles (ventricular rate 120–180 bpm) with no discernible P-wave.
- Occasional or intermittent bizarre QRS complexes (AVC) as a result of one of three reasons:
  - A short coupling interval or
  - Ashman's phenomenon or
  - An extremely rapid ventricular rate.

Atrial Fibrillation with Advanced Atrioventricular Block (Fig. 9.31)

Definition: AF with advanced AV block is AF with a slow ventricular rate as a result of an abnormality prolonged refractory period in the AV junction.

ECG Criteria

- Grossly irregular ventricular cycles with no discernible P-wave.
- Ventricular rate slower than 80 bpm as a result of an abnormally prolonged refractory period in the AV junction (Advanced AV block).
- Occasional AV junctional escape beats because of advanced AV block.

Note: Relatively slow ventricular rate in AF the rhythm resemble Bradyarrhythmias. If ventricular rate is slower than 50 bpm. Then underlying disorder of AF with advanced AV block is often sick sinus syndrome (SSS).

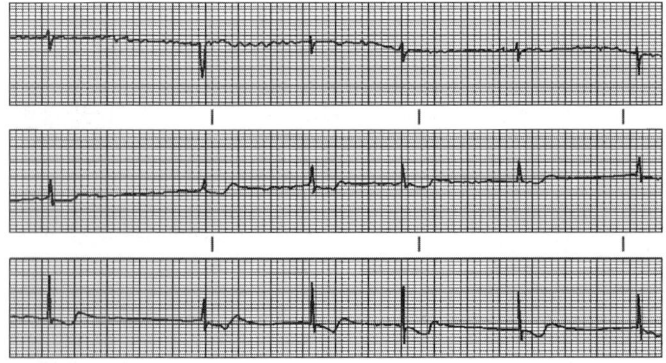

Fig. 9.31 Atrial fibrillation with advanced atrioventricular block (rate of 38–45 bpm) producing intermittent atrioventricular junctional escape beats

ASHMAN PHENOMENON (FIG. 9.32)

Definition: Ashman phenomenon is a form of aberrant ventricular conduction that occurs during atrial fibrillation when a long R-R interval is followed by a short R-R interval.

ECG Criteria

- Atrial fibrillation
- Wide QRS in between AF
  (AF followed by supraventricular impulse which are aberrantly conducted in ventricles resulting wide QRS).

Difference between Ashman Phenomenon and PVC

Ashman phenomenon	Premature ventricular contraction (PVC)
• RBBB pattern	• Wide bizarre complex
• No pause	• Pause present
• Long-short cycle sequence	• No such sequence

Note:
- Asman phenomenon
  - Is not PVC
  - Is abberency (aberrant ventricular conduction)
  - RBBB pattern.
- Significant
  - To regenerate VT
  - If this phenomenon present AF, not used digoxin
  - Use amiodaron.

Significance with Definition

When refractory period of bundle branch are unequal, an impulse which occur with a critical prematurity, will find one bundle branch recovered and the other refractory.

It will thus be conducted to one branch only, resulting in bizarre QRS pattern of BBB aberrant conduction commonly results in RBBB pattern. Aberrant conduction tends to occur when a long ventricular cycle is followed by a short cycle is terminated by an aberrantly conducted beat. This phenomenon is knows as Ashman phenomenon.

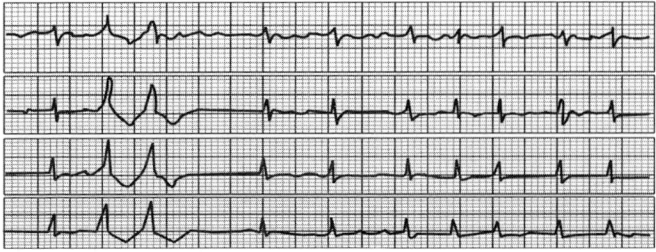

Fig. 9.32 Ashman phenomenon

It signify effectiveness of digoxin therapy, so no need for withdrawal of digoxin.

VENTRICULAR EXTRASYSTOLES (VES) OR, VENTRICULAR PREMATURE CONTRACTION (VPC) OR VENTRICULAR ECTOPIC (FIGS 9.33 AND 9.34)

Definition: VPC is the premature occurrence of a bizarre and broad QRS complex originating from any position of the ventricles.

ECG Criteria

- Absence of P-wave
- Wide, bizarre QRS complex (>0.12 sec)
- *ST and T wave*: Opposite the major deflexion of QRS complex
- A compensatory pause following the ectopic beat.

Note: VPC or VES is an abnormal QRS complex that originates from an ectopic focus in the ventricles. A VPC that interrupts normal sinus rhythm produces a long pause, termed compensatoty pause between the VPC and the next normally conducted sinus beat. The compensatory pause is confirmed by measuring the distance between the two normally conducted sinus beats that surround the VPC. This measured interval should equal twice the normal R-R interval (2 × R-R).

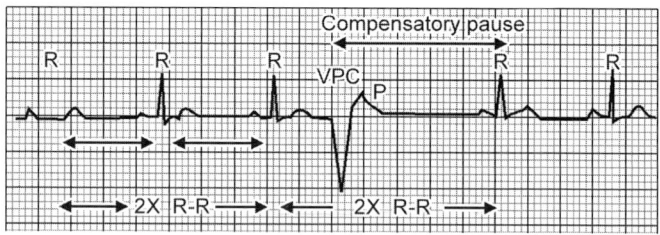

Fig. 9.33 Ventricular extrasystole

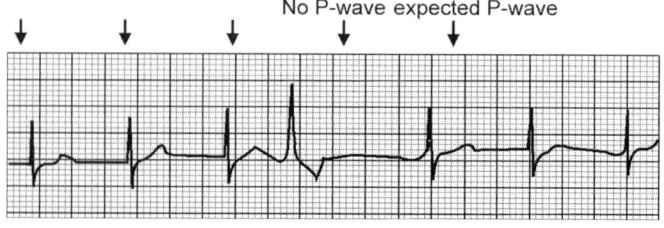

Fig. 9.34 Ventricular extrasystole with compensatory pause

Types of Ventricular Ectopic: (Patterns of VES)

- *Interpolated VES*: Means when ventricular ectopics occur between two normal sinus beat without compensatory pause.
- *Uniform or unifocal VES:* Similar configuration of ectopics in all leads and originates from a single ventricular focus (QRS-similar)
- *Multiform or multifocal VES*: Variable configuration of ectopics in the same lead, because the ectopics originate from different focus of the ventricle (QRS-variable)
- *Ventricular bigeminy:* Every one normal beat followed by VES
- *Ventricular trigeminy:* Every two normal beats followed by VES
- *Ventricular Quadrigeminy*: Every three normal beats followed by VES
- *Couplet*: Two VES in a row, multifocal
- *Triplet*: Three VES in a row (runs of ectopic)
- *Grouped VES*: 2–5 consecutive ventricular ectopics.

Lown's Grading of Ventricular Ectopic

Grading is done according to severity of ectopic (in acute myocardial infarction)
- Grade   O : No PVC
- Grade   1
    - A : Isolated PVC (<30/hour, <1/minute)
    - B : Isolated PVC (<30/hour, >1/minute)
- Grade   2 : Frequent PVCs (>30/hour)
- Grade   3 : Multiform PVCs
- Grade   4
    - A : Repetitive PVC, couplet
    - B : Repetitive PVCs, salvos (3 or more consecutive VES)
- Grade   5 : R on T
- Grade   6 : Non-sustained VT

Causes of Ventricular Ectopic

As follows:
- Normally in young adults
- Also in anxiety, excess caffeine, alcohol
- AMI
- Myocarditis
- Cardiomyopathy
- Valvular heart disease
- Mitral valve prolapse
- Hypertensive heart disease
- Electrolyte imbalance (hypokalemia)
- Digoxin toxicity
- Hypoxaemia.

Note: VES originating in left ventricle resembles RBBB pattern
VES originating in right ventricle resembles LBBB pattern.

Characteristics of VES

- Rate : Usually within normal range.
- Rhythm : Essentially regular with premature beats, if the VES is an interpolated VES, the rhythm will be regular.
- P-wave : Absent or with retrograde conduction to the atria, may appear after the QRS.
- PR interval : None with the VES because the ectopic originates in the ventricles.
- QRS : Greater than 0.12 sec, wide and bizarre T-waves usually in opposite direction of the QRS.

Treatment of VES

- *Asymptomatic case or absence of heart disease*: No treatment and blocker may be used.
- *With organic heart disease:* Treatment of primary cause.
- Antiarrhythmic drug does not improve.

Note: VES may be found in normal people, incidence increases with age.
- VES in normal heart is prominent at rest but disappear with exercise. No treatment require.
- Multifocal VES or couplet VES always abnormal it indicates serious myocardial disease.

PATTERNS OF VENTRICULAR PREMATURE COMPLEX OR VENTRICULAR EXTRASYSTOLE

Interpolated Ventricular Extrasystole (Fig. 9.35)

Definition: Interpolated VES is a VES sandwiched between two consecutively occurring sinus beats without pause.

ECG Criteria

- VES occurs between two normal sinus beats without a compensatory pause.
- P-R interval of the sinus beat following the interpolated VES, is slightly longer than normal P-R interval.

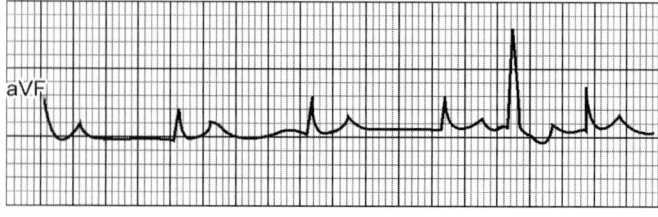

Fig. 9.35 Interpolated ventricular extrasystole

Diagnostic Criteria

- VES sandwiched between two consecutively occurring sinus beats.
- R-R interval of two consecutively occurring sinus beats that contain an interpolated VES.
- Sinus P-P cycle is not disturbed by an interpolated VES.

Note: Interpolated VES is more common in healthy individuals than in patients with cardiac disease it is a true extra heart beat because the underlying sinus rhythm continues without missing any QRS complex of the sinus origin.

Multiform VES: (Multifocal) (Fig. 9.36)

Definition: Multifocal VES are VES originating from two or more locations in the ventricles.

ECG Criteria

- Ventricular extrasystole display varying QRS configurations in the same ECG leads.
- Compensatory pause following the ectopic beat.

Diagnostic Criteria

- VES originating from two or more foci in the ventricles and producing two or more different QRS configurations
- Constant or varying coupling intervals
- Full compensatory pause following a VES in sinus rhythm
- Long ventricular pause following a VES in AF or atrial flutter.

Note:
- Multifocal VES usually occur among older adults with diseased hearts.
- Multifocal VES are frequently observed in advanced digitalis intoxication, particularly in the presence of underlying AF.

Uniform or Unifocal VES

ECG Criteria

- All VES or VPCs are similar in configurations in the same ECG leads
- Compensatory pause following the ectopic beat.

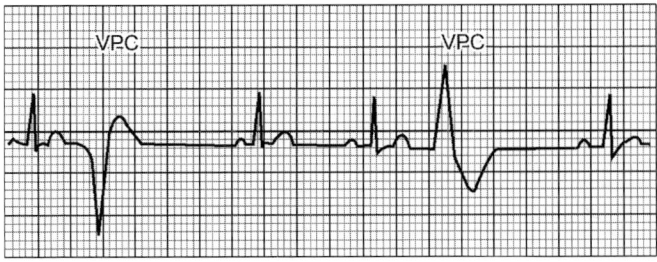

Fig. 9.36 Multiform ventricular extrasystole

Bigeminy VES (Fig. 9.37)

ECG Criteria

- Each VES alternate with a normal sinus beat repeatedly
- VES is coupled or associated with the preceding beat by a 'fixed coupling interval'.

Trigeminy VES (Fig. 9.38)

ECG Criteria

Each VES alternates with two normal sinus beats repeatedly, or a normal beat alternates with two VES or VPCs repeatedly.

Couplet VES (Fig. 9.39)

ECG Criteria

- Two VES in a row
- *Configuration*: Multiform VES.

Triplet VES (Fig. 9.40)

ECG Criteria

- Three VES in a row
- *Configuration*: Uniform or multiform VES.

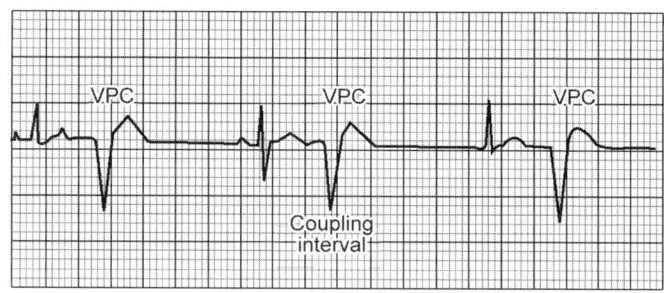

Fig. 9.37 Bigeminy and unifocal ventricular extrasystole

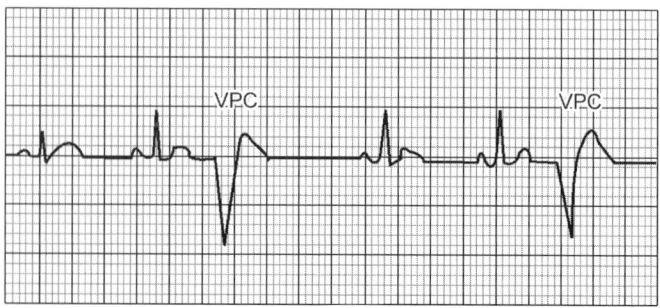

Fig. 9.38 Trigeminy ventricular extrasystole

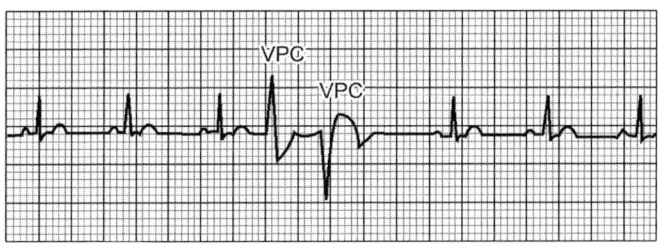

Fig 9.39 Couplet ventricular extrasystole

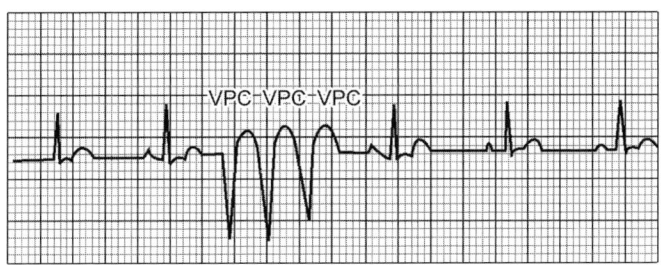

Fig. 9.40 Triplet ventricular extrosystole

Note: Arbitrarily, three or more VES or VPCs in a row is termed ventricular tachycardia.

R-on-T Phenomenon (Fig. 9.41)

Definition: R-on-T phenomenon means R wave of ventricular ectopic occur on or near the peak of previous T-wave.

This is also called malignant ectopic it may induce VT or VF.

ECG Criteria

The VES occurs on or near the peak of the previous T-wave.

Note: This is the vulnerable period during ventricular depolarization and may predispose to ventricular tachycardia or ventricular fibrillation.

Note:
- VES that is so premature (very short coupling interval) that it is imposed upon the T-waves of the preceding sinus impulse, exhibits the R-on-T phenomenon (Fig. 9.42).
- They may precipitate VT or VF particularly in the course of an acute myocardial infarction (AMI) or with very long QT intervals.
- VT and VF most commonly occur without a preceding R on T beat and most R on T beats do not precipitate a sustained ventricular tachyarrhythmia.

Grouped VES

Definition: Grouped VES are two to five consecutively occurring VES.

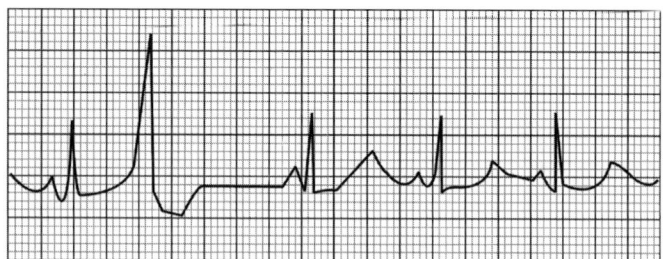

Fig 9.41 R-on-T phenomenon

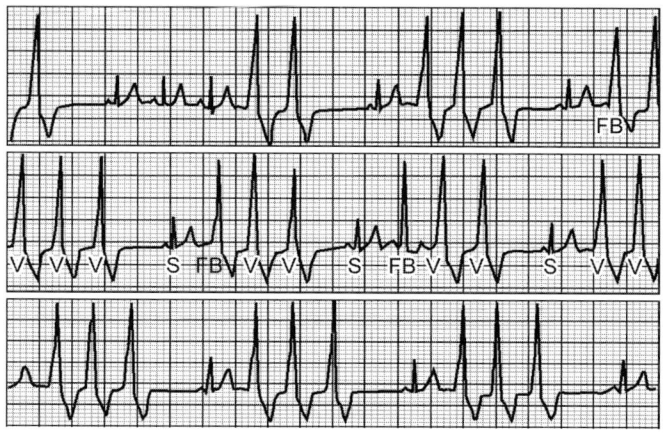

Fig. 9.42 Sinus rhythm (marked S) with grouped ventricular premature contractions (marked V). Note occasional ventricular fusion beats (marked FB)

ECG Criteria

- Two to five consecutively occurring VESs
- The configuration of the VES may be identical or may vary
- Inter-ectopic intervals (R-R interval between consecutively occurring VES) may be constant but more commonly vary
- Grouped VES are usually followed by a long ventricular pause
- Underlying cardiac rhythm may be sinus or ectopic (e.g. AF).

Note: A long ventricular pause following bizarre and brood QRS supports the diagnosis of grouped VES, particularly when the underlying rhythm is AF.

Characteristics of VES

- Rate : Usually within normal range, but depends on underlying rhythm.
- Rhythm : Regular with premature beats. If the VES is an interpolated VES, the rhythm will be regular.

- P-wave : Usually absent or with retrograde conduction to the atria, may appear after the QRS.
- PR-interval : None with the VES because the ectopic originates in the ventricles.
- QRS duration : Greater than 0.12 sec, wide and bizarre. T-waves usually in opposite direction of the QRS.

VENTRICULAR TACHYCARDIA (FIG. 9.43)

Ventricular tachycardia (VT) or extrasystolic VT is a series of three or more consecutive VES in a row at a rate faster than 100 beats/min.

Definition: When there is three or more consecutive ventricular ectopic impulses at a rate of 100 bpm or greater, the atria usually remain under the control of the sinus node, the arrhythmia is known as VT.

ECG Criteria

- Wide (>0.12 sec), bizarre QRS complexes
- Heart rate (R-R): 140–220 beats/minute
- P-wave dissociated from QRS complexes (AV—dissociation) (Absence of P and T waves)
- Occasional sinus capture beat present (normal P-QRS-T complex in between VT)
- Occasional fusion (Dressler) beats present (conducted sinus impulse fuses with impulse from tachycardia
- QRS—in chest leads (V_1 - V_6) either all positive or all negative (ventricular concordance).

Note: VT may be classified.
- *Sustained VT*: May degenerate into ventricular fibrillation causing cardiac arrest
- *Non-sustained VT*: Consists of short salvos of three or more VES in a row.

Cause of Ventricular Tachycardia

- AMI
- Chronic ischemic heart disease, specially poor left ventricular function

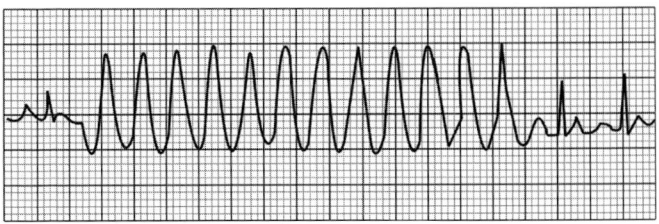

Fig. 9.43 Ventricular tachycardia

- Myocarditis
- Cardiomyopathy
- Ventricular aneurysm
- Mitral valve prolapse
- Electrolyte imbalance (hypokalemia, hypomagnesemia)
- Idiopathic.

Classification of VT (According to Different Ways)

- According to etiology
    - Primary—due to disease processes
    - Secondary—due to metabolic and hemodynamic dearrangement
- According to morphology
    - Monomorphic
    - Polymorphic
    Without long QT polymorphic VT or with long QT syndrome Torsades de-pointes.
- According to duration
    - Sustained
    - Nonsustained
- According to site of action
    - RV → LBBB + RAD type
    - LV → RBBB + LAD type.

Specific Forms of VT

- According to duration
    - Salvos (3–5 impulses)
    - Nonsustained VT (6 impulses, 29 sec)
    - Sustained VT (>30 sec)
- According to ECG pattern
    - Uniform morphology VT (monomorphic)
    - *Polymorphic VT*: Torsad de pointes
    - RV outflow pattern- bidirectional tachycardia
- According to Hemodynamically
    - Benign
    - Potentially malignant
    - Malignant.

Differentiation between VT and SVT with Aberrant Conduction

In ECG, points suggesting VT are as follows:
- History of MI
- QRS > 0.14 sec
- Extreme left axis deviation
- AV dissociation (dissociated P-wave may be seen)
- Capture beat (normal sinus in the middle of VT)
- Fusion beat (the conducted sinus impulse fuses with impulse from tachycardia)

- Ventricular concordance (either all positive or all negative in chest leads)
- Bifid R in V_1 with a tall first peak in V_1 and deep S in V_6
- R-R interval is regular
- No response to carotid sinus massage or $\frac{1}{V}$ adenosine (but, it terminates SVT).

NONSUSTAINED VENTRICULAR TACHYCARDIA (FIG. 9.44)

Definition: Nonsustained VT is six or more consecutively occurring VES lasting up to 29 sec

ECG Criteria

- Six or more consecutively occurring VES lasting up to 29 sec
- Ventricular rate of 140–180 bpm
- VES may be unifocal or multifocal
- Nonsustained VT often occurs intermittently
- The interectopic interval (VT cycle) are often not constant
- Underlying rhythm may be sinus or any ectopic rhythm (e.g. AF).

Note:
- A short episode of nonsustained VT should be distinguished from consecutively occurring aberrant ventricular conduction (AVC), particularly in the presence of underlying AF.
- Nonsustained VT becomes sustained VT when the patients clinical condition further deteriorates.

SUSTAINED VENTRICULAR TACHYCARDIA (FIG. 9.45)

Definition: Sustained VT is VT lasting longer than 29 sec.

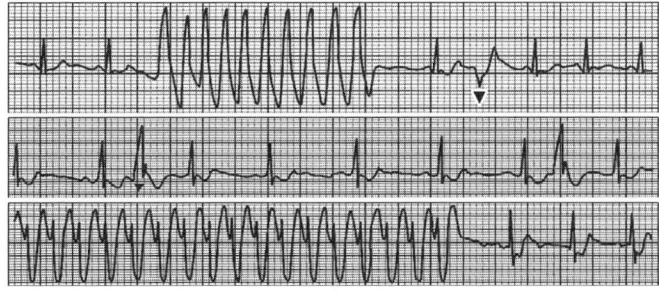

Fig. 9.44 Sinus rhythm with multifocal ventricular premature contractions (marked V) and intermittent nonsustained ventricular tachycardia (rate of 155–166 bpm) originating from two foci. Note that all ventricular premature contractions are interpolated

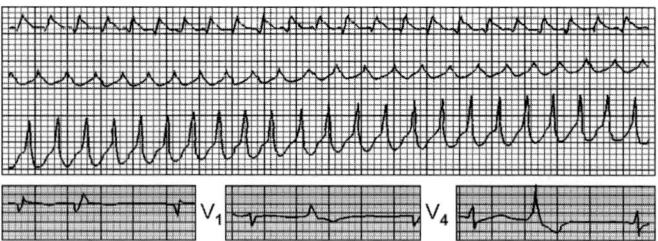

Fig. 9.45 Sustained ventricular tachycardia with a rate of 187 bpm

ECG Criteria

- Consecutively occurring VES (VT) lasting longer than 29 sec
- *Ventricular rate*: 140–180 bpm
- VT may be unifocal or multifocal
- *VT cycle*: Usually regular. Often irregular when the tachycardia is multifocal in origin.
- VT may occur in the presence of underlying sinus rhythm or any ectopic rhythm (e.g. AF).

Note: Differential diagnosis between sustained VT and any form of SVT with bizarre or broad QRS complexes (due to LBBB, RBBB, AVC) is often difficult.

Cause of VT

- Sustained VT
  - Sustained monomorphic VT
    - Prior MI
    - Ventricular aneurysm
  - Sustained polymorphic VT
    - Transient myocardial ischemia
- Repetitive recurrent VT
  - Proarrhythmic drugs
  - Ischemia
  - Heart failure, i.e. DCM
  - Myocarditis
  - Electrolyte disturbance
  - Drugs.

Causes of Monomorphic VT

- Acute or chronic IHD
- Idiopathic DCM and HCM
- Electrolyte disturbance
- Physical and emotional stress
- RV dysphasia
  - Arrhythmogenic RV dysphasia (ARVD)
  - RV cardiomyopathy (RVCM)
- VT following congenital heart disease surgery
  - Tetralogy of fallot (OF)
  - The great arteries (TGA).

Differences between VT and SVT with Aberrant Conduction

	VT	SVT with aberrancy
Regularity of rhythm	Slightly irregular	Clock-like regularity
P-QRS relation ship	P-wave not seen unrelated	P-wave may be seen related
QRS	>0.14 sec bizarre	0.12–0.14 sec triphasic
Pattern in V_1–V_6	rS in V_1–V_6	Rs R' in V_1, Rs in V_6
QRS in V_6	rS R < S	Rs R > S
QRS axis	Left ward	Normal
Hemodynamics	Compromised	Stable
Organic heart disease	Often present	Absent
Respond to carotid sinus pressure	No response	Slowing or termination

Bidirectional Ventricular Tachycardia (Fig. 9.46)

Definition: Bidirectional VT is VT with two different QRS complex alternating on every other beat.

ECG Criteria

- VT having different QRS configurations that alternate on every other beat
- *Ventricular rate*: 140–180 bpm
- The R-R intervals (ventricular cycles) are precisely regular in unifocal bidirectional VT
- Two different R-R intervals (ventricular cycle) alternate in bifocal bidirectional VT
- The underlying atrial mechanism is almost always an ectopic rhythm AF (atrial flutter). Leading to AV dissociation.

Note: The most common underlying cause of bidirectional VT is advanced digitalis intoxication. The prognosis is grave.

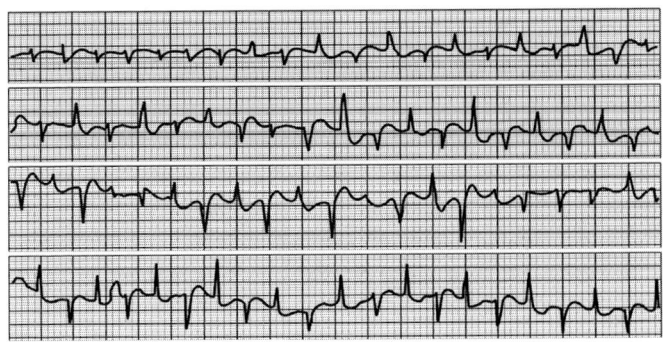

Fig. 9.46 Atrial fibrillation with bidirectional ventricular tachycardia

Monomorphic VT (Fig. 9.47)

Definition: VT may originate from an ectopic focus in either ventricle. When the QRS of VT are of the same shape and amplitude, the rhythm is called monomorphic VT.

Characteristics of Monomorphic VT

- Rate : 101–250 bpm
- Rhythm : Regular
- P-wave : May be present or absent
- PR interval : None QRS duration: >0.12. Often difficult to differentiate between the QRS and T-wave

Polymorphic VT (Fig. 9.48)

Definition: When the QRS complexes of VT vary in shape and amplitude from beat-to-beat, the rhythm is called polymorphic VT. In polymorphic VT, the QRS appear to twist from upright to negative or negative to upright and back.

Characteristic of Polymorphic VT

- Rate : 150–300 bpm. Typically 200–250 bpm
- Rhythm : May be regular or irregular
- P-wave : None
- PR interval : None
- QRS duration : >0.12 sec, gradual alteration in amplitude and direction of the QRS complexes. A typical cycle consists of 5–20 QRS complexes.

Classification

Polymorphic VT

- Normal QT
- Long QT syndrome (LQTS)

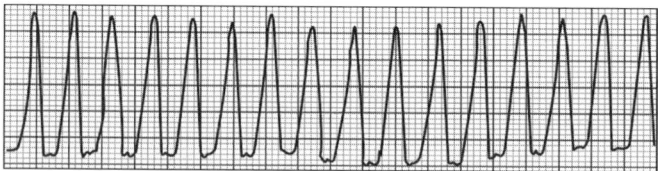

Fig. 9.47 Monomorphic ventricular tachycardia

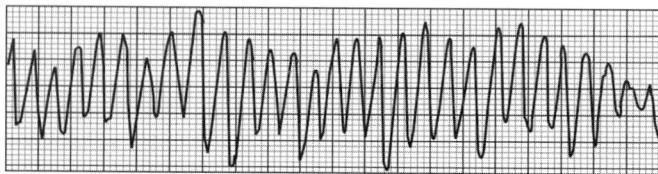

Fig. 9.48 Polymorphic ventricular tachycardia

- Acquired (Iatrogenic)
- Congenital (Idiopathic)

Note:
- Polymorphic VT that occurs in the presence of a long QT interval is called Torsades de pointes (TdP)
- TdP means "twisting of the points"
- Long QT syndrome is an abnormality of the hearts electrical system
- The electrical problem in heart is caused by defects in sodium and potassium channels that affect repolarization
- These electrical defects prolong the QT interval, predisposing affected persons to TdP.

Common Causes of Wide Complex Tachycardia

- VT
- SVT with aberrant conduction
- WPW syndrome.

Treatment of VT

- Nonsustained VT (NSVT)
  In normal heart (6%) : No treatment
  With heart disease   : β-blocker. If with myocardial infarction and ejection fraction 30% or less Implantable cardioventer defibrillator (ICD) may be helpful.
- Sustained VT
  - If patient hemodynamically unstable
  - (Hypotension, systolic <90 or heart failure)—then DC shock.
  - If stable
    IV amiodaron bolus followed by IV infusion
    IV lignocaine 100 mg bolus (1-2 mg/kg).
    It is followed by lignocaine infusion- 2-4 mg/minute for 24-36 hours.
  - If fails–DC shock
  - To prevent recurrence—β-blocker, amiodaron
  - Correction of hypokalemia, hypomagnesemia, Hypoxemia and acidosis
  - If all fail
    - Autonomic implantable cardioverter defibrillator (AICD) device, or
    - Radiofrequency ablation of focus (RFA).

ACCELERATED IDIOVENTRICULAR RHYTHM (FIG. 9.49)

Definition: Accelerated idioventricular rhythm (AIVR) is six or more consecutively occurring VES with a slow ventricular rate (41–100 bpm).

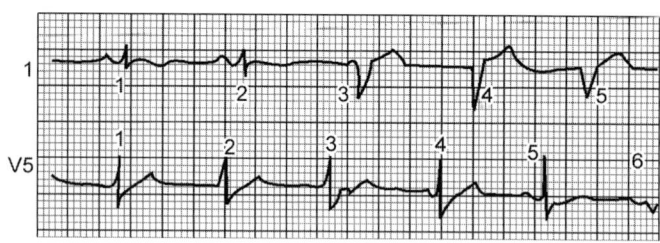

Fig. 9.49 Accelerated idioventricular rhythm

AIVR is often called 'idioventricular tachycardia' or 'non-paroxysmal VT' or 'Slow VT'.

ECG Criteria

- Wide, bizarre QRS complexes
- P-wave dissociated from QRS complexes (AV dissociation) (Absence of P)
- *Heart rate*: Less than 100 beats/minute
- Occasional fusion (Dressler) beats present.

Note: Accelerated idioventricular rhythm is an enhanced ectopic ventricular rhythm where by the pacemaker site in the ventricles fires rate is 40–100 beats/minute that faster than the intrinsic ventricular pacemaker rate of 15–40 beats/minute. It is most commonly seen within the first 48–72 hours of acute MI.

Diagnostic Criteria

- Six or more consecutively occurring VES with a relatively slow ventricular rate (41–100 bpm)
- QRS complex is uniform, but it may vary
- *Ventricular cycle*: Regular but it may be irregular, when AIVR is short in duration.
- AIVR may occur in the presence of underlying sinus rhythm or any ectopic atrial rhythm (e.g. AF, atrial flutter, tachycardia).

Note:
- An AIVR exists when three or more ventricular escape beats occur in a row at a rate 41–100 bpm
- AIVR is usually considered a benign escape rhythm that appears when the sinus rate slows and disappears when the sinus rate speed up
- Episodes of AIVR usually last a few seconds to a minute
- Fusion beats are often seen at the onset and end of the rhythm.

Characteristics of AIVR

- Rate : 41–100 bpm (faster than intrinsic ventricular pacemaker rate of 15–40 bpm)

- Rhythm : Essentially regular
- P-wave : Usually absent or, with retrograde conduction to the atria, may appear after QRS
- PR interval : None
- QRS duration : >0.12 sec, T-wave frequently in opposite direction of the QRS complex.

Note:
- AIVR is most commonly seen within the first 48–72 hours of AMI and frequently after successful reperfusion during AMI (thrombolysis or angioplasty) and also after cardiac surgery.
- It is benign arrhythmia asymptomatic, transient self-limiting and does not require treatment.

TORSADES DE POINTES (FIG. 9.50)

Definition: Torsades de pointes is a type of polymorphic ventricular characterized by twisting of the points of QRS in ECG which shows rapid irregular complex from upright to inverted position, it is multiformed VT initiated by VES with prolonged QT intervals and broad T-waves so, polymorphic VT along with QT prolongation is known as Torsades de pointes.

ECG Criteria

- *QRS:* Wide, bizarre, irregular of different or changing amplitude from upright to inverted position (different configuration of QRS)
- *QT:* Prolonged.

Note: ECG looks like VT and different configuration of QRS.

Causes of Torsades de Pointes

- Electrolyte imbalance: Hypokalemia
  Hypocalemia
  Hypomagnesemia
- *Drugs*:
  - Class I a antiarrhythmic drugs
    Quinidine (most common)
    Disopyramide
    Procainamide
  - Class III antiarrhythmic drugs
    Amiodarone
    Sotalol

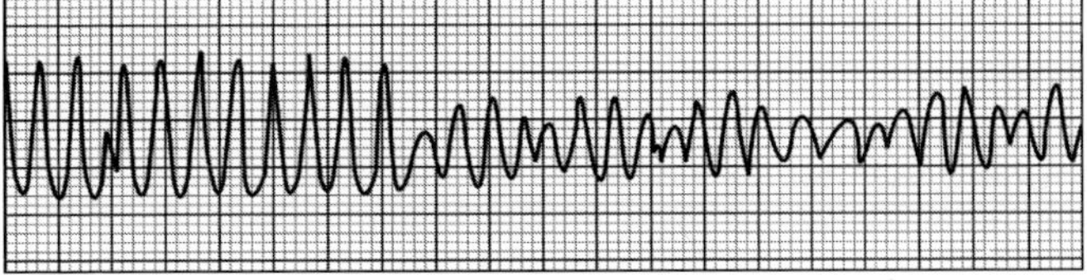

Fig. 9.50 Torsades de pointes

- Psychotropic drugs
  - Tricyclic Antidepressants
- MI and myocarditis
  - Chlorpromazine
  - Phenothiazine
- Bradycardia — SSS, CHB
- CNS disease
  - Subarachnoid hemorrhage
  - Ruptured berry aneurysm
- Congenital syndrome
  - Jervell-lange-Nielson syndrome (Autosomal recessive)
  - Romano-Ward syndrome (Autosomal dominant)

Clinical Features

- Palpitation
- Syncope
- Death.

Management of Torsades de Pointes

- Electrolyte imbalance—corrected
- Causative drugs—stopped
- IV magnesium—8 mmol for 15 minute, then 72 mmol every 24 hours
- Cardiac pacing (atrial, ventricular or dual chamber)
- If no pacing is available—isoprenaline infusion (it is avoided in congenital QT syndrome)
- If all fails and history of sudden death—automatic implantable cardioverter defibrillator (AICD)
- In congenital—β-blocker is helpful
- Others treatment—left stellate ganglion block, AICD
- If AMI and ventricular arrhythmia—give Inj. lignocain
- If primary ventricular arrhythmia—Inj. lignocain with β-blocker
- If secondary ventricular arrhythmic—Inj. lignocain with amiodarone.

Note:
- TdP may progress to ventricular fibrillation and sudden death
- It is more common in women, triggered by multiple drugs and hypokalemia.

Diagnostic Criteria

- Multiformed VT initiated by a VES with the R on T phenomenon in the presence of a prolonged QT interval with a broad T-wave.

- Multiformed VT—irregular, with components of ventricular flutter and/or VF
- *Ventricular rate*: 140–180 bpm (may be faster or slower)
- The broad T-waves may be upright or inverted
- The underlying cardiac rhythm may be sinus or any atrial mechanism (AF, atrial flutter or tachycardia)
- Multiformed VT often transforms to VF.

VENTRICULAR FLUTTER (FIG. 9.51)

Definition: Ventricular flutter is a regularly occurring undulation (waveform) originating from any portion of the ventricles.

ECG Criteria

- Large amplitude QRS complex
- Rhythm regular
- Absence of P, ST, T-wave
- *Heart rate (R-R):* 180–300 beats/minute.

Note: The ST and T wave are not seen in ventricular flutter, whereas in VT, these ST, T can be seen. This flutter is a precursor of ventricular fibrillation. It is difficult to separate QRS, ST, T-wave. This is 'sine-like wave from' which beat seen in lead I.

Diagnostic Criteria

- Regularly occurring undulation (waveform) with no boundary between the QRS, S-T segments, and T-wave, leading to a continuous loop
- *Usual rate*: 140–180 bpm (may be 180–300 bpm)
- No discernible P-wave or any other atrial activities
- Ventricular flutter often transforms from or to VF or VT and at times to unstable VER or ventricular standstill, leading to chaotic ventricular rhythm.

VENTRICULAR FIBRILLATION (FIG. 9.52)

Ventricular fibrillation (VF) is very rapid, chaotic and grossly irregular multiformed electrocardiographic complexes of various amplitudes originating anywhere in the ventricles.

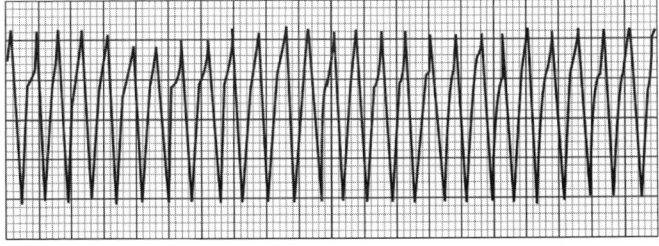

Fig. 9.51 Ventricular flutter

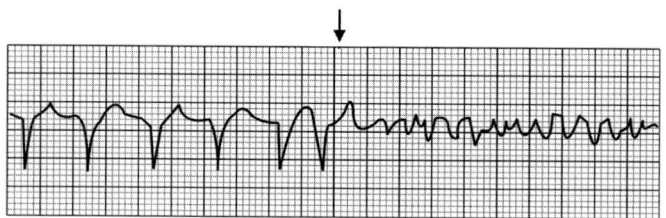

Fig. 9.52 Ventricular fibrillation

Here impulse occurs irregularly at rate of 300–500 bpm. Ventricular contraction is uncoordinated and ventricular filling and emptying ceases. Cardiac output falls to zero. VF is the more common causes of sudden death.

Definition: VF is the type of ventricular arrhythmia characterized by rapid chaotic irregular, ineffective and uncoordinated ventricular activation with no mechanical effect.

ECG Criteria

- Wide, bizarre QRS complex
- *Rhythm*: Irregularly irregular
- P, QRS, T-wave replaced by fibrillatory (f) wave
- Heart rate—up to 500 beats/minute.

Note: Ventricular fibrillation represents completely disorganized electrical and mechanical activity in the heart (cardiac arrest), and if allowed to continue, results in death.

Causes of VF

As follows:
- AMI, unstable angina cardiomyopathy
- Electrolyte imbalance—hypokalemia
   hypomagnesemia
- Electrocution
- Drowning
- Drug overdose (digitalis, adrenaline, isoprenaline).

Clinical Findings

- *Pulse*: Absent (disappearance of arterial pulse)
- *BP*: Not recordable or absent
- *Respiration*: Ceases or absent
- Patient may be unconscious
- *Pupil*: Dilated, no reaction to light
- *Heart sounds*: Absent.

Note:
- VF is invariably fatal immediate treatment is necessary if death is to be prevented
- Sinus rhythm can usually be restored by defibrillation

- Effective circulation and ventilation must be obtained within 4 minutes to prevent, if irreversible brain damage.

Diagnostic Criteria

- Very rapid, chaotic and grossly irregular multiformed electrocardiographic complexes with various amplitudes
- No discernible P-wave or any other atrial activities
- *Ventricular rate*: Impossible to determine but faster than 140–180 bpm
- No discernible S-T segment, T-wave or clear-cut QRS
- VF is often preceded or followed by VT, ventricular flutter, unstable VER, or ventricular standstill, leading to chaotic ventricular rhythm.

Characteristics of VT

- Rate : Cannot be determined because there are no discernible waves or complexes to measure
- Rhythm : Rapid chaotic with no pattern or regularity
- P-wave : Not discernible
- PR interval : Not discernible
- QRS duration : Not discernible

Types

- *Coarse VF*: VF with waves that are 3 mm or more high is called 'coarse' VF (Fig. 9.53).
- *Fine VF*: VF with low amplitude waves (<3 mm) is called 'fine' VF (Fig. 9.54).
- *Primary VF*: Is the VF that occurs within first 4 hours in the setting of AMI which results from micro-reentry mechanisms in the infarct zone. Incidence 3–5%.

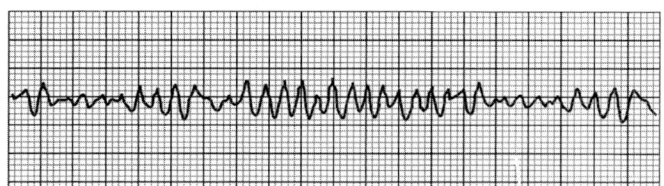

Fig. 9.53 Coarse ventricular fibrillation

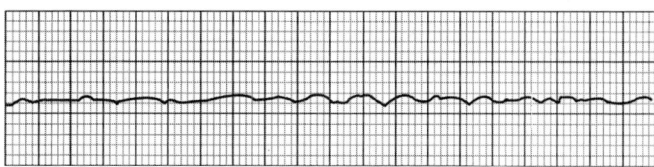

Fig. 9.54 Fine ventricular fibrillation

Triggering Mechanisms of Primary VF

- Electrolyte imbalance
- Acidosis
- Increased FFA
- Increased intracellular calcium.

Secondary VF: These are the occurrence of symptomatic sustained VT or VF in the later phase of hospital cause of AMI patients occurs as a result of chronic arrhythmogenic focus develop in the damaged ventricles.

It is most common in patients with large anterior wall MI.

Treatment of VF

- Immediate defibrillation: 200 joules.
  If no response, DC shock with 200 joules
  If still no response, DC shock with 360 joules
- If 3 shocks unsuccessful $\frac{1}{v}$ adrenaline, followed by CPR (cardiopulmonary resuscitation)
- If defibrillator is not available—CPR should be given
- The patient who survives from VF in the absence of identifiable cause is at high-risk of sudden death. This case is treated with implantable cardioverter defibrillator (ICD).

VENTRICULAR PARASYSTOLE (FIG. 9.55)

Definition: Ventricular parasystole is a cardiac rhythm originating from any location in the ventricles independent of any underlying cardiac rhythm.

ECG Criteria

- VPC or VES are present. These are called parasystolic VPCs
- Distance between two VPC is a multiple of the shortest R-R interval between two parasystolic beats
- Varying coupling intervals between VPC and normal beats
- Occasional fusion (Dressler) beats present
- Unchanged QRS complex of VPCs
- The usual rate ranges from 30 to 50 bpm.

Note: In ventricular parasystole:
- Some QRS are normal, i.e. sinus stimulated
- Some QRS is ventricular in origin, i.e. VES or VPC

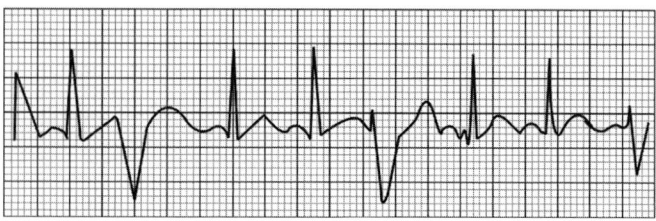

Fig 9.55 Ventricular parasystole

- Some QRS complexes are preceded by P-wave and have mixed configuration of QRS complex between the normal QRS and VPC. These are fusion (dressler) beat or complex. This represent the fusion of a sinus and an idioventricular beats.
- Ventricular parasystole is a rather uncommon ventricular arrhythmia. The configuration of the QRS complex is essential the same as that of an ordinary VES, but the former produces an independent ventricular rhythm in the presence of any underlying rhythm.

CHAOTIC VENTRICULAR RHYTHM (FIG. 9.56)

Definition: chaotic ventricular rhythm is a multifocal ventricular rhythm consisting of periods of grouped VES, VT VF, ventricular flutter, VER and ventricular standstill (Arrest).

Diagnostic Criteria

- Various multifocal and multiformed ventricular rhythms
- The predominant cardiac rhythms consists of ventricular flutter, VF and unstable VER (ventricular escape rhythm)
- The underlying atrial mechanism is often AF with advanced AV block
- Ventricular dissociation and ventricular standstill are the usual final events in dying hearts.

VENTRICULAR ESCAPE RHYTHM (FIG. 9.57)

Definition: Ventricular escape rhythm (VER) is a slow and regular escape rhythm originating from any location in the ventricles.

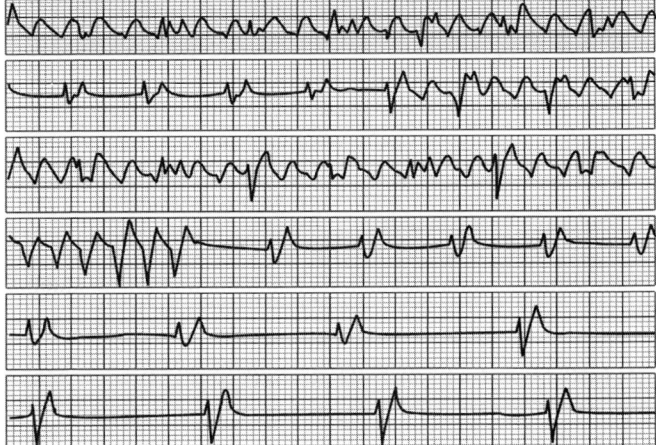

Fig. 9.56 Chaotic ventricular rhythm consisting of areas of ventricular tachycardia, ventricular flutter, and ventricular escape rhythm arising from different foci

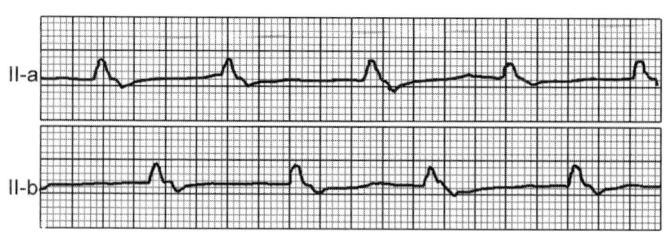

Fig. 9.57 Ventricular escape rhythm with a rate of 30 bpm

The VER occurs after a pause in which a supraventricular pacemaker failed to fire. Thus, escape beat is late, appearing after the next expected sinus beat, VER is a protective mechanism. It protects the heart from more extreme slowing or even asystole.

Diagnostic Criteria

- Regular and slow rhythm with broad QRS
- *Ventricular rate*: 20–40 bpm (may be slower or faster)
- Underlying cardiac rhythm is advanced or complete AV block in most cases
- In rare cases, broad QRS may be followed by a retrograde P-wave
- The underlying atrial mechanism may be sinus or ectopic, e.g. AF.

Note:
- Pure from of VER is rather unusual, and in most cases, VER is observed as a result of advanced or complete AV block
- AV junctional escape rhythm with LBBB or RBBB closely mimics VER.

Characteristics of VER

- Rate   : Depends on underlying rhythm. Ventricular rate is 20–40 bpm.
- Rhythm   : Essentially regular with late beats ventricular escape beat occurs after the next expected sinus beat
- P-wave   : Usually absent
- P-R interval : None with the ventricular escape beat
- QRS duration : > 0.12 sec wide bizarre T-wave frequently in opposite direction of the QRS.

VENTRICULAR STANDSTILL (ARREST) OR, CARDIAC STANDSTILL OR ASYSTOLE (FIG. 9.58)

Definition: Ventricular standstill or asystole is a total absence of ventricular activity. No QRS complex for a few seconds or longer. No ventricular rate or rhythm, no pulse and no cardiac

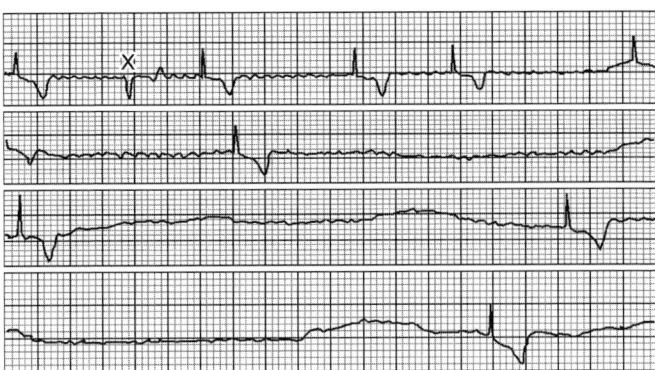

Fig. 9.58 Atrial fibrillation with advanced atrioventricular block and areas of ventricular standstill

output if atrial electrical activity is present, the rhythm is called P-wave asystole.

Characteristics of Asystole

- Rate : Ventricular usually not discernible but atrial activity may be seen (P-wave asystole)
- Rhythm : Ventricular not discernible
- P-wave : Not discernible
- PR interval : Not measurable
- QRS duration : Absent

Cardiac Arrest Rhythms

- Ventricular fibrillation
- Pulse less VT
- Asystole
- Pulse less electrical activity.

10

Heart Block

INTRODUCTION

Conduction disturbances may occur anywhere in the heart and are ordinarily expressed as a heart block in general impaired conduction, which is divided into 5 categories according to the location of the block.
1. *Sinoatrial block:* Conduction disturbances at the sino-atrial junctional tissues.
2. *Intra-atrial block:* Block within the atria.
3. *Atrioventricular block:* At the AV junctional tissues.
4. *Intra-His block:* Within the His bundle.
5. *Intra-ventricular block:* Within the ventricles or bundle branch system.

DEFINITION

Heart block is a delay or obstruction in the conduction of the electrical impulses in the heart. Block in AV node or His bundle result in atrioventricular block (AV block) and block lower in conducting system produces bundle branch block it defects in either initiation or conduction of cardiac impulses.

Site

- *Anywhere in conducting system (Fig. 10.1)*
  - SA node
  - AV node

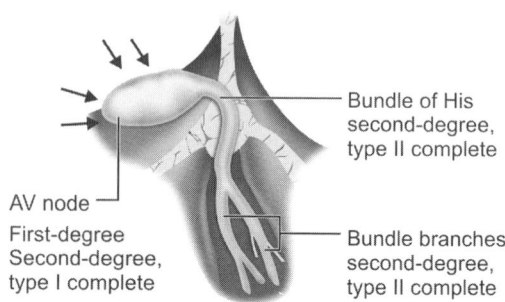

Fig. 10.1 Locations of AV block

- His bundle
- Branches of His bundle
- *The muscle of the heart.*

CLASSIFICATION

- SA block (sinoatrial block) in SA node
- AV block (atrioventricular block) in AV node
  - First degree AV block
  - Second degree
    - Mobitz type I (Wenckebach phenomenon)
    - Mobitz type II
  - Third degree or complete heart block (CHB)
- Intraventricular block- in the ventricles
  - Right bundle branch block (RBBB)
  - Left bundle branch block (LBBB)
    - Left anterior hemiblock (LAHB)
    - Left posterior hemiblock (LPHB)

What is Hemiblock?

Hemiblock means when there is block involving one of the fascicle of left bundle branch. it is diagnosed by seeing the axis deviation in ECG. When Left axis deviation—called left anterior hemiblock (LAHB) when right axis deviation—called left posterior hemiblock (LPHB).

Note: There may be more block either two or three in that case it is called bifascicular or trifascicular block.

CAUSES OF HEART BLOCK

- Ischemia
- Infarction
- Injury
- Drugs
- Hypertrophy
- Aging.

CLASSIFICATION BY DEGREE

Name of block	Type of block
First degree AV block	Incomplete
Second degree AV block Type-I	Incomplete
Second degree AV block Type-II	Incomplete
Third degree AV block	Complete

CLASSIFICATION BY SITE/LOCATION

Site	Name of block
• AV node	First-degree AV block Second-degree AV block (type-I) Third-degree AV block
• Infranodal (sub-nodal) – Bundle of His – Bundle branches	Second-degree AV block (type-II) Third-degree AV block Second-degree AV block (type-II) (common) Third-degree AV block

SINOATRIAL BLOCK

Introduction

SA block indicates impaired conduction of electrical impulses from SA node into the atria. No depolarization at the atria and absence of the entire P-QRS-T complex. So the duration of the interval between two normal beats in multiple of the previous P-P interval in SA block, the pacemaker cells within the SA node initiate an impulse but it is blocked as it exists the SA node (Fig. 10.2).

Definition

An impulse from the sinus node fails to activate the atrial.

ECG Criteria

- Normal sinus beat followed by absence of PQRS- T complex
- Duration of two normal beats = 2 previous P-P interval (long P-P interval is double than short P-P interval).

Causes

- Increased vagal tone (may like sick sinus syndrome)
- Drugs—digoxin
- Inferior myocardial infarction/ischemic heart disease (MI/IHD)—involving SA node
- Degeneration from aging.

Diagnosis

As follows:
- *Clinically:* Drop beat and no heart sound at the time of drop beat

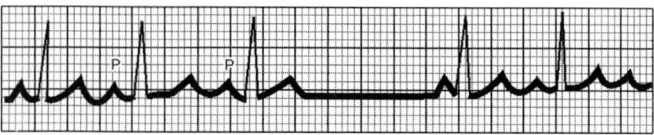

Fig. 10.2 Sinoatrial block

- *ECG:* Complete absence of one complex (P-QRS-T)
- *Holter monitoring:* Show the block.

Treatment

As follows:
- If asymptomatic—no treatment
- Withdraw the offensive drug, if any
- If any syncopal attack or sick sinus syndrome—permanent pacemaker (PPM).

Differential Diagnosis

- Sinus arrest (sinus pause)
- Sinus stand still.

Characteristics

- *Rate:* Usually normal but varies because of the pause
- *Rhythm:* Irregular
- *P-waves:* Positive (upright) in lead II
- *P-R interval:* 0.12–0.20 see and constant from beat to beat
- *QRS duration:* 0.10 sec or less unless an intraventricular conduction delay exists.

SINUS ARREST OR SINUS PAUSE OR SINUS STANDSTILL

Introduction

In sinus arrest, the pacemaker cells of the SA node fail to initiate an electrical impulse for one or more beats. When SA node fails to initiate an impulse, an escape pacemaker site (the AV junction or ventricles) should assume responsibility for pacing the heart. If they do not, you will see absent PQRST on the ECG (Fig. 10.3).

Definition

The sinus node fails to initiate an impulse, after a pause, junctional or ventricular escape occurs. So prolonged failure of discharged from SA node followed by escape rhythm. So sinus arrest is defined as a failure of impulse formation in the SA node leading to an absence of P-waves.

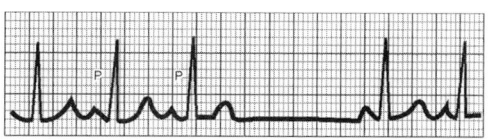

Fig. 10.3 Sinus pause

ECG Criteria

- Normal sinus beat followed by absence of P-QRS-T complex
- P-P interval surrounding the pause is not a exact multiple of previous P-P intervals.

Characteristics

- *Rate:* Normal but varies because of the pause
- *Rhythm:* Irregular
- *P-waves:* Positive (upright) in lead II
- *P-R interval:* 0.12–0.20 sec and constant
- *QRS duration:* 0.10 sec or less

Note: In sinus arrest P-P (R-R) is not exactly the double of next normal beat.

AV BLOCK: FIRST DEGREE

Introduction

AV block indicates a delay or obstruction in the transmission of impulses from the atria to the ventricles.

First degree AV block is a partial block in the AV node (AV junction) which causes prolongation of the P-R interval to greater than 0.2 sec. Every atrial depolarization is followed by conduction to the ventricles, but with delay.

Definition

First-degree AV block (1° AV block) is the prolongation of the P-R interval due to an increased relative refractory period in the AV junction (Fig. 10.4).

ECG Criteria

- Prolonged P-R interval (> 0.2 sec) in all leads but constant
- *QRS:* Normal rhythm: Normal.

Causes

- Acute MI (mostly inferior)
- Acute rheumatic carditis
- *Drugs:* Digoxin, B-blocker

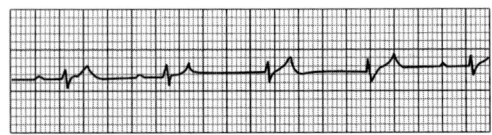

Fig. 10.4 First-degree AV block

- Increased vagal tone, normal in athlete (due to increased vagal tone)
- Aging (atherosclerosis)
- Hyperkalemia.

Clinical features: Usually asymptomatic

Note: Markedly prolonged PR interval may progress to Wenckebach's, atrioventricular heart block.

Treatment

- No treatment but the patient must be closely monitored
- Treatment of the primary causes: Done.

Characteristics

- *Rate:* Within normal range
- *Rhythm:* Regular
- *P-waves:* Normal in size and shape positive before each QRS in Leads II, III aVF
- *P-R interval:* Prolonged (>0.120 see) but constant
- *QRS duration:* 0.10 sec or less if broad (with LBBB or RBBB).

ATRIOVENTRICULAR BLOCK: SECOND DEGREE [MOBITZ TYPE I (WENCKEBACH)]

Definition

Mobitz type I AV block is characterized by a progressive increment of the P-R intervals as a result of a progressive increment of the refractor period in the AV junction untill a blocked P-wave occurs (Fig. 10.5).

Progressive prolongation of P-R interval until a P-wave fails to conduct. P-R interval before the blocked P-wave is much longer than the PR interval after the blocked P-wave.

ECG Criteria

- Progressive lengthening of P-R interval followed by absence of QRS complex (dropped beat)
- *P-P interval:* Constant
- Progressive shortening of R-R interval until block (non-conducted beat) occurs.

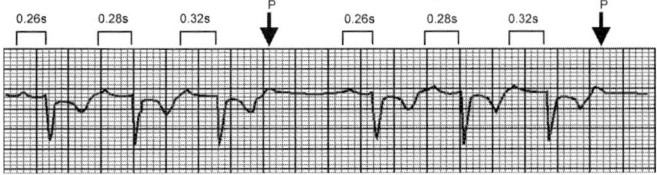

Fig. 10.5 Mobitz type I

- After non-conducted beat, next conducted beat has a shorter P-R interval than the preceding conducted beat.

Note: In this block, some but not all atrial impulses are totally blocked in the AV node and fail to conduct to the ventricles so that some p waves are not followed by QRS complexes.

Causes

- Digoxin
- Acute inferior MI
- *Physiological:* In athlete, during rest, sleep (due to increased vagal tone)

Site of block is in higher areas of AV node (proximal to bundle of His).

Clinical features: Asymptomatic, pulse—irregular (drop beat occurs).

Features of primary diseases.

Treatment

- No treatment but the patient must be closely monitored
- Primary cause should be treated.

Prognosis: It is benign condition, prognosis is good.

Characteristics

- *Rate:* Atrial rate > ventricular-rate
- *Rhythm:* Atrial—regular, Ventricular—irregular
- *P-waves:* Normal, some P-waves are not followed by a QRS (more Ps than QRSs)
- *PR interval:* Lengthens with each cycle until P-wave appears without a QRS
- *QRS duration:* 0.10 sec or less but is periodically dropped.

AV BLOCK: SECOND DEGREE (MOBITZ TYPE II ATRIOVENTRICULAR BLOCK)

Introduction

The conduction delay in Mobitz type II AV block occurs below the AV node, either of the bundle of His or, more commonly. At the level of the bundle branches (Fig. 10.6).

Definition

Mobitz type II AV block is the periodic or intermittent occurrence of blocked P-waves without Wenckebach phenomenon. This type of block is more serious than Type I AV block and frequently progresses to third-degree AV block.

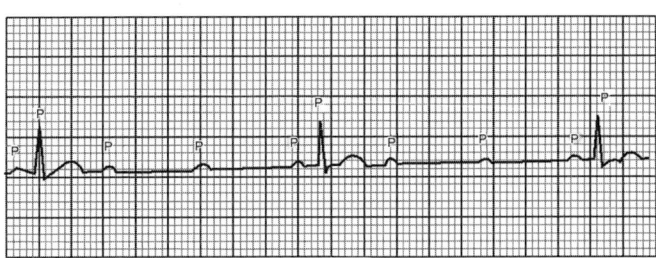

Fig. 10.6 Mobitz type II

ECG Criteria

- P-waves followed by QRS complexes and sudden intermittent blocked P-waves that are not followed by QRS complexes
- P-P interval constant
- P-R intervals of normally conducted beats (P, QRS, T) maintains constant length
- A : V ratio—2:1, 3:1, 3: 2, 4:1, 4:3, 5:1.

Note: In this serious type of AV block, an atrial impulse (P wave) suddenly fails to conduct to the ventricles.

A:V ratio: The relation between number of P-wave to the number of QRS complex, i.e. P-waves: QRS complexes.

Site of block: Lower area is the AV junction (distal to the bundle of His).

Causes: Anterior myocardial infarction. It is not seen in digoxin toxicity.

Prognosis

It is more serious than mobitz type 1.

There may be—
- Complete heart block (CHB)
- Stokes Adams syndrome
- Heart failure.

Treatment

- If associated with anterior MI, temporary pacing (TPM) followed by permanent pacemaker (PPM) is required (because complete heart block may develop)
- If associated with inferior MI-
  - If asymptomatic—close monitoring and follow- up
  - If symptomatic—Inj. atropine 0.6 mg $^1/_v$ if fails- TPM. Majority will resolve in 7–10 days.

Characteristics

- *Rate:* Atrial rate > ventricular rate
- *Rhythm:* Atrial—regular, ventricular—irregular
- *P-waves:* Normal, some P-waves are not followed by QRS (Ps>QRSs)
- *P-R interval:* Within normal limit or slightly prolonged but constant
- *QRS duration:* Usually 0.10 sec or greater periodically absent after P-waves.

ATRIOVENTRICULAR BLOCK: THIRD DEGREE (COMPLETE HEART BLOCK) (FIG. 10.7)

ECG Criteria

- Ventricular rate (heart rate) < 40 beats/min
- P-R interval variable
- P-P interval constant or equal
- R-R interval constant
- Atrial rate (P-P) is faster than ventricular rate (R-R)
- Abnormal shaped QRS complexes.

Note: If escape rhythm is junctional in origin (narrow QRS), then ventricular rate is 40–60 beats/ min. If ventricular in origin (wide QRS) then ventricular rate is 15–40 beats/min.

Causes

Commonest Cause

- Acute CHB
  - AMI (commonly inferior)
- Chronic CHB
  - Degenerative fibrosis and calcification of distal His-Purkinje system (Lev's disease in elderly)
  - Degenerative fibrosis of proximal His-Purkinjee conductive tissue (Lenegre's disease in younger)

Other Causes

- Cardiomyopathy (ischemic or idiopathic)
- Myocarditis

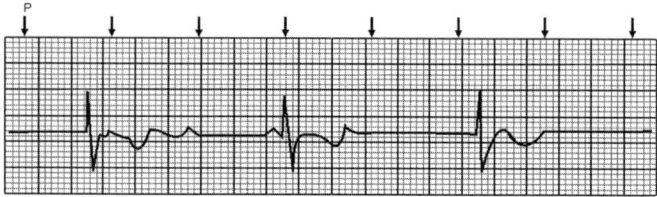

Fig. 10.7 Complete heart block

- Drugs
  - Digoxin
  - B-blocker
  - Amiodarone
- Cardiac surgery
  - Aortic valve replacement
  - Ventricular septal defect (VSD) repair
  - CABG (coronary artery bypass grafting)
- *Infection:* Endocarditis, Chaga's disease, Lyme's disease
- *Collagen disease*
  - Systemic lupus erythematosus (SLE)
  - Rheumatoid arthritis
- Infiltrative disease
  - Sarcoidosis
  - Amyloidosis
  - Hemochromatosis
- Congenital CHB: Common in child of mother with SLE due to transplacental transfer of anti-Ro antibody/Sjögren's syndrome A antigen (SS-A)
- *Neuromuscular:* Duchenne muscular dystrophy
- Radiofrequency AV node ablation.

Escape Rhythm

When there is complete dissociation between atria and ventricles, no impulse is transmitted from atria to the ventricle. In that case ventricular activity is maintained by pacemaker from other site like AV junctional or ventricular. This is called escape rhythm.

Determination Site of Complete Heart Block

Ventricular activity is maintained by junctional origin (AV node or bundle of His) or ventricular escape rhythm.

So, CHB can result from block at the level of–
- AV node
- Within bundle of His Narrow complex escape rhythm
- Distal to bundle of His (ventricular origin, wide complex escape rhythm).

Note: In a narrow complex escape rhythm:

QRS	: Junctional origin (more proximally in AV node or in bundle of His) Narrow (< 0.12 sec)
Ventricular rate	: High (50 – 60 bpm)
Patient	: Asymptomatic
In wide complex rhythm	: Ventricular origin (distally in His-Purkinje system)
QRS	: Wide (>0.12 sec)
Ventricular rate	: Slow (15–40 bpm)
Patient	: Symptomatic (dizziness syncope or black outs)

Symptoms

As follows:
- May be asymptomatic
- Dizziness, giddiness, black outs
- Sudden loss of consciousness without warning or syncope (Stokes-Adam's attack)
- Pre-syncope
- Transient amnesia
- Palpitation
- Symptoms related to decreased cardiac output
- Misdiagnosed epilepsy.

Signs

As follows:
- *Pulse:*
  - Bradycardia (20–40 bpm)
  - Large volume with systolic flow murmur
  - Does not increase with exercise
  - Or, Inj. atropine except congenital CHB
- *BP:*
  - High systolic
  - Normal diastolic
  - High pulse pressure
- *Neck vein (JVP):* Cannon wave (Large a wave) when the atria contracts against closed tricuspid valve, backward pressure produces cannon wave.
- *Heart sound-S_1:* Variable intensity of S_1 along with atrial sound due to loss of AV synchrony.
  S_2: Split normally or paradoxically.
- *Murmur:* Systolic flow murmur due to increased stroke volume.
- When ventricular rate > atrial rate produces very loud sound (bruit de cannon) and appearance of giant 'a' wave.

Treatment

As follows:
- *If Asymptomatic:* No Rx
- *Symptomatic:* PPM (VDD)
- *CHB and AF*
  - PPM, avoid atrial pacing mode VVI
  - Prophylaxis for prevention of thromboembolism.

Characteristics

- *Rate:* Atrial rate > ventricular rate
- *Rhythm:*
  - Atrial—regular
  - Ventricular—regular
  - No relationship between the atrial and ventricular rhythms

- *P-wave:* Normal
- *P-R interval:* Variable
- *QRS duration*
  - Narrow or wide
  - *Narrow:* Junctional pacemaker
  - *Wide:* Ventricular pacemaker.

A Quick Look at P-waves and AV Blocks

- *AV block:* P-wave conduction
- *First-degree:* All P-wave conducted but delayed
- *Second degree:* Some P-wave conducted others blocked
- *Third degree:* No P-wave conducted.

AV Block-Quick Summary

	Mobitz type I	*Mobitz type II*
Ventricular rhythm	Irregular	Irregular
PR interval	Progressively lengthening	Constant
QRS width	Usually narrow	Usually wide

	Mobitz type II 2:1 block	*Complete heart block (CHB)*
Ventricular rhythm	Regular	Regular
P-R interval	Constant	Variable
QRS width	Narrow or wide	Narrow or wide

STOKES-ADAMS SYNDROME (ATTACK)

It is a syndrome characterized by episodes of syncopal attack or fit during CHB due to ventricular asystole.

It also Occurs in–

- CHB
- $2°$ HB Mobitz type II
- Ventricular tachycardia (VT)
- Ventricular fibrillation
- SA disease.

Clinical Features

- Syncope or blackout with or without preceding dizziness
- During attack
  - Unconscious
  - Looks pale and may have convulsion
- If asystole persists
  Cyanosis, no pulse, fixed and dilated pupil, incontinence urine, plantar extensor
- Consciousness recovers rapidly followed by flushing
- *Mode of death:* Ventricular asystole or ventricular fibrillation (VF).

Treatment

- Confirmation of diagnosis in patients with syncope
- Between episodes
  - BBB (bundle branch block)
  - 2° HB
  - CHB
- During attack
  - A chest blow over the cardiac apex due to restore the heart action
  - If fail or no response—cardiopulmonary resuscitation (CPR)
- *Prevention:* Permanent pacemaker (PPM)

Difference between Stokes-Adams attack and epilepsy

Stokes-Adam's attack	Epilepsy
No aura or warning	Present
Unconsciousness—transient	Prolonged
During attack—very pale	Tonic/clonic phase
Recovery—rapid	Prolonged, very drowsy
Hot flushes—during recovery	Absent

ATRIOVENTRICULAR DISSOCIATION (AV DISSOCIATION)

Definition

The AV dissociation is a type of arrhythmia in which atria and ventricles are activated and contract independently.

It is minor, transient arrhythmia (Fig. 10.8).

Causes

- AMI
- Acute rheumatic carditis
- Myocarditis
- Digitalis toxicity
- In normal people.

ECG Changes

- Variable PR interval
- P: Hidden in T-wave or QRS or appear after QRS
- Ventricular rate—same like atrial rate or slightly high.

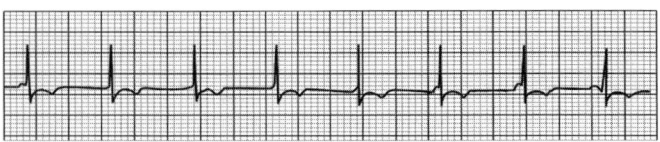

Fig. 10.8 Common type of AV dissociation

Site of Pacemakers in AV Dissociation

Two pacemakers:
1. One from SA node or atria—that control atria activator
2. Another from AV junction or ventricle—controls ventricular activation.

Difference between CHB and AV-dissociation

CHB	AV-dissociation
P—more than QRS complex	QRS—more than P wave
For total AV block, ventricular rate is much slower than atrial rate	Ventricular rate is same or slightly higher than atrial rate
Long ECG lead will fail to show any fusion or capture beat	Long ECG lead will show capture or fusion beats

Treatment

Treatment is directed towards the underlying heart disease and precipitating causes.

Range of Therapy

- *Pacemaker implantation:* AV dissociation due to CHB
- *Anti-arrhythmic drugs:* Due to VT, PVC.

Note: When the atrial and ventricular rates are almost the same, the term is called "isorhythmic AV dissociation". Then atria and ventricles beat independently. It is minor, usually transient arrhythmia.

COMPLETE RIGHT BUNDLE BRANCH BLOCK

Definition

Right bundle branch block (RBBB) is characterized by delayed activation of the right ventricle as a result of a block in the right bundle branch system (Fig. 10.9).

ECG Criteria

- Wide QRS complex (> 0.12 sec)
- rSR or M-pattern in V_1, V_2 or tall R in V_1, V_2
- Downsloping ST and inverted T in V_1, V_2
- Wide or slurred S wave in V_5, V_6 (also I, aVL).

Causes

As follows
- Normal variant (common)
  - 1% young adult
  - 5% elderly
- Acute myocardial infarction

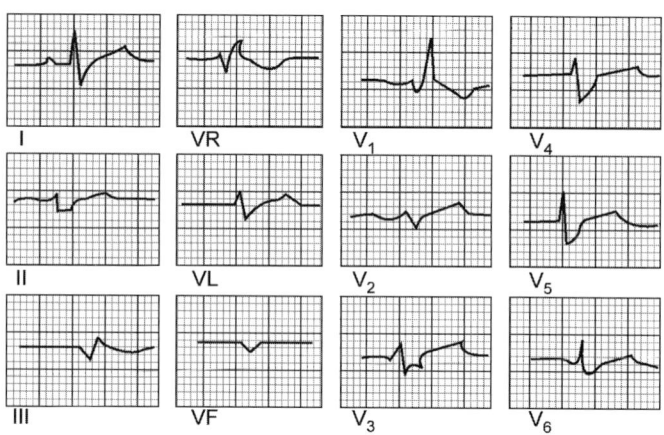

Fig. 10.9 Complete right bundle branch block (RBBB)

- Congenital heart diseases-
  - ASD (atrial septal defects)
  - TOF (Fallot's tetralogy)
  - PS (pulmonary stenosis)
  - VSD (ventricular septal defects)
- Right ventricular hypertrophy (RVH)
- Chronic cor pulmonale
- Pulmonary embolism
- Cardiomyopathy
- Fibrosis in conduction system

Note: In RBBB the initial ventricular septal activation is normal because the conduction disturbance involves only the terminal ventricular activation force.

INCOMPLETE RIGHT BUNDLE BRANCH BLOCK (FIG. 10.10)

ECG Criteria

- QRS duration between 0.10-0.12 sec
- rSR or M-pattern in V_1, V_2 or tall R in V_1, V_2
- Wide or slurred S wave in V_5, V_6 (also I, aVL)
- Downsloping ST and inverted T in V_1, V_2.

Causes of Tall R in V_1

- RBBB
- RVH
- WPW syndrome
- Normal variant
- Post MI
- Duchenne muscular dystrophy.

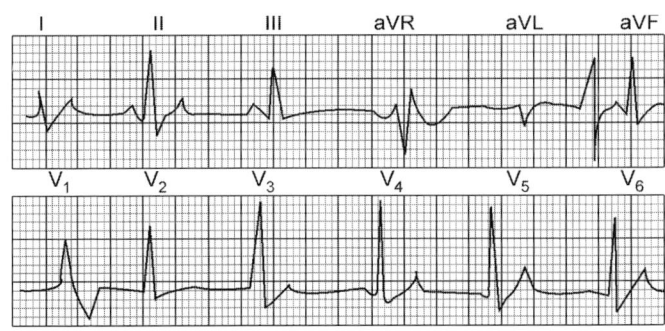

Fig. 10.10 Incomplete right bundle branch block (RBBB)

COMPLETE LEFT BUNDLE BRANCH BLOCK (FIG. 10.11)

Definition

Left bundle branch block (LBBB) is characterized by delayed activation of the left ventricle as a result of a block in the left bundle branch system (above the bifurcation of the fascicles).

ECG Criteria

- Wide QRS complex (> 0.12 sec): Wide L_1 to all Leads—a clue for diagnosis
- RSR or rSR or M-pattern in V_5, V_6 (also I, aVL)
- Downsloping ST and inverted T in V_1, V_2
- Wide or deep S wave in V_1, V_2.

Causes

- Coronary artery disease
- AMI
- LVH
- Aortic valve disease- AS, AR.
- Cardiomyopathy
- Hypertension
- Myocarditis.

Diagnosis

On auscultation, there is reverse splitting of second heart sound.

Note:
- LBBB is always pathological
- In presence of LBBB, AMI is difficult to diagnose
- When LBBB occurs in AMI, CHB may develop
- RBBB may be a normal variant
- Old anterior MI may be difficult to diagnose in presence of LBBB
- Small q in V_1 to V_2 may be present normally in LBBB.

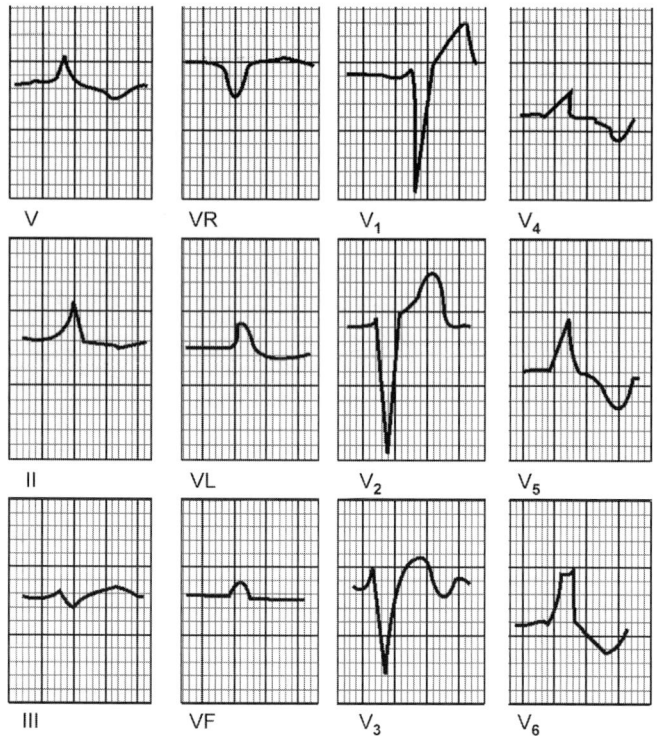

Fig. 10.11 Complete left bundle branch block

Treatment

- Treatment of primary cause
- In acute Ml
  - If New LBBB present
  - TPM (temporary pacemaker) is indicated

INCOMPLETE LEFT BUNDLE BRANCH BLOCK (FIG. 10.12)

ECG Criteria

- QRS duration between 0.10–0.12 sec
- RSR or rSR or M-pattern in V_5, V_6 (also I, aVL)
- Downsloping ST and inverted T in V_1, V_2 (I, also aVL)
- Broad and deep S wave in V_1, V_2.

LEFT ANTERIOR FASCICULAR BLOCK OR LEFT ANTERIOR HEMIBLOCK

Definition

Left anterior hemiblock (LAHB) is characterized by marked left axis deviation (LAD) of the QRS Complexes as a result of a block. In the anterior (superior) division (fascicle) of the left bundle branch system (Fig. 10.13).

Heart Block 159

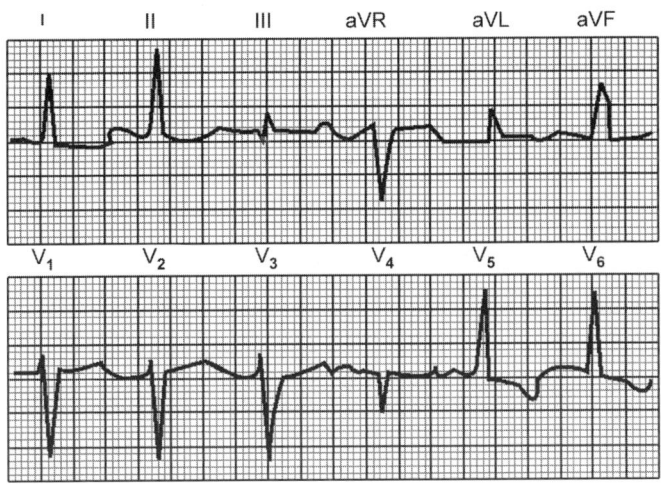

Fig. 10.12 Incomplete left bundle branch block

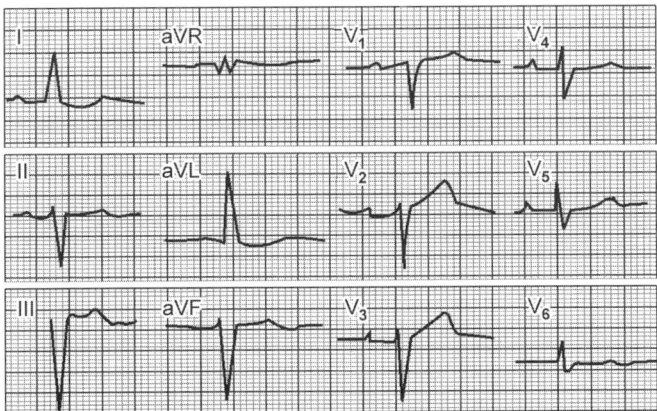

Fig. 10.13 Left anterior hemiblock

ECG Criteria

- QRS duration normal
- Left axis deviation (LAD) (usually $\geq -60°$)
- Small q-wave and large R-wave in I, aVL
- Small r-wave and deep S-wave in II, III, aVF
- Late intrinsicoid deflection in aVL (>0.045s)
- Increased QRS voltage in limb leads.

Diagnostic Pearls

There are various other causes of LAD of the QRS complexes (e.g. diaphragmatic Ml). This aspect should be carefully considered before making the diagnosis of LAHB. LAHB co-exists with RBBB Leading to bifascicular block.

Note:
- Left bundle divides into–
  - *Anterior fascicle:* Spreads in anterior and superior part of the left ventricle.
  - *Posterior fascicle:* Spreads posterior and inferior part of the left ventricle.
- RBBB with LAHB- RBBB with left axis deviation (LAD).

LEFT POSTERIOR FASCICULAR BLOCK OR LEFT POSTERIOR HEMIBLOCK

Definition

Left posterior hemiblock (LPHB) is characterized by marked right axis deviation (RAD) of the QRS complexes as a result of a block in the posterior (inferior) division (fascicle) of the left bundle branch system (Figs 10.14 and 10.15).

ECG Criteria

- QRS duration normal
- Right axis deviation (usually ≥ - 120°)
- Small q-wave and large R-wave in II, III, aVF
- Small r-wave and deep S-wave in I, aVL
- Late intrinsicoid deflection in aVF (>0.045s)
- Increased QRS voltage in limb leads
- No evidence of RVH.

Note: Bifascicular block = RBBB + LAFB or LPHB

Note:
- RBBB with LPHB → RBBB with RAD

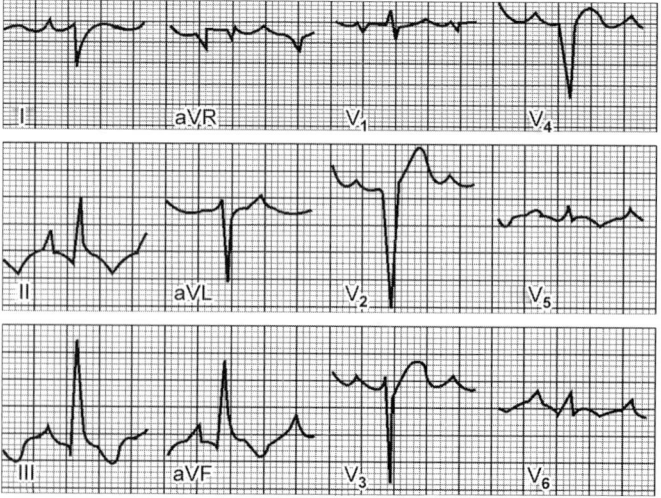

Fig. 10.14 Left posterior hemiblock

Heart Block

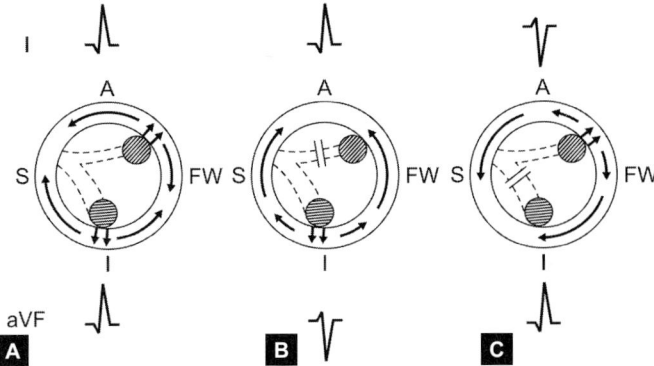

Figs 10.15A to C Left-fascicular blocks and cancellation. Top. QRS complexes in lead I. Bottom. QRS complexes in lead aVF. A. Normal, B. Left anterior fascicular block (LAFB), C. Left pasterior fascicular block (LPFB). A, anterior regions of the left ventricle; FW, left-ventricular free wall; I, inferior regions of the left ventricle; S, interventricular septum. Dashed lines, fascicles; wavy lines, sites of fascicular block; small crosshatched circles, papillary muscles; outer rings, endocardial and epicardial surface of the left ventricular myocardium; arrows, directions of activation wave fronts

- Combination of RBBB with LAHB or RBBB with LPHB is called bifascicular block
- LAHB is common but LPHB is rare.

Treatment of Bifascicular Block

- In asymptomatic case-No treatment
- Complete heart block (CHB) with acute anterior MI → TPM may be needed.

INTERMITTENT BUNDLE BRANCH BLOCK
Definition

Intermittent BBB is characterized by the intermittent occurrence of LBBB or RBBB that may be related to the heart rate (rate-dependent) or unrelated to the heart rate (rate-independent) (Fig. 10.16).

Diagnostic Criteria

- Diagnostic criteria of RBBB and LBBB
- Rate dependent BBB is much more common than rate independent BBB.

Diagnostic Pearls

When LBBB or RBBB occurs alternatively with a normal QRS complex, the ECG finding superficially mimics ventricular

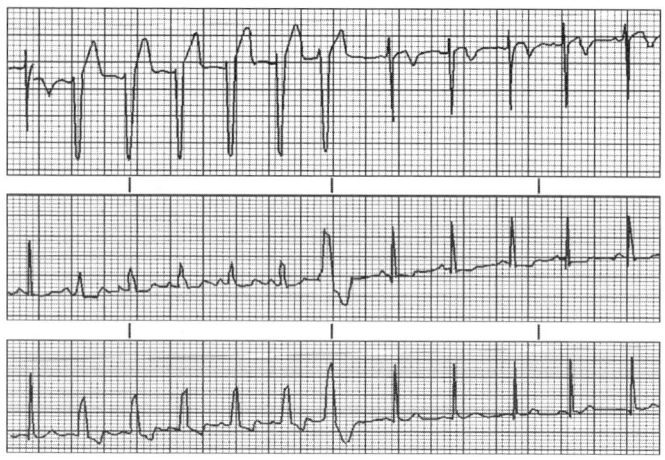

Fig. 10.16 Intermittent left bundle branch block (rate-dependent) and a ventricular premature contraction

premature contractions (VPC) causing ventricular bigeminy. VT may be closely simulated when LBBB or RBBB occurs periodically.

11

Myocardial Ischemia, Injury, Infarction

BASIC PRESENTATION

The infarcted region consists of a central core of necrotic tissue, surrounded by a zone of injured tissue which is surrounded by a zone of ischemic tissue (Fig. 11.1A). So, in the echocardiogram

- *Myocardial ischemia:* Inverted, symmetrical and pointed T-wave (Fig. 11.1B)
- *Myocardial injury (spasm):* Elevated, coved or convex-upward ST segment (Fig. 11.1C)
  If subepicardial injury → ST elevation
  If subendocardial injury → ST depression
  During exercise testing exercise tolerance test ST depression is an important indicator of coronary artery disease.
- *Myocardial infarction or necrosis*
  – Appearance of Q or QS complex (pathological Q-wave)
  – In addition to Q-waves, loss of height of R-wave indicate infarction
  – Poor 'R' wave progression in V_1–V_4 indicate old anteroseptal infarction (Figs 11.1D and E)

Note: Myocardial ischemia: Denotes a temporary reduction of the blood supply to the myocardium.

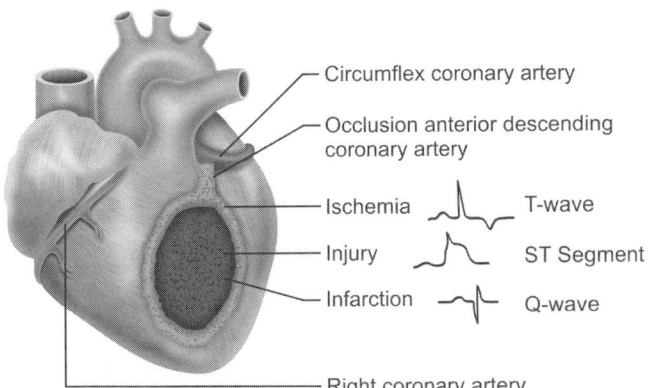

Fig. 11.1A Diagram of myocardial and ECG changes of acute ischemia injury and infarction

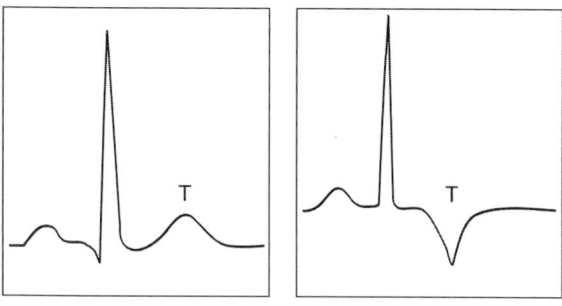

Fig. 11.1B Ischemia

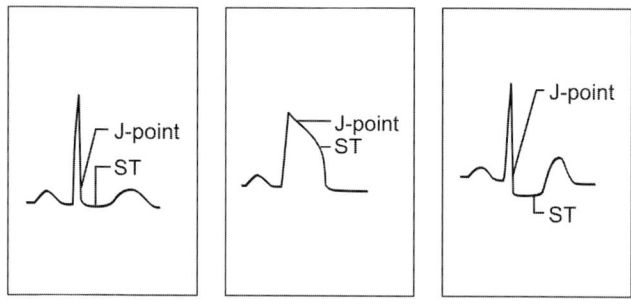

Fig. 11.1C Injury

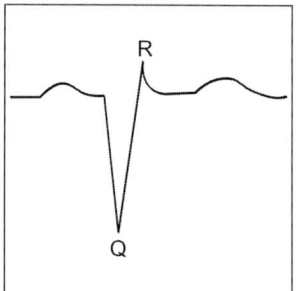

Fig. 11.1D Infarction

Myocardial injury: Denotes an acute reduction in the coronary blood supply causing injury to ventricular heart muscle.

Myocardial infarction: Denotes death or necrosis of ventricular heart muscles when the compromised coronary blood supply is not re-established.

INSUFFICIENT MYOCARDIAL PERFUSION

A decrease in coronary blood supply is typically caused by the sudden occlusion of flow owing to thrombosis or spasm.

Myocardial Ischemia, Injury, Infarction

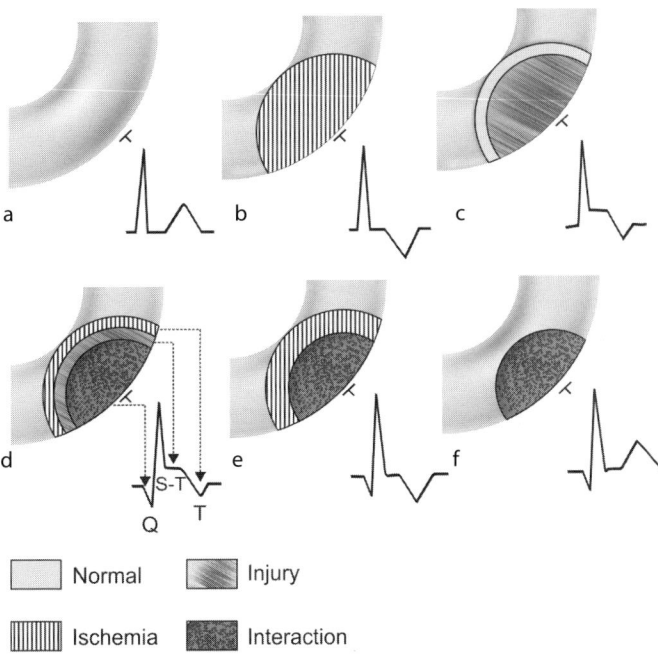

Fig. 11.1E Myocardial ischemia, injury, and infarction compared with a normal myocardium. During acute myocardial infarction the electrocardiogram discloses all three stages including ischemia (outer layer of heart) injury (middle layer of heart) and necrosis center of heart as shown in diagram D (a = normal myocardium, b = myocardial ischemia c = myocardial injury and ischemia, d = myocardial infarction, e = subacute myocardial infarction, f = old myocardial infarction

Electrical Processes

Cause	Affected	ECG altered
Increased demand	Recovery	ST segment
Decreased supply	Recovery activation	ORS, ST. T

An increase in demand is manifested by changes only in the ST segments, but a decrease in perfusion can produce a broad array of changes in the ST, T and QRS when reperfusion does not rapidly return permanent changes of infarction are produced in the QRS (Fig. 11.1F).

Grade 1: T waves only, "ischemia"
Grade 2: T-waves + ST segments, "injury"
Grade 3: T-waves + ST segments + QRS complexes, "tomb stoning"

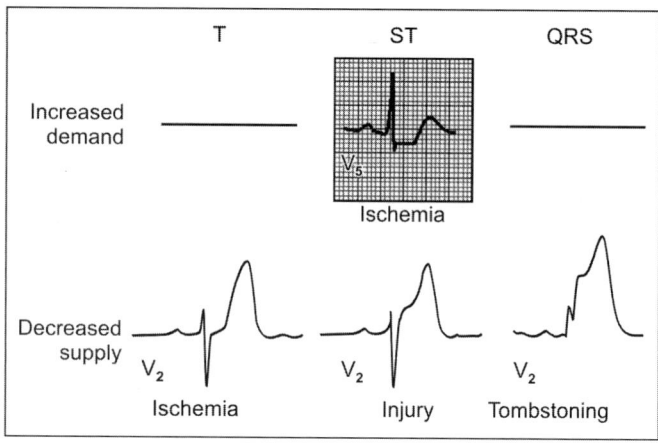

Fig. 11.1F ST-segment change indicating increased demand (above) and decreased supply (below)

ECG Changes in Response to Increased Demand and Decreased Supply

Cause	Electrical process primarily affected	Terms	ECG waveforms altered	
			Primary changes	**Secondary changes**
Increased demand	Recovery	Ischemia	ST segment	QRS complex and T-wave
Decreased supply	Recovery and activation	Ischemia (grade 1)	T-wave	–
		Injury (grade 2)	ST segment	QRS complex and T-wave
		Tomb stoning (grade 3)	QRS complex	–

LOCATION OR SITE OF MYOCARDIAL ISCHEMIA OR INFARCTION

Site	Leads showing main changes
• High lateral	I, aVL
• Inferior	II, III, aVF
• Anterior	$V_1 - V_6$
• Anteroseptal	$V_1 - V_3$ or $V_1 - V_4$
• Anterolateral	$V_4 - V_6$ (also I, aVL)
• Lateral	I, aVL, V_5, V_6
• Posterior	V_1, V_2 (mirror image change)
• Subendocardial	Any leads
• Extensive anterior	I, aVL, $V_1 - V_6$

Localization of Myocardial Infarction/Ischemia with Affected Coronary Artery

Ischemia infarct terms	Diagnostic lead	LV quadrant(s)	LV segment(s)	Affected coronary artery	Level
Antero-septal	V_1–V_3 (elevation)	Septal	Apical	LAD	Mid-distal
Extensive anterior	V_1–V_4 (elevation)	Septal	Apical/middle	LAD	Proximal
	I, aVL (elevation)	Anterior	Apical/middle		
	V_4–V_6 (elevation)	Lateral	Apical		
	II, III, aVF (depression)	Inferior	Apical		
Mid-anterior	I, aVL (elevation)	Anterior	Basal/middle	Diagonal or marginal	Proximal
	II, III, aVF (depression)				
Lateral	V_1–V_2 (depression)	Lateral	Basal	LCX	Mid-distal
Extensive lateral	V_1–V_2 (depression)	Lateral	Basal/middle	LCX	Proximal
	V_3–V_4 (depression)	Anterior	Basal		
Extensive antero-lateral	aVR > V_1 (elevation)	Septal	Basal/middle/apical	Left main	Proximal
		Anterior	Basal/middle/apical		
		Lateral	Basal/middle/apical		
Inferior	II, III, aVF (elevation)	Inferior	Basal/middle	Posterior descending	Proximal
Inferolateral	II, III, aVF (elevation)	Inferior lateral	Basal/middle	RCA	Mid
	V_1–V_2 (depression)				
Extensive inferior	II, III, aVF (elevation)	Inferior (and RV)	Basal/middle basal	RCA	Proximal
	V_1^a (elevation)				

V_1 is also V_2R

LAD, left-anterior descending; LCX, left circumflex artery; RCA, right coronary artery

MYOCARDIAL ISCHEMIA

ECG Criteria

- T inversion in leads; or
- ST depression in leads
- No Q-wave
- No ST elevation

Characteristics of Normal and Abnormal ST Segment

- *Normal ST segment*
  - It leaves the baseline
  - It blends with the proximal limb of T-wave
  - ST segment—visible and iso-electric

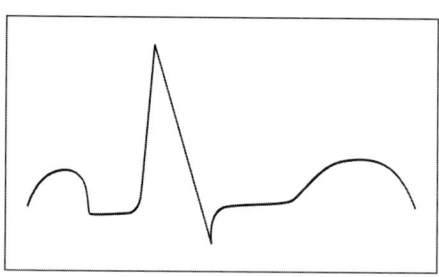

- *Junctional ST depression (physiological)*
  - Distal limb of P-wave, P-R segment, ST segment and proximal limb of T-wave form a parabola
  - Horizontally depressed ST segment at the level of TP line is less than 0.08 s
  - It is not possible to separate T-wave form ST segment

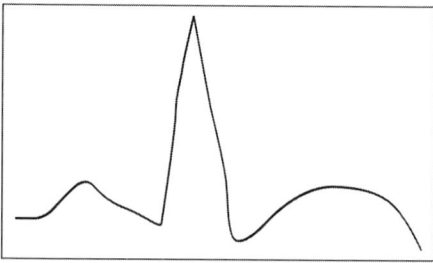

- *Junctional ST depression (pathological)*
  - It does not form parabola
  - ST persists for more than 0.08 s below TP line
  - T-wave separated from ST
  - It occurs in ischemia

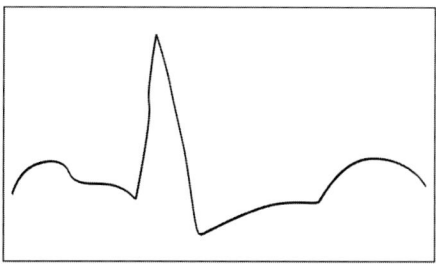

- *Horizontal ST depression*
    - It remains horizontal (i.e. 0.12 s or 3 mm or longer)
    - Sharp angle between ST and T-wave
    - Earliest change in myocardial ischemia

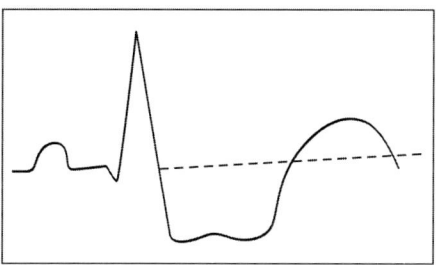

- *Depressed ST with upward sloping*
    - Junction ST depression—proximal part of ST and its junction with QRS is depressed but others upward
    - May be physiological (normal person)
    - Pathological—in myocardial ischemia

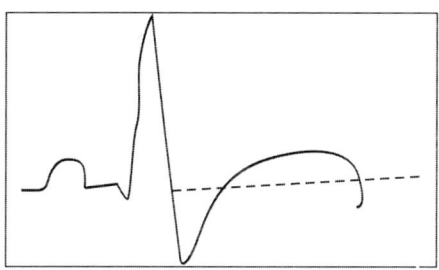

- *Plane ST segment depression*
    - It depressed in plane and horizontal or in coving manner
    - Sharp angled ST-T junction
    - T-wave separates from ST
    - In mild to moderate ischemia

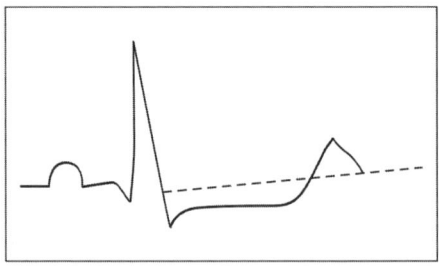

- *Sagging ST segment*
  - It is sagged downwards and cup-shaped
  - It is abnormal in acute coronary insufficiency

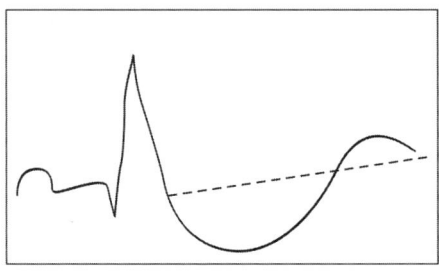

- *ST depression with down slopping*
  - It is depressed below iso-electric line
  - It slopes downwards
  - Indicated severe coronary in sufficiency

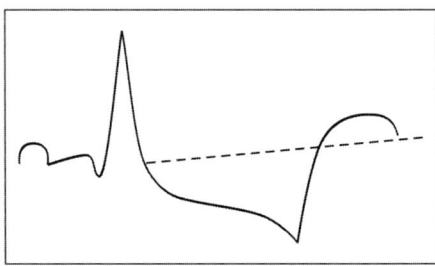

Difference between Pseudodepression and True (Ischemic) Depression of ST

Pseudodepression

- ST display a continuous ascent with upward concavity
- Down sloping of PR due to T-waves
- T-wave of atrial repolarization may continue through ventricular depolarization and is still evident after QRS as pseudodepression of ST.

True Depression

- J point is depressed
- ST segment horizontal or downsloping
- No change in PR segment

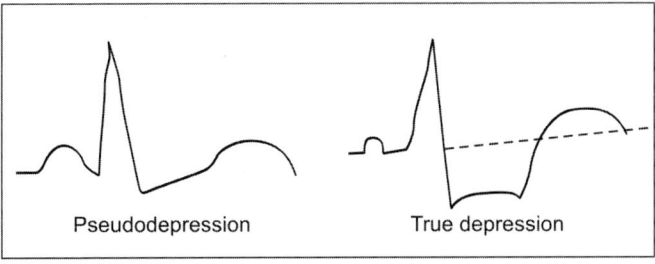

Difference between Pseudoelevation and True Elevation of ST

Pseudoelevation

Due to imposition of T on the PR, the TP line and the ST that represent the baseline and maintain iso-electricity appear elevated- called pseudoelevation of ST.

True Elevation

- J point elevated
- ST segment elevated above the baseline
- Convex contour of ST with sagging of T wave upwards

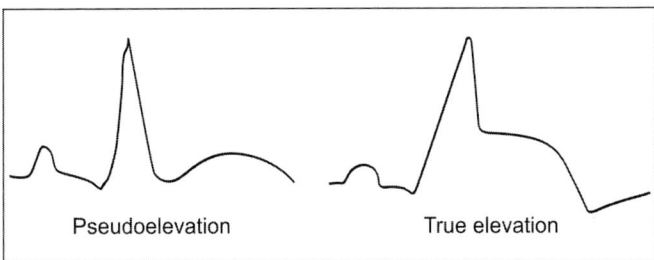

Important Causes of ST and T Changes

- *Physiological*
  - Positional
  - Hyperventilation and anxiety
  - Temperature variation
  - High carbohydrate meal
  - Neurogenic influences
  - Tachycardia induced
- *Drugs*
  - Digitalis
  - Anti-arrhythmics
  - Psychotropic drugs (Phenothiazines tricyclics)
- *Noncardiac*
  - Electrolyte disturbance
  - Cerebrovascular accidents
  - Shock

- Anemia
- Pulmonary infarction/infections
- Endocrinal disorders
- Acute abdominal disorders
- *Myocardial diseases*
  - *Ischemic:* Myocardial ischemia MI
  - Myocarditis, cardiomyopathies
  - Amyloidoses, sarcoidosis
  - Hemochromatosis
  - Neoplasms
  - Connective tissue disorders
  - Neuromuscular disorders

ELECTROCARDIOGRAPHIC PHASE OF MYOCARDIAL INFARCTION

Four Phases (Figs 11.2A to D)

1. *The hyperacute phase:* (early changes)
   - Increased amplitude of R-wave
   - Slope elevation of the ST segment
   - *Tall and widened T-waves:* Due to necrosis of myocardium (Myocytes), releasing potassium which causes hyperkalemia
   - Reciprocal ST segment depression of leads of injured surface
   - Increased ventricular activation time (VAT) [normal, < 0.04 mm]
   - No Q-wave or present
   - *Duration:* 0–6 hours
   - *Significance:*
     - Critical phase
     - Ventricular fibrillation common
     - Myocardial injury occurs but still no infarction or necrosis
     - Few hours persist
     - If treated, myocardial blood supply improved

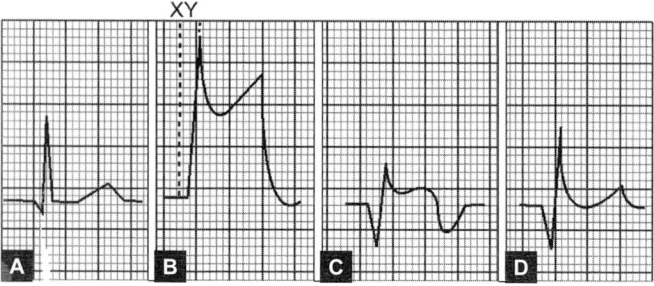

Figs 11.2A to D The phases of a myocardial infarction. (A) Normal; (B) Hyperacute phase; (C) Fully evolved phase; (D) Chronic stabilized

2. *The acute phase (full evolved phase):* Later change
   - Pathological Q-wave
   - ST elevation convexity upwards (coving pattern) with symmetrical pointed T-wave inversion
   - Reduces the amplitude of R-wave
   - *Duration:* 6 hours to 7 days
3. *Recent (subacute) phase:* Late pattern
   - Pathological Q-wave
   - ST elevation or returns to the base line
   - T—Biphasic or depression
   - *Duration:* 7 days to 28 days
4. *The chronic stabilized phase or old MI:* Very late pattern
   - Pathological Q-wave
   - ST segment returns to the base line
   - Inverted T gradually become upright (positivity)
   - QRS-reduced
   - *Duration:* > 28 days

EVOLUTION OF ACUTE MI

During acute chest pain due to infarction, ECG changes do not appear simultaneously but take sometime to appear, ECG taken immediately may be normal but a subsequent ECG taken few hours later may show changes (Fig. 11.3).

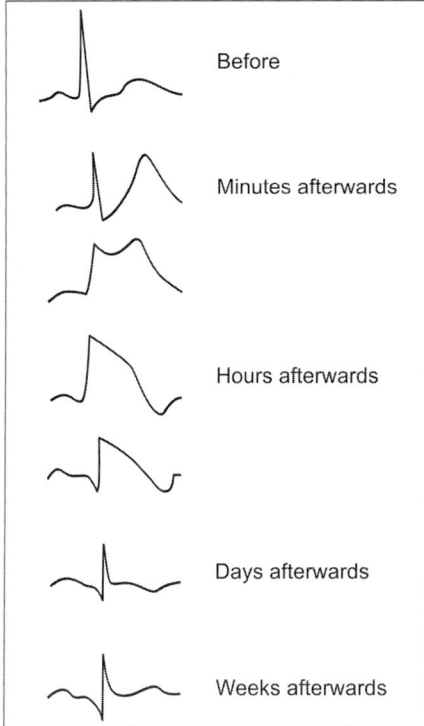

Fig. 11.3 Electrocardiographic evolution of myocardial infarction

Classic ECG Criteria for Acute MI (Fully Evolved)

- ST elevation (with upward convexity)
- T-inversion
- Q-wave (pathological)

ECG Criteria in Old MI

- Pathological Q-wave
- ST–in baseline
- T–normal or inverted

Note
- *T inversion:* Due to ischemia
- *ST elevation:* Due to myocardial injury
- *Q-wave:* Due to myocardial necrosis.

Serial ECG Changes during Evolution of MI

- *The early change:* If ECG is normal it is pre-infarct complex (Hyper acute phase)
  Duration: Few minutes to few hours (0–6 hours)
  ECG complex:
    - ST elevation appears
    - T-wave obscured by ST elevation
    - Height of R-wave-reduced
    - Superimposition of ST elevation on old infarction signifies a fresh infarction in a region of previous involvement
    - Lasts for few hours
- *Later changes:* The acute phase
  Duration: Few hours to few days (6 hours – 7 days)
  ECG complex
    - Abnormal Q-wave or QS appear
    - Ordinarily Q develops while ST is still elevated
    - Normal R may be replaced by QS; Or
    - R may be smaller
    - It is preceded by a abnormal Q
- *Late pattern:* Subacute phase
  Duration: Few days to few weeks (7 days–4 weeks)
  ECG complex:
    - Deep symmetrical inversion T appear
    - ST returns to baseline
    - This stage indicates transmural ischemia
    - It was masked by strong current of injury
- *Very late pattern:* Chronic or old
  Duration: After several weeks to several (>4 week) months
  ECG complex
    - ST returns to baseline
    - Abnormal Q and inverted T persists
    - May persists for months or years
    - It is called changes of an old infarction

ST Segment Elevation Other than AMI

- Early repolarization syndrome
- Prinzmetals angina
- Myopericarditis
- Ventricular aneurysm
- Hyperkalemia
- A cardiac tumor.

Correlation of MI with Side of Occlusion of a Coronary Artery

Infarction	Site of coronary occlusion
Anterior infarction	Left coronary artery (LCA)
Inferior infarction	• Right coronary • Right or left circumflex artery
Strict posterior or posterolateral infarction	Left circumflex artery Right or left circumflex artery

ECG Predictors of Left Anterior Descending (LAD) Occlusion in Anterior MI

Site of occlusion	ECG findings
Proximal to first septal perforator (S_1)	ST ↑ (V_1) > 2.5 mm • Complete RBBB • ST ↑ aVR • ST ↑ V_5
Proximal to first diagonal branch (D_1)	Q-wave in aVL
Proximal to S_1/D_1	ST ↓ in inferior leads > 1 mm
Distal to S_1	Q-waves in $V_4 - V_6$
Distal to D_1	ST ↓ aVL

- ST ↑ = ST elevation
- ST ↑ = ST depression

ECG Findings in Culprit Vessel

Culprit vessels	ECG findings
Right coronary artery (RCA)	ST ↑ in III > II ST ↓ in lead I T-wave upright in V_{4R}
Left circumflex artery (LCX)	ST ↑ in II > III ST ↑ in lead I T-wave inverted in V_{4R}

ECG Criteria of AMI in the Presence of LBBB

Criteria

- ST ↑ ≥ 1 mm and concordant with a predominantly negative QRS

- ST $\downarrow \geq 1$ mm lead V_1, V_2 or V_3
- ST $\uparrow \geq 5$ mm and discordant with a predominantly negative QRS

Sensitivity and Specificity of ECG in MI

- *Causes of false negative cases:* Infarct present but ECG does not show diagnostic changes
  - Second infarction
  - Left ventricular hypertrophy (LVH)
  - Lateral and posterior wall MI
  - Wolff-Parkinson-White (WPW) syndrome
  - Non-specific ST-T changes in absence of Q
- *Causes of false positive cases:* Infarction absent but ECG shows diagnostic changes
  - Q-wave present but infarction absent:
    - LVH
    - WPW syndrome
    - Chronic obstructive pulmonary disease (COPD)
    - Fascicular blocks
    - Infiltrative heart disease
  - Q-wave absent ST present but infarction absent
    - Right ventricular hypertrophy (RVH)
    - Drugs electrolytes disturbances
    - Secondary ST-T changes in presence of BBB
    - COPD
    - Acute pulmonary embolism
    - Hyperventilation
    - Myocarditis

Site of Myocardial Infarction by ECG

Site of infarction	ECG leads
Left ventricle	
• Anterior wall	V_1-V_3, V_4 also
– Anteroseptal	V_4-V_6 and I, aVL
– Anterolateral	V_1-V_6
– Anteroapical	V_5-V_6
– Apical	I, aVL, V_1-V_6
– Extensive anterior	I and aVL
– High anterior or high lateral	II, III, aVF
• Inferior wall	II, III, aVF and V_1-V_2
– Inferoposterior	II, III, aVF and V_1-V_2 and V_5-V_6
– Inferoposterior lateral	II, III, aVF and V_5-V_6
– Inferolateral	Mirror image changes in right precordial leads
• Posterior wall	
– True posterior	V_3R, V_1-V_2
– Posterolateral	V_1, I and V_5-V_6
Right ventricle	V_{3R-6R} and V_1 or V_2 or both

Subendocardial Ischemia

Definition

Subendocardial ischemia is myocardial ischemia involving primarily the subendocardial zone of the left ventricle (Fig. 11.4).

ECG Criteria

- Increased amplitude of T-waves in two or more ECG leads facing the ischemic zone
- Often associated with broad T-waves
- Often associated with a prolonged Q-T interval

Note:
- Subendocardial ischemia is usually a transient ECG phenomenon but a persisting subendocardial ischemia may lead to acute MI
- It should be differentiated from hyperkalemia and CNS disorders.

Subepicardial Ischemia

Definition

Subepicardial ischemia is myocardial ischemia involving primarily the subepicardial zone of the left ventricle (Fig. 11.5).

ECG Criteria

- Deeply and symmetrically inverted T-waves in two or more ECG leads facing the Ischemic zone
- Little or on prolongation of T-wave width or Q-T interval

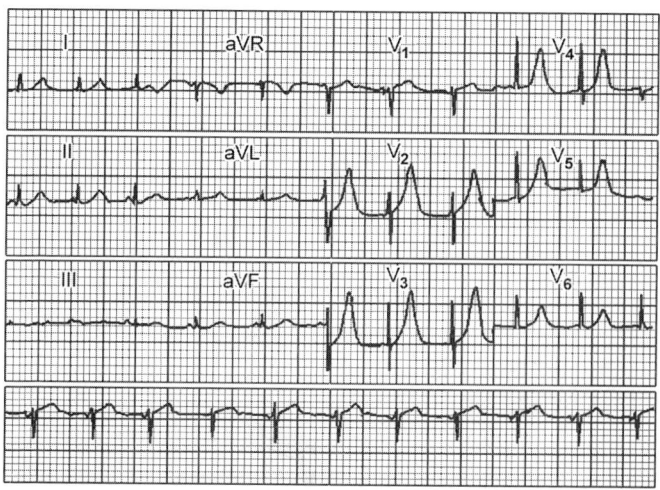

Fig. 11.4 Diffuse subendocardial ischemia

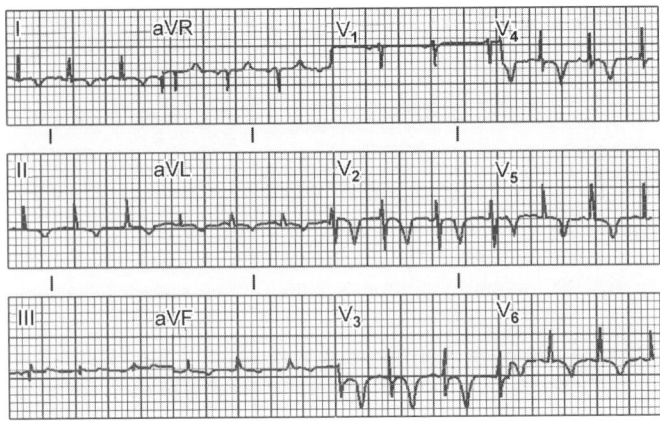

Fig. 11.5 Diffuse subepicardial ischemia

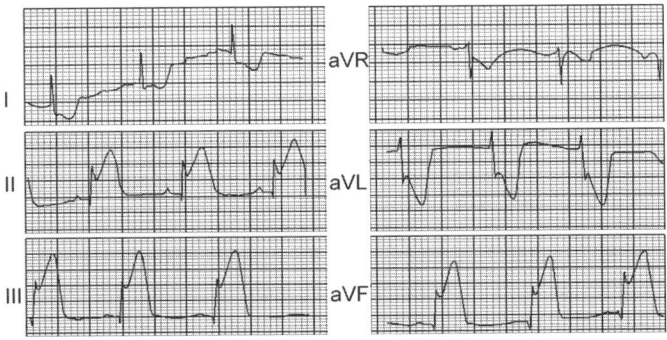

Fig. 11.6 Diaphragmatic (inferior) subepicardial injury

Note: When subendocardial and subepicardial ischemia occur simultaneously the end result is the same as a pure subepicardial ischemia.

Subepicardial Injury

Definition

Subepicardial injury is myocardial injury primarily involving the subepicardial zone of the left ventricle (Fig. 11.6).

ECG Criteria

- ST elevation ($\geq$ 1 mm up sloping or horizontal) in two or more ECG leads facing injured zone
- Reciprocal ST depression in other ECG leads in the opposite area from the injured zone.

Note:
- It is often a transient phenomenon but persisting ST segment elevation frequently leads to acute MI
- When ST elevation involves practically every ECG lead diffusely acute pericarditis is likely the diagnosis

- It should be distinguished from the early repolarization pattern in which 'J point elevation' is the main ECG findings.

Coronary Artery Spasm

Definition

Coronary artery spasm involves one or more coronary arteries and is associated with chest pain coronary artery spasm may or may not be associated with underlying fixed coronary artery lesion (Figs 11.7A and B).

ECG Criteria

- ST elevation in two or more ECG leads facing the involved associated and chest pain
- Coronary artery spasm may occur spontaneously, but it may be provoked by various maneuvers, including the cold pressor test
- Coronary artery spasm may involve only one artery but multiple arteries may be involved
- ECG findings may return to normal when spasm subsides.

Note: Coronary artery spasm may lead to acute MI and sudden death in severe cases.

Extensive Anterior Myocardial Infarction

Definition

Extensive anterior myocardial infarction (EAMI) involves the entire anterior wall of the left ventricle (Fig. 11.8).

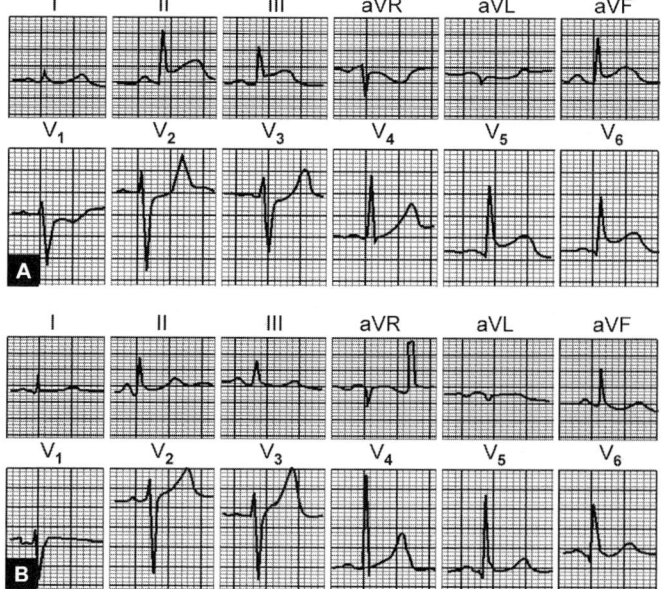

Figs 11.7A and B Coronary artery spasm

ECG for Medical Diagnosis

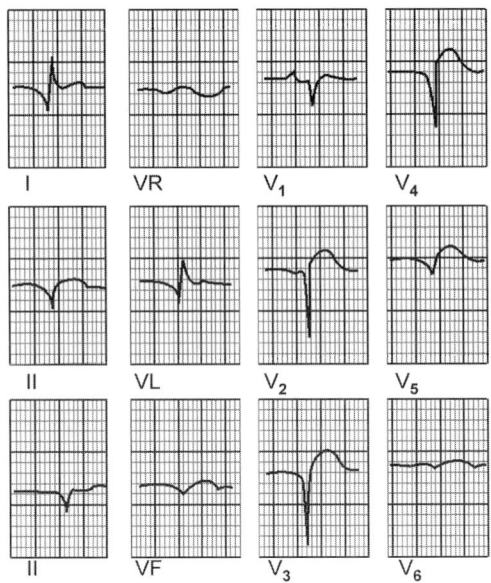

Fig. 11.8 Extensive anterior infarction

ECG Criteria for Extensive Anterior MI

- ST elevation in $V_1 - V_6$, I, aVL
- T inversion in $V_1 - V_6$
- Q-wave in $V_1 - V_5$, I, aVL
- ST elevation with T inversion during first 72 hours.

Note: Extensive anterior Ml is frequently called massive anterior Ml. It is actually a combination of anteroseptal, anterior, anterolateral and high lateral MI.

Anteroseptal Myocardial Infarction

Definition

Anteroseptal myocardial infarction (ASMI) involves the ventricular septum of the left ventricle (Fig. 11.9).

ECG Criteria

- ST elevation in $V_1 - V_3$ or V_4
- T inversion in $V_1 - V_3$ or V_4
- Q wave in $V_1 - V_3$ or V_4
- ST ↑ and T ↓ during first 72 hours

Anterior Myocardial Infarction

Definition

Anterior MI involves the anterior wall of the left ventricle (Fig. 11.10).

Myocardial Ischemia, Injury, Infarction

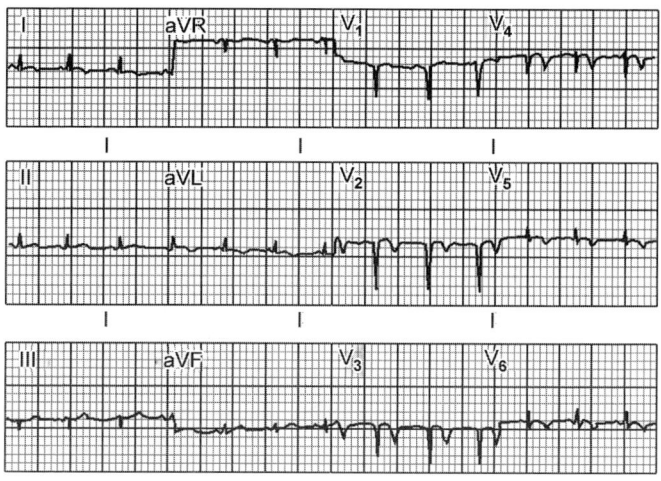

Fig. 11.9 Anteroseptal myocardial infarction with diffuse anterior ischemia

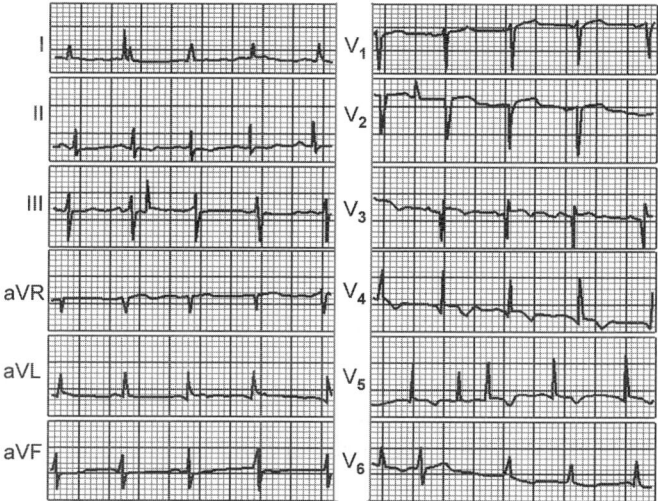

Fig. 11.10 Anterior myocardial infarction

ECG Criteria

- ST elevation in $V_1 - V_6$
- T inversion in $V_1 - V_6$
- Q-wave in $V_1 - V_6$
- ST elevation and T inversion during the first 72 hours.

Note: In AMI the ventricular septal activation is normal. Thus lead V_1 shows the expected small R-wave in AMI.

Anterolateral Myocardial Infarction

Definition

Anterolateral MI involves the lateral wall of the left ventricle (Fig. 11.11).

ECG for Medical Diagnosis

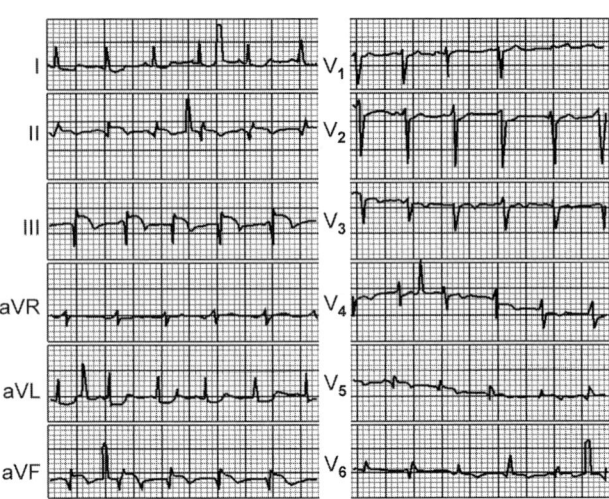

Fig. 11.11 Anterolateral myocardial infarction associated with acute diaphragmatic (inferior) myocardial infarction

ECG Criteria

- ST elevation in $V_4 - V_6$
- T inversion in $V_4 - V_6$
- Q-wave in $V_4 - V_6$
- ST ↑ and T ↓ during first 72 hours

Note: ALMI is often called lateral MI.

High Lateral Myocardial Infarction

Definition

High lateral myocardial infarction (HLMI) involves the higher portion of the left ventricular lateral wall (Fig. 11.12).

ECG Criteria

- ST elevation in I, aVL
- T inversion in I, aVL
- Q wave in I, aVL
- ST ↑ and T ↓ during the first 72 hours

Note: HLMI often coexists with posterior MI inferior MI and anterolateral MI.

Inferior Infarction (Diaphragmatic MI)

Definition

Inferior MI involves the inferior wall of the left ventricle (Fig. 11.13).

Myocardial Ischemia, Injury, Infarction

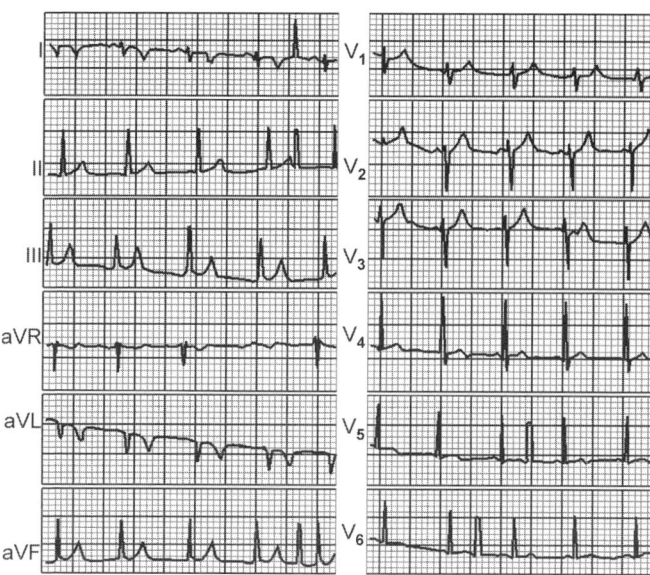

Fig. 11.12 High lateral myocardial infarction

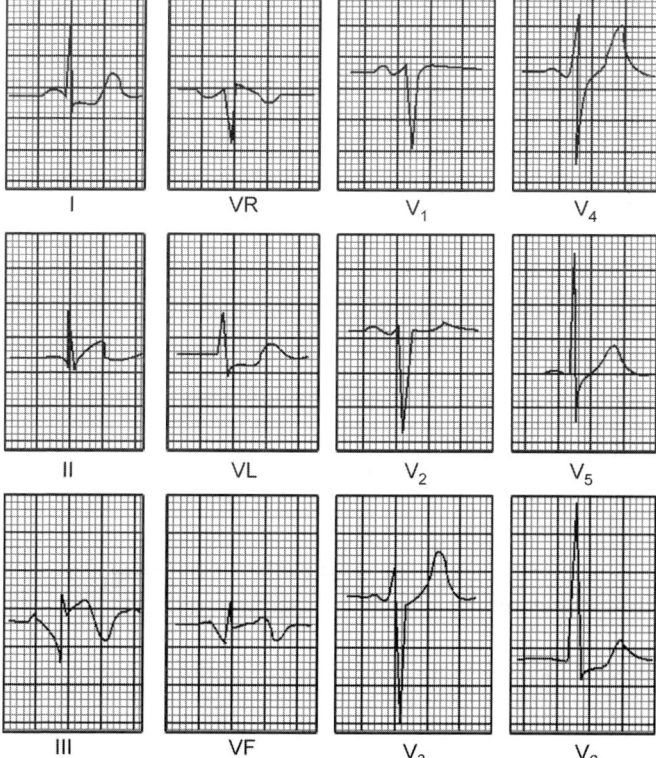

Fig. 11.13 Inferior infarction

ECG Criteria

- ST elevation II, III, aVf
- Q-wave in II, III, aVF
- T inversion in II, III, aVF
- ST ↑ and T ↓ during the first 72 hours

Note: Inferior MI coexists with posterior MI and lateral MI. The QS waves are not reliable findings to diagnose inferior MI.

Posterior Wall Myocardial Infarction

The right precordial leads V_1 to V_3 and especially lead V_2 are orientated to anterior wall and reflect the inverse change or mirror-image of this presentation for posterior wall MI.

Definition

Posterior myocardial infarction involves the posterior wall of the left ventricle (Fig. 11.14).

ECG Criteria Note

Lead V_2 Showing

- Tall, widened R-wave
- ST depressed and concave upward
- Tall, widened, upright, T-wave and symmetrical during the first 72 hours

Mirror-image of Lead V_2 Showing

- Deep, broad Q-wave R/S ratio in $V_1 > 1$
- ST segment coved and elevated is a diagnostic
- Inverted, symmetrical T-wave criteria for true posterior MI

Note: Ventricular aneurysm
- Pathological Q-wave
- ST segment elevation   persistent 3 months or
- T-wave inversion   more from acute attack

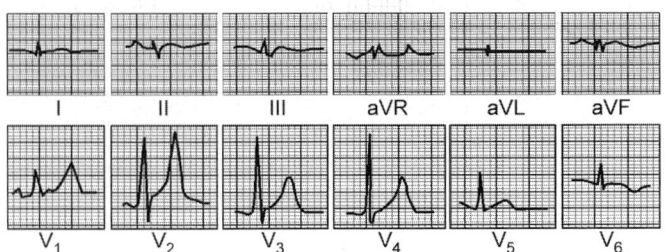

Fig. 11.14 The features of inferolateral MI with posterior wall MI

Note:
- Posterior MI fails to produce abnormal Q-wave because there are no ECG leads facing the posterior wall
- PMI coexists with inferior MI and lateral MI

Inferoposterolateral Myocardial Infarction

Definition

Inferoposterolateral MI involves the inferior-posterior and lateral walls of the left ventricle diffusely (Fig. 11.15).

ECG Criteria

- ST elevation tinversion and Q-wave in II, III, aVF and $V_4 - V_6$
- Tall R-wave in $V_1 - V_3$
- Reciprocal ST depression in $V_1 - V_3$ with upright T-wave during first 72 hours.

Note: Often high lateral wall of the left ventricle is involved together.

Non-Q-wave Myocardial Infarction (Subendocardial Infarction)

Definition

Non-Q-wave MI or subendocardial infarction involves the subendocardial zone of the left ventricle. It has other EGC terms, including non-transmural MI or non-ST elevation MI (Fig. 11.16).

ECG Criteria

- Deeply inverted and symmetrical T-wave persists
- ST depression persist horizontally to downsloping of 1 mm or more
- Non-Q-wave (No abnormal Q)
- Elevation of troponin 1 enzyme or creatine phosphokinase (CPR) with MB- isoenzyme.

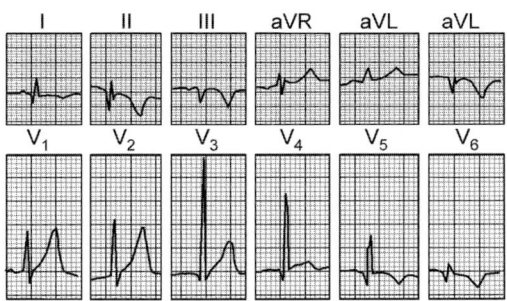

Fig. 11.15 Diaphragmatic posterolateral myocardial infarction

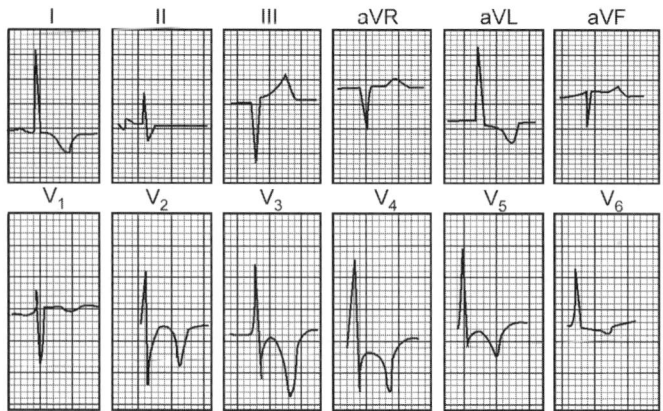

Fig. 11.16 Subendocardial infarction

Note: When the ECG changes are transient (<30 min) without Troponin-I or CPK elevation then the diagnosis of angina pectoris is not non-Q-wave MI. Then persisting ST and/or T-wave in version without serum troponin-I or CPK elevation are difficult to label clinically. Then, it is called unstable angina.

Clinical Importance

- Thrombolytic therapy is not indicated
- Higher risk of re-infarction
- Early mortality is less
- Complication are uncommon
- Frequent follow-up adequate preventive measures.

Transmural Myocardial Infarction (Q-wave Infarction) (Fig. 11.17)

ECG Criteria

- Q-wave
- ST elevation
- T-wave inversion
- R-wave lower

Note: Transmural myocardial infarction denotes death of myocardial tissue extending from the outer (subepicardial) portion of the ventricular wall to the inner (subendocardial) portion of the ventricular wall.

N.B. Q-wave infarction means infarction of full thickness myocardium (Transmural MI).

Right Ventricular Myocardial Infarction

Definition

Myocardial infarction involving the right ventricle (Fig. 11.18).

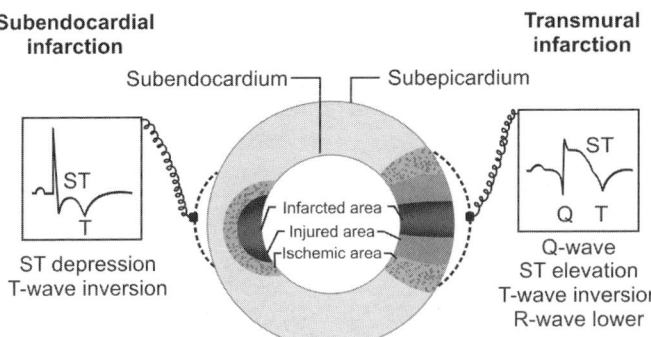

Fig. 11.17 Subendocardial and transmural infarction

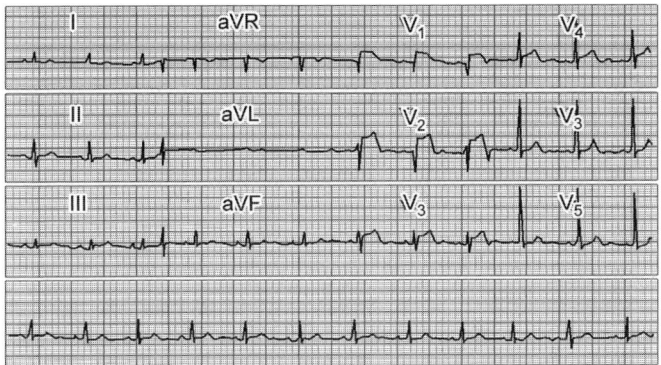

Fig. 11.18 Acute right ventricular MI

ECG Criteria

- ST elevation ($\geq$ mm) in $V_1 - V_3$
- ST elevation ($\geq$ 1 mm) in V_1 and V_{3R-6R}
- ST elevation in $V_1 - V_6$ (marked in V_1 and least in V_6)
- Often associated with acute inferior MI of the left ventricle

Note:

- In right ventricular MI abnormal Q-waves are not produced
- An early stage of ECG in acute anteroseptal MI (ASMI) superficially resembles right ventricular MI but ASMI eventually produces the characteristic abnormal Q.
- Taking additional right precordial leads (V_{3R-6R}) is beneficial in the diagnosis of right ventricular MI.

Left Bundle Branch Block Associated with Acute Anterior MI

Definition

Acute anterior MI occurs in the presence of preexisting LBBB or LBBB as a result of acute anterior MI (Fig. 11.19).

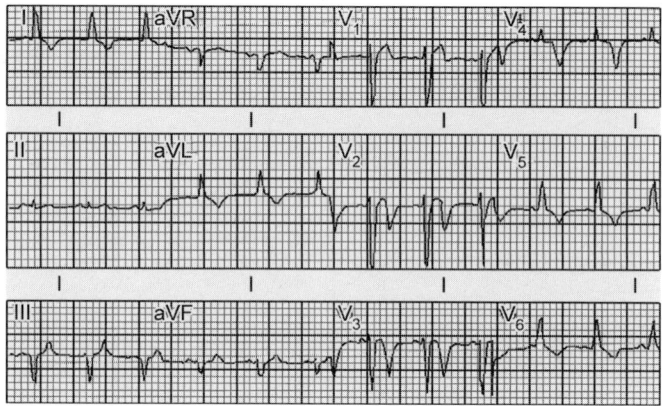

Fig. 11.19 Left bundle branch block associated with acute anterior myocardial infraction

ECG Criteria

- Primary T-wave change replacing the secondary T-wave change (symmetrically and deeply inverted T-waves replacing biphasic or slightly inverted T-waves in I, aVL and $V_2 - V_6$
- Upright or tall T-wave replacing the biphasic or slightly inverted T-wave in I, aVL, $V_2 - V_6$
- ST elevation replacing the ST segment depression in $V_2 - V_6$
- Reappearance of Q in I, aVL and $V_2 - V_6$ in presence of LBBB
- Diagnostic criteria of LBBB appears

Note: Old MI is often difficult or even impossible to recognize in the presence of LBBB.

TYPES OF MI: MINNESOTA CRITERIA

As follows:
- Hyperacute MI—from onset of MI up to 6 hours
- Acute MI—6 hours to 7 days
- Recent MI or subacute MI—7 days to 28 days
- Old MI or chronic MI—after 28 days.

Significance of Pathological Q, ST Elevation and T Inversion in MI

- *T inversion:* Due to ischemia
- *ST elevation:* Due to myocardial injury
- *Q-wave:* Due to myocardial necrosis.

Significance of the Hyperacute Phase

It is the most critical phase. VF is common in this period. There is myocardial injury but still no infarction or necrosis. This phase may persist for few hours, if treated properly, myocardial blood supply is improved.

Mechanism of Tall T in Hyperacute MI

It is due to necrosis of the myocardium (myocytes), releasing potassium which causes localized hyperkalemia and leading to tall T.

Difference between Q-wave and Non-Q-wave MI

Features	Q-wave MI (Transmural or subepicardium)	Non-Q-wave MI (subendocardial)
Prevalence	47%	53%
Coronary occlusion	80–90%	15–25%
Infarction size	Moderate to large	Small
Residual ischemia	10–20%	40–50%
Early reinfarction	5–8%	15–25%
Thrombolysis	Indicated	Not indicated
Complication	common	Uncommon
One month mortality	10–15% more	3–5% less
Two year mortality	30%	30%

Note:
- ST elevation may not occur before 6 hours.
- Fully evolved phase is usually seen after 24 hours
- *Pathological Q:* Broad > 1 mm deep > 2 mm or and > 25% of the amplitude of R-wave is suggestive of MI
- Q-wave may appear after 8–16 hours (commonly after 24 hours)
- ST segment returns to normal after a few days.
- T-wave may remain upright for weeks to months
- Q-waves usually remain permanently in most of the cases (90% case)
- If ST remain elevated after few months of acute MI, it is ventricular aneurysm
- MI may be ST elevation MI (STEMI) and non-ST elevation MI (NSTEMI)
- Acute MI may be masked in presence of LBBB, WPW syndrome and pacemaker

Note: MI may be difficult to diagnose if following disease are present:
- WPW syndrome
- LBBB and LVH
- Cardiomyopathy
- Hyperkalemia
- COPD and RVH
- Chest deformity.

Dresslor's Syndrome (Postmyocardial Infarction Syndrome)

Definition

Dresslor's syndrome is a late complication of myocardial infarction that occurs usually a few weeks or even months (2–10 weeks) after acute MI.

It is characterized by (5**P**)
- **P**ain (chest pain)
- **P**yrexia
- **P**leurisy
- **P**ericarditis (pericardial effusion)
- **P**neumonitis (pulmonary infiltrate).

Mechanism

It is due to autoimmune reaction to necrosed myocardium antimyocardial antibody may be found in blood. Recurrence is common confuses with new MI or unstable angina.

Treatment

As follows:
- Aspirin (600–900 my) every 4–6 hours high doses
- In severe or recurrent cases—corticosteroid
- Anticoagulant should be discontinued unless strong evidence for high-risk of thromboembolism.

Enzymatic Changes with Time in AMI

Enzyme	Rise (hrs)	Peaks at (hrs)	Persists for
Troponin I and T	2–4	12–14	7 days (up to 2 wks)
CPK – MB	4–6	12	2–3 days
AST/ SGOT	12	24	3–4 days
LDH	12	3–4 days	7–10 days

ECG Changes in Myocardial Ischemia

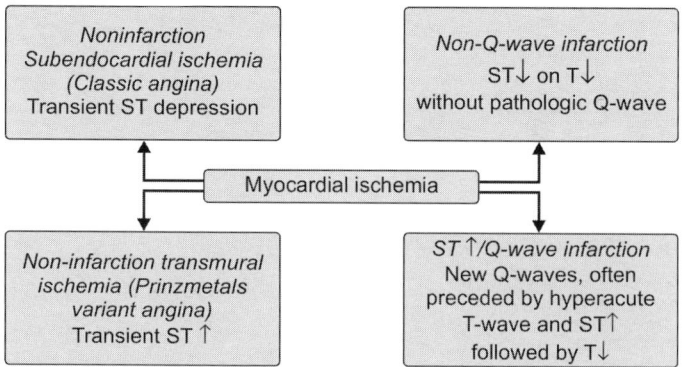

ACUTE CORONARY SYNDROMES

Definition

Acute coronary syndrome (ACS) is the constellation of clinical symptoms which include STEMI (ST elevation myocardial infarction) and non-STEMI (unstable angina, non-QWMI).

Or,

Acute coronary syndrome (ACS) is the clinical condition developed due to acute myocardial ischemia due to disruption of atherosclerotic plaque resulting thrombus formation which is associated with increased risk of cardiac death and myocardial infarction.

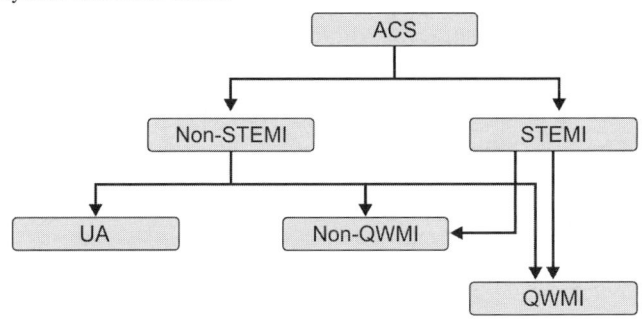

The initiating event is disruption of the pre-existing atheromatous plaque either by erosion or rupture resulting in platelet activation and fibrin deposition leading to thrombus formation.

Diagnosis

Diagnosis or assessment of patients with suspected acute coronary syndrome is made on:
- *Clinical assessment:* Presentation, history, clinical sign and symptoms
- ECG findings
- Measurement of biochemical cardiac markers.

ECG Findings for Diagnosis

ST Elevation Myocardial Infarction (STEMI)

ECG
- ST elevation in corresponding leads
- New onset left bundle branch block
- Evolution of Q-wave

Cardiac markers

CK-MB: Positive, troponin 1 or T : positive

Non-ST Elevation Myocardial Infarction (NSTEMI)
Non-Q-wave MI

ECG
- ST depression more than 1 mm
- Transient ST elevation
- T-wave inversion
- Nonspecific ECG changes.

Cardiac markers:
- *CK-MB:* Positive
- *Troponin 1 or T:* Positive

Unstable Angina (UA)

ECG
- Transient ST elevation/ST depression
- T inversion
- Non-specific ECG changes
- Normal ECG
- Associated findings-T changes, arrhythmias conduction defects

Cardiac marker
- *CK-MB:* Within normal limit
- *Troponin 1 or T:* Normal limit.

Diagnosis of ACS

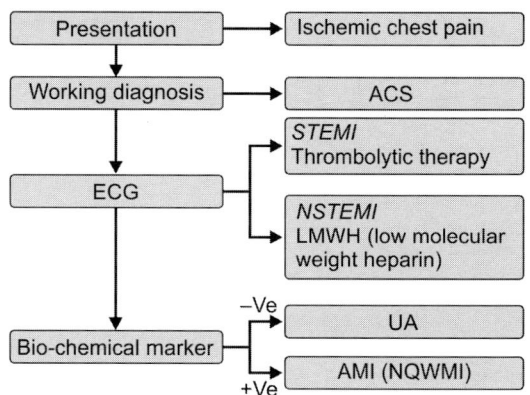

Assessment and Classification of ACS

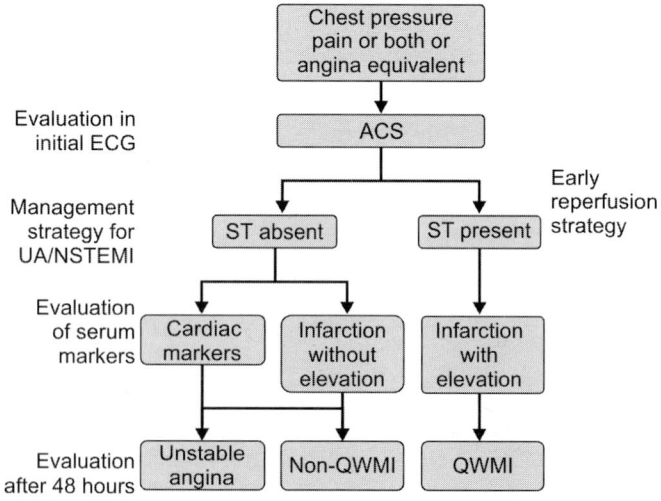

Biochemical Cardiac Markers

- *Creative kinase (CK-MB):*
  - *Rises:* Within 6 hours of onset of infarction
  - *Peak:* 12–24 hours
  - *Normal:* After 72 hours
- *Troponin I and T:*
  - *Appear:* Within 3 hours of onset of infarction
  - *Normal:* After 2 weeks
- Myoglobin
- AST (SGOT)
- LDH

CK-MB and troponin I or T are the most important cardiac biomarkers for the diagnosis of ACS.

Diagnosis of ACS

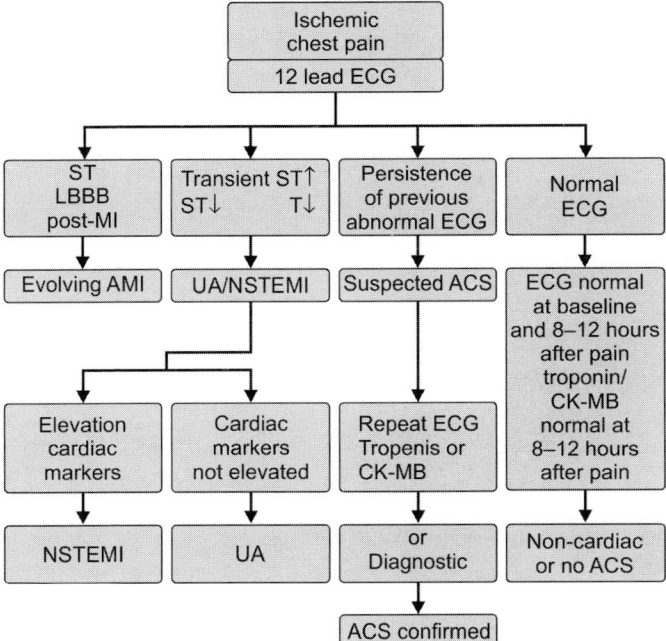

Nonocclusive thrombi are often responsible for non-Q-wave or subendocardial infarcts. As the name implies, such infarcts and the ischemia associated with them do not involve the full thickness of the myocardial tissue; instead, unlike Q-wave MI, they are limited to the subendocardium with no epicardial involvement. Whether a coronary syndrome manifests as unstable angina or as an MI depends on the extent and duration of the ischemia (Fig. 11.20).

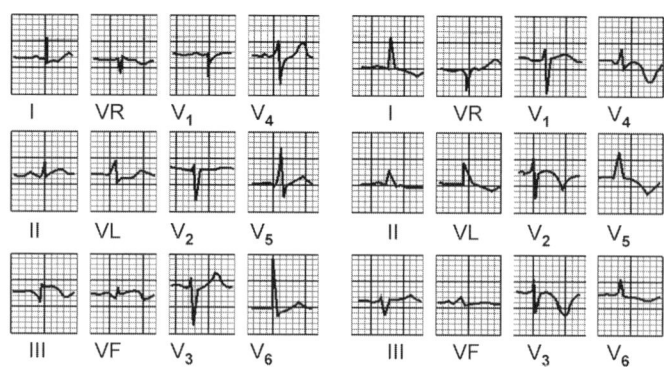

Fig. 11.20 Acute coronary syndrome

Outline of Management of ACS

Control symptoms	Nitrates, sedative analgesics
Anti-ischemic therapy	Nitrates and β-blocker, calcium antagonists
Anti-thrombotic therapy	• Anti-platelet: Aspirin clopidogreal Gp IIB/IIIa receptor blocker • *Anti-coagulant:* Heparin LMWH
Thrombolysis	Thrombolytics–streptokinase
Management of complication	Antiarrhythmic drugs; DC shock, pacemakers
Revascularization	Percutaneous coronary intervention (PCI) Primary PTCA Surgical–CABG
Risk factor management	Life style, smoking diet, exercise statins

Clinical and Hemodynamic Subsets in AMI and Management (Forrester Classification)

Clinical subsets	Hemodynamic subsets	Management
No pulmonary congestion or tissue hypoperfusion	PCW < 18 CI > 2.2	Conventional
Pulmonary congestion only	PCW <18 CI > 2.2	Diuretics and vasodilators
Tissue hypoperfusion only	PCW < 18 CI > 2.2	IV fluid if needed inotropes
Pulmonary congestion Tissue hypoperfusion	PCW < 18 CI < 2.2	Diuretics, vasodilators Inotropes IABP

12

Drugs and Electrolytes Effects

DIGITALIS EFFECT

Introduction: ECG is significantly affected by cardiac drugs.

Digitalis effect depresses ST segment shortens Q-T interval and lengthens the P-R interval. But, digitalis toxicity causes higher degrees of A-V block and numerous arrhythmias (Fig. 12.1).

ECG Criteria

- ST segment depression (Sagging)/reverse tickmark/rounded concave like thumb impression in V_4–V_6
- T-wave inverted or flattened
- Q-T interval shortening (< 0.42 sec)
- *P-R interval*: Modest increase.

Note: Here, ECG changes of digitalis effects are finding in patients who are taking digoxin and are not indicative of toxicity.

DIGITALIS TOXICITY (DIGOXIN TOXICITY)

Introduction: It causes higher degrees of AV block and numerous arrhythmias with extracardiac effects clinically (Fig. 12.2).

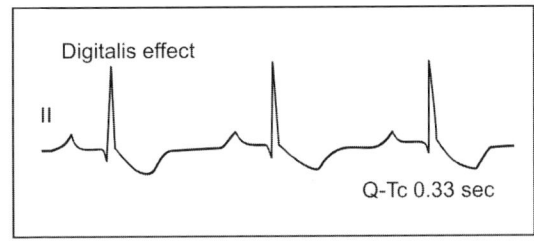

Fig. 12.1 Diagram of digitalis effect

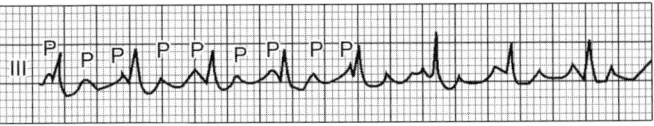

Fig. 12.2 Atrial tachycardia with block secondary to digoxin toxicity

Arrhythmias of Digoxin Toxicity

Atrial Arrhythmias

- Sinus bradycardia
- SA block
- Atrial premature complexes (APCs)
- Atrial tachycardia with AV block.

AV Junctional Arrhythmias

- First degree AV block
- Second degree AV block (Mobitz type 1)
- Complete heart block
- Junctional premature contraction (JPC)
- Junctional rhythm (rate 40–60)
- Accelerated junctional rhythm (rate 60–150).

Ventricular Arrhythmias

- Ventricular premature complex (VPC)
- Bigeminy VPC
- Ventricular tachycardia (VT)
- Ventricular flutter
- Ventricular fibrillation (VF).

Extracardiac Effect of Digoxin Toxicity

- Anorexia, nausea, vomiting
- Diarrhea, abdominal pain
- Visual disturbance
- Drowsiness
- Confusion, delirium
- Depression
- Hallucination
- Gynecomastia.

Treatment of Digoxin Toxicity

- Discontinuation of digoxin or treatment of underlying arrhythmias
- Potassium supplementation (Correction of hypokalemia)
- *Pacemaker, if necessary*: If severe bradycardia or complete heart block (CHB)
- Digoxin-specific antibody—in life-threatening case or in digoxin poisoning.

QUINIDINE EFFECTS (FIG. 12.3)

Introduction: Quinidine enhances the U-waves, widens the QRS and may cause fatal ventricular, fibrillation.

Combined, digitalis and quinidine simulate the pattern of hypokalemia in ECG.

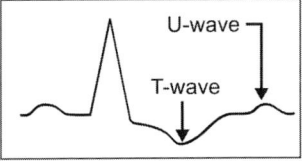

Fig. 12.3 ECG effects of quinidine therapy

ECG Criteria

- Widening of P-wave and QRS complex
- Q-T interval prolongation (> 0.43 sec), very important
- ST depression
- T-wave inversion ⎤
- U-wave prominent ⎦ in I aVL, V_4-V_6

Causes

- *Atrial arrhythmia*: SA block, intra-atrial block
- AV block
- *Ventricular arrhythmia*
  - VPCs idioventricular rhythm
  - VT
  - VF
- Torsade-de-pointes (Tdp).

Drugs that affect different sites of heart (with Vaughan-William classification) (Fig. 12.4).

POTASSIUM EFFECT

Hyperkalemia (Figs 12.5 and 12.6)

ECG Criteria

- Tall, symmetrical peaked T-wave (Tent-like) in chest leads
- Virtual disappearance of ST segment
- P-R prolongation
- P-wave disappearance (atrial arrest) or wide, small
- QRS widening and fusion with tall T-wave.

Effect of Hyperkalemia on Heart

- Any arrhythmia even VT, VF, ventricular flutter, ventricular stand still (straight line)
- Hyperkalemia cause hyperpolarization of cell membranes, leading to decreased cardiac excitability, hypotension, bradycardia and eventual asystole/cardiac arrest
- If K^+ is > 7 mmol/L—causes cardiac arrest in systole.

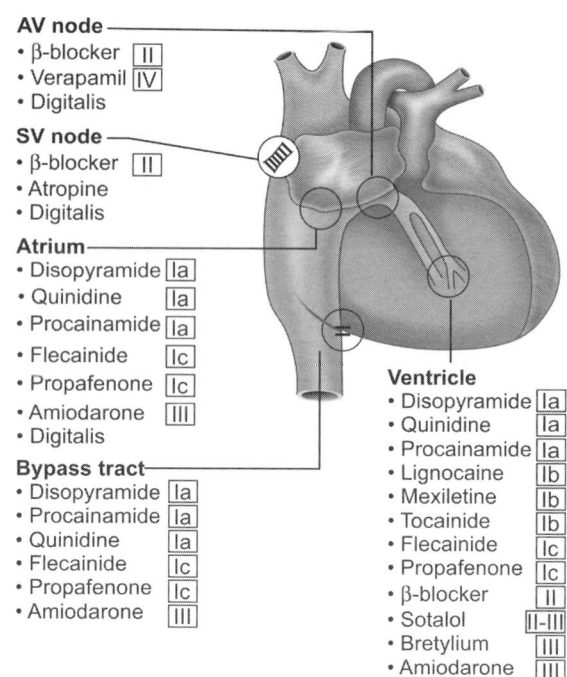

Fig. 12.4 Drugs that affect different sites of heart (diagram) with Vaughan William classification

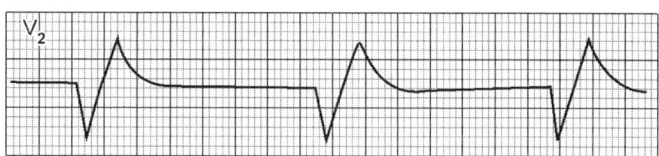

Fig. 12.5 ECG changes in hyperkalemia

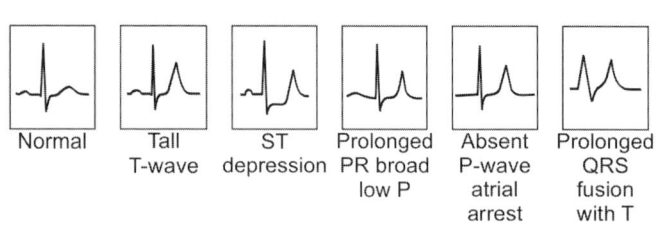

Fig. 12.6 ECG patterns of hyperkalemia sequentially as potassium level increases

Treatment

- Discontinuation of potassium, potassium containing food and offending drugs
- Administration of calcium for toxic arrhythmia: Inj. 10% Ca-gluconate 10–20 mL over 10 minutes

- *Glucose with insulin*: Inj 50 mL of 50% glucose + Inj insulin 10 units
- *Bicarbonate:* Intravenous (IV) sodium bicarbonate 500 mL 6–8 hourly
- Na-K exchange resin
- Treatment of primary causes
- If all fail, hemodialysis or peritoneal dialysis.

Features of Hyperkalemia

- It may be asymptomatic.
- Muscular weakness—may be severe causing flaccid paralysis, loss of tendon jerk
- Paralytic ileus (abdomen distended)
- Tingling around the lip or finger
- Sudden death-due to cardiac arrest or arrhythmia.

Common Causes of Hyperkalemia

- High potassium intake
- Renal diseases—ARF, CRF
- Endocrine diseases—Diabetic ketoacidosis, Addison's diseases
- *Drugs*:
  - Potassium-sparing diuretics (spironolactone amiloride)
  - ACE inhibitor
  - Non-steroidal anti-inflammatory drug (NSAID)
- Hemolysis
- Acute Leukemia
- Acidosis
- Digoxin poisoning
- Transfusion of stored blood.

POTASSIUM EFFECT: HYPOKALEMIA (FIGS 12.7 AND 12.8)

Definition: Hypokalemia is characterized by ECG abnormalities and cardiac arrhythmias due to a serum potassium of less than 3.2 mEq/L.

ECG Criteria

- Prominent P-wave (increased amplitude and wide)
- Prolongation of P-R interval
- Lowering and inversion of T-wave
- Prominent U-wave (most common)
- ST depression
- Premature beats and sustained tachyarrhythmias
- Prolongation of the QTc interval.

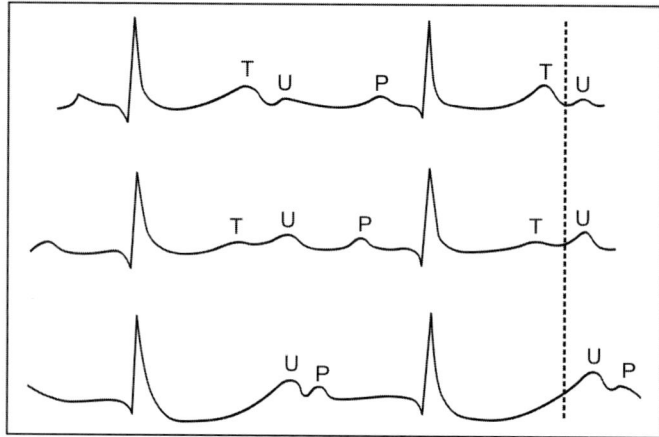

Fig. 12.7 ECG changes in hypokalemia

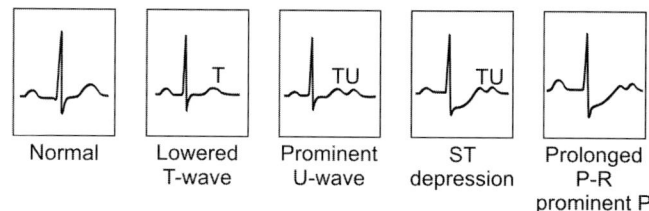

Fig. 12.8 ECG patterns of hypokalemia sequentially as potassium level decreases

Effects of Hypokalemia

- May be asymptomatic (if S potassium > 2.5 mmol/L)
- If severe, muscular weakness, paralysis loss of plantar reflex, paralytic ileus, arrhythmia increase digoxin toxicity.

Effects of Hypokalemia on Heart

- *Arrhythmia*: VT VF
- Aggravates digoxin toxicity
- Cardiac arrest (in diastole).

Causes of Hypokalemia

- *Diuretis*: Thiazide, frusemide most common
- *Gastrointestinal loss*: Diarrhea, vomiting, purgative abuse
- *Renal loss*: Renal tubular necrosis
  RTA type I and II
  Bartter's syndrome
  Liddle's syndrome
  Gitelman's syndrome
- *Endocrine cause*: Cushing's syndrome, Conn's syndrome

- *Other*: Heart failure
  Liver failure
  Nephrotic syndrome
  Drugs
  Insulin therapy
  Alkalosis.

Treatment

- If serum potassium is > 2.5 mmol/L—oral potassium
- If severe or S. potassium is < 2.5 mmol/L—potassium is given in infusion K-should never be given in direct IV
- Treatment of primary cause.

Note:
- When the prominent U-wave is fused with T-wave, ECG shows a prolonged Q-T interval
- Peaked P-wave due to advanced hypokalemia (pseudo-p-pulmonales) may mimic true P-pulmonale due to COPD.

CALCIUM EFFECT

Hypercalcemia

Definition: Hypercalcemia is characterized by ECG abnormalities and cardiac arrhythmia due to excessive amounts of calcium in the body (Fig. 12.9A).

ECG criteria: Shortens QT interval, prominent U-wave, shortening ST segment prolonged PR interval and QRS complex.

Note:
- Atrial or ventricular arrhythmias, especially in patients taking digoxin, may occur with hypercalcemia'
- VPCs and VT or VF occur in advanced case
- There is synergistic action between digitalis and calcium
- QT interval tends to be short in healthy children and young adults as a normal variant.

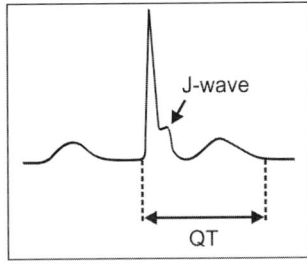

Hypercalcemia

Fig. 12.9A ECG changes in hypercalcemia shortening of the QT interval primarily by shortening of the ST segment. A J wave may also be seen

Hypocalcemia

Definition: Hypocalcemia is characterized by ECG abnormalities and cardiac arrhythmias due to depleted levels of calcium in the blood (Fig. 12.9B).

EGC Criteria

- Prolonged QT interval
- Prolonged ST segment
- Flattening or inversion T (Less common)
- Significant cardiac arrhythmic
- Hypocalcemia co-exists with hyperkalemia.

Note:
- QT interval prolonged in many clinical conditions including:
  - Quinidine toxicity
  - Congenital QT syndrome
  - CNS disorders
- Remember that hypocalcemia produces prolonged QT and prolonged ST
- It causes atrial or ventricular arrhythmia even Torsades de pointes.

HYPERMAGNESEMIA

Excessive amounts of magnesium (> 2.5 mEq/L) in blood is called hypermagnesemia

ECG criteria: Like hyperkalemia

Thus, the early change in hypermagnesemia is often a prolonged P-R interval followed by a widened QRS when the magnesium concentration rises.

HYPOMAGNESEMIA

Depleted levels of magnesium (< 1.5 mEq/L) in blood is called hypomagnesemia.

ECG criteria: ECG change like hypokalemia.

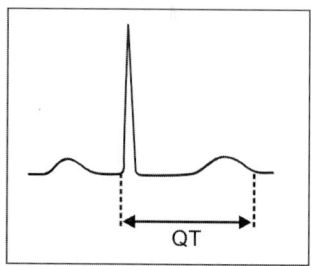

Fig. 12.9B Hypocalcemia, lengthening of the QT interval primarily by lengthening of the ST segment

ECG CHANGES ASSOCIATED WITH ELECTROLYTE DISTURBANCES

Electrolyte disturbance	P-wave	PR	QRS	ST	T	QT heart rate
Hyperkalemia	Disappear as level increases	Normal or prolonged	Widen as level increases	Disappear as level increases	Tall, peaked or tented	Slow
Hypokalemia	+	+	Widen as level decreases	Depressed	Flattened U-wave present	Prolonged
Hypercalcemia	+	Prolonged	+	Shortened	+	Shortened
Hypocalcemia	+	+	+	Long flattened	+	Prolonged
Hypermagnesemia	+	Prolonged	Widened	+	Tall or elevated	+
Hypomagnesemia	Diminished voltage (amplitude)	+	Widen as level decreases diminished voltage	Depressed	Flattened U-wave present	Prolonged

13

Miscellaneous Conditions

HYPOTHERMIA
Introduction

- In significant hypothermia, characteristic, ECG changes are observed
- Atrial tachyarrhythmias, particularly atrial fibrillation (AF), may be encountered in hypothermia
- Hypothermia induced ECG changes may resemble an early repolarization pattern, acute pericarditis, an early phase of acute myocardial infarction (MI) and various intraventricular conduction disturbances (Fig. 13.1).

ECG Criteria

- Sinus bradycardia (35°–37°C)
- Prolongation of P-R and QT interval (30°–35°C), QRS complex, ST segment
- *Osborn or O-wave or J-wave (<30°C) present:* This wave appears at the end of ventricular depolarization (at the end of QRS)
- *Arrhythmias:* APC, AF, VPC, VF, VT
- Tracing may be low voltage.

CEREBROVASCULAR ACCIDENT PATTERN
Introduction

- Various central nervous system (CNS) disorders, including cerebrovascular accident (CVA), brain tumors, heat stroke,

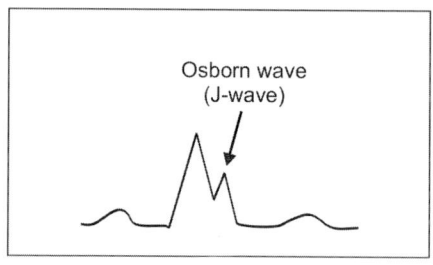

Fig. 13.1 ECG changes in hypothermia

head trauma, delirium and coma may produce various ECG abnormalities.
- Among CNS disorders, subarachnoid hemorrhage is prone to produce ECG abnormalities more frequently (Fig. 13.2).

ECG Criteria

- Abnormal, widened T-wave that may be deeply inverted or tall and peaked
- Prominent U-wave
- Prolonged QT interval
- ST elevation
- Various supraventricular tachyarrhythmias.

Note: Diffusely inverted broad T-wave with a prolonged QT interval are considered to be a unique feature of subarachnoid hemorrhage, but in an early stage the ST elevation is a pronounced changes.

PERICARDITIS

Introduction

Since pericarditis is also diffuse in nature, the ECG abnormalities involve many leads (Fig. 13.3).

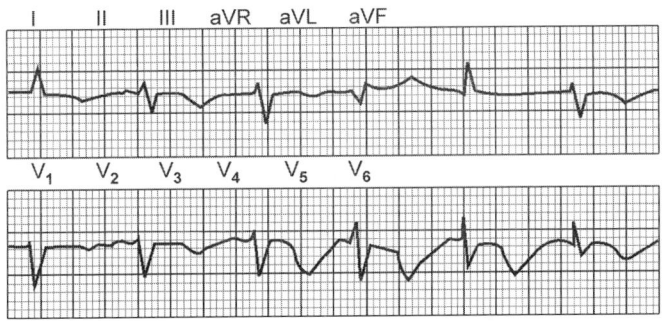

Fig. 13.2 ECG hanges in cerebrovascular accident pattern

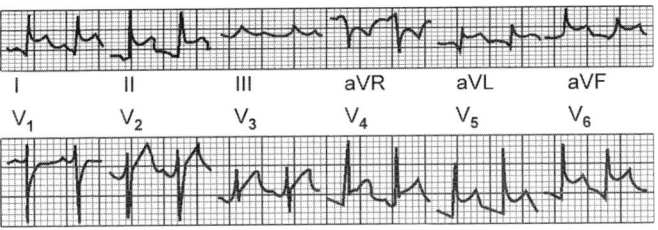

Fig. 13.3 ECG changes in pericarditis

ECG Criteria

During early phase:
- ST elevated concave upward with
- Upright T-wave V_4-V_6 　　　 in I, II, aVL, aVF
- Sinus tachycardia.

Subsequent ECG Changes

When pericarditis resolves (during late stage)
- ST returns to baseline
- T inversion that remains for weeks to months before returning to baseline

Causes of Acute Pericarditis

As follows:
- Following acute myocardial infarction (AMI) (Usually in 2nd or 3rd day)
- Viral (Coxsackie B, Echovirus)
- Acute rheumatic fever (ARF)
- Tuberculous pericarditis
- Bacterial
  - *Staphylococcus aureus*
  - *Haemophilus influenzae*
- Fungal
- Uremia
- Malignancy (Carcinoma of bronchus, breast, lymphoma, leukemia)
- Collagen disease—systemic lupus erythematosus (SLE). Scleroderma
- Trauma
- Radiation
- Drugs—doxorubicin, cyclophosphamide.

Presentation of Acute Pericarditis

As follows:
- Chest pain
  - Retrosternal
  - Sharp or stabbing in nature radiate to the shoulder and neck
- Pain is aggravated by movement. Lying down and deep breathing, exercise and swallowing
- Pain may be relieved by sitting or bending forward.

Clinical Findings

Pericardial Rub

- It is a high pitched, harsh, scratching, grating, leathery sound, to and fro in quality

- Better heard over the left lower parasternal area with the patient leaning forward
- Augmented by pressing the stethoscope
- It is usually heard in systole but may be present in diastole
- It is present after holding the breath (to differentiate from pleural rub).

How to Differentiate Acute Pericarditis from Acute Myocardial Infarction by ECG?

In acute myocardial infarction (AMI)- ST elevation with upward convexity, in pericarditis- ST elevation with upward concavity.

Management

As follows:
- To relieve pain—NSAID (Indomethacin, ibuprofen, aspirin)
- In severe or recurrent case—corticosteroid
- If no response to steroid—azathioprine or colchicine
- Pericardiotomy.

Note:
- Low voltage of QRS is very common in chronic pericarditis (constrictive pericarditis) and massive pericardial effusion.
- The terms 'Postcardiotomy syndrome' and 'Postpericardiotomy syndrome' are commonly used to describe pericarditis resulting from any trauma, including cardiac surgery (CABG).

PERICARDIAL EFFUSION

ECG

- Low voltage ECG
- Inverted T-wave in most leads
- Ventricular or potential electrical alternans, i.e. alteration of the QRS height every other beat, in which height of R and T alternates from beat-to-beat
- Sinus tachycardia (Fig. 13.4).

Note:
- Small QRS + Tachycardia + Electrical alternans → pericardial effusion
- In myxedematous pericardial effusion the QRS amplitude becomes so low that the ECG tracing appears to be the isoelectric line in many leads.

CHRONIC OBSTRUCTIVE PULMONARY DISEASE

In chronic obstructive pulmonary disease (COPD), a strain is placed on the right atrium and right ventricle as well as a shift of the position of the heart occurring inside the chest (Fig. 13.5).

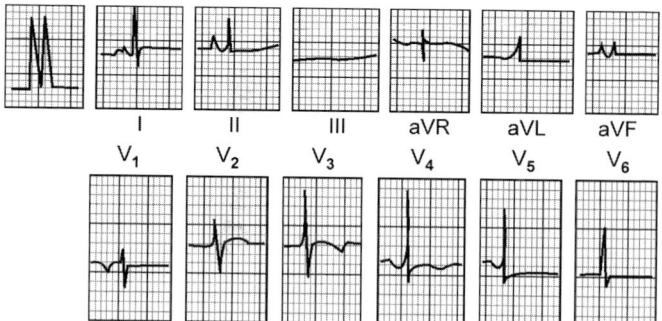

Fig. 13.4 ECG changes in pericardial effusion

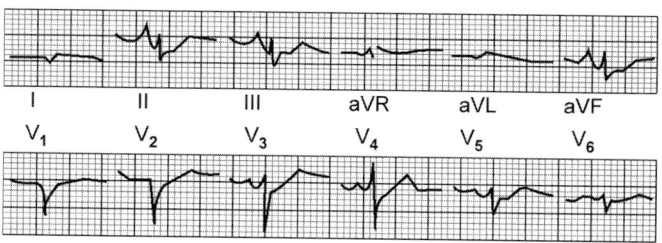

Fig. 13.5 ECG changes in chronic obstructive pulmonary disease

ECG Criteria

- Low voltage of QRS in limb leads
- *P-pulmonale:* Tall; peaked P-wave in II, III, aVF
- *Right axis deviation (RAD)*
- *Right ventricular hypertrophy (RVH):* Tall R in V_1 or V_2 with depressed ST segments and inverted T-wave
- Poor R-wave progression (PRWP) in chest leads
- *Multifocal atrial tachycardia (occasionally):* APCs and MAT

THE S_1, S_2, S_3 SYNDROME

ECG Criteria

- Prominent S-wave in lead, II, III
- S-wave > R-wave in at least one of the three leads.

Causes

- Normal variant
- Right ventricular dominance
  Right ventricular hypertrophy (RVH) of congenital heart disease, e.g.
    - Tetralogy of Fallot (TOF)
    - Pulmonary atresia
    - VSD with pulmonary hypertension

- Acute anterior wall MI
- The straight back syndrome.

PRE-EXCITATION SYNDROMES

'Pre-excitation' is abnormal early excitation of the ventricles. It occurs through accessory conducting fibers that activate the ventricles early. This cause's ventricular depolarization (QRS) to begin earlier than if an impulse had traveled through the normal AV conducting system and thus avoids the 'delay' in the AV node.

Three Types

1. Wolff-Parkinson-White (WPW) syndrome: (a) Type A, (b) Type B (Figs 13.6 to 13.8)

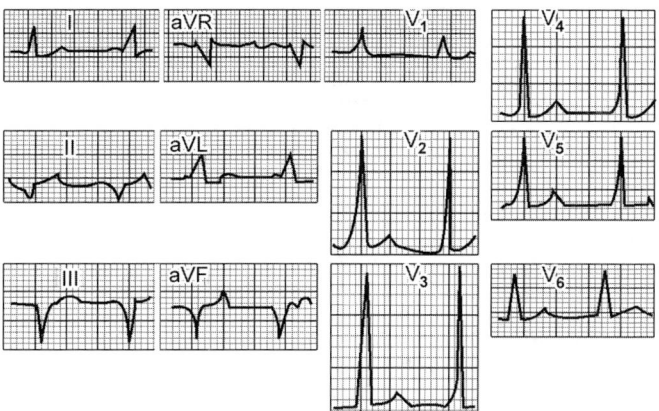

Fig. 13.6 Wolff-Parkinson-White syndrome

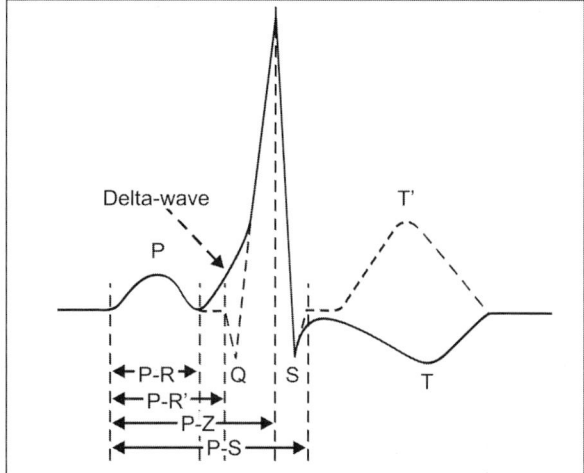

Fig. 13.7 Wolff-Parkinson-White syndrome

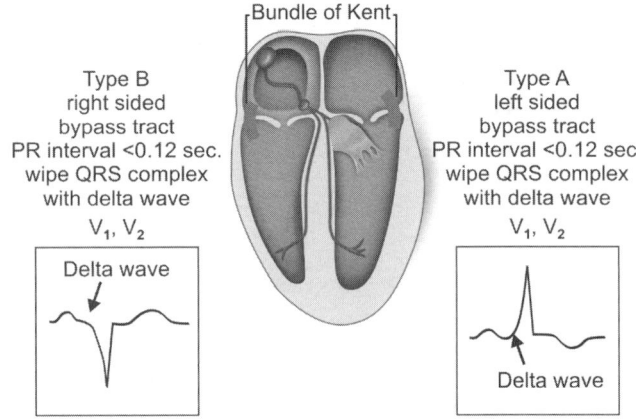

Fig. 13.8 Wolff-Parkinson-White syndrome. Type A indicates a left-sided bypass tract with predominantly positive QRS complexes in leads V_1, V_2. Type B indicates a right-sided bypass tract with predominantly negative QRS complexes in leads V_1, V_2

2. Lown-Ganong-Levine (LGL) syndrome or James bypass tract
3. Mahaim bypass tract syndrome.

Types of Accessory Pathways

Three Types

1. Bundles of Kent
2. James bypass tract
3. Mahaim's fiber—are AV bypass tract within conduction system
   PR-normal, QRS abnormal

Wolff-Parkinson-White Syndrome

Definition

Wolff-Parkinson-White (WPW) syndrome is characterized by a short P-R interval with a broad QRS due to a delta wave (initial slurring of the QRS) that is directed anteriorly and either inferiorly or superiorly (In case of Type-A) or is directed posteriorly and either inferiorly or superiorly (In case of Type-B).

ECG Criteria

- P-R interval short (<0.12 sec.)
- QRS wide and
- Slurred, thickened, initial upstroke of the QRS called delta wave
- Depression of ST segment with inversion of T-wave due to secondary repolarization change

- Q may be present in lead II, III, aVF (may be confused and inferior MI)
- Tall R in V_1 or V_2 (Type A)
- Deep Q in V_1 or V_2 (Type B)

Wolff-Parkinson-White (WPW) is a syndrome in which there is an accessory track or pathway that by passes the AV node and connects the atria and ventrical (By bundle of Kent). It may be associated with congenital anomaly, commonly Ebstein anomaly.

Types of WPW Syndrome

It is of two types
1. *Type A*: Accessory pathway on the left side (in ECG, tall R in V_1 and V_2)
2. *Type B*: Accessory pathway on the right side (in ECG, deep Q in V_1 and V_2) accessory pathway is called the bundle of Kent.

Presentation of WPW Syndrome

- May be asymptomatic—50%
- May present with palpitation
- Paroxysmal attack of atrial and SVT most common—due to re-entry circuit
- Atrial fibrillation (AF) or atrial flutter
- Syncope
- Sudden death—due to AF
- Rarely VT, VF.

Note: In presence of WPW syndrome, the following disease may be difficult to diagnose.

Type A Confuses with:

- Right bundle branch block (RBBB)
- Right ventricular hypertrophy (RVH)
- True posterior MI.

Type B Confuses with:

- Left bundle branch block (LBBB)
- Left ventricular hypertrophy (LVH)
- Inferior myocardial infarction.

Treatment of WPW Syndrome

As follows:
- *If asymptomatic:* No treatment is required
- *If symptomatic:*
  - Transvenous radiofrequency catheter ablation of accessory pathway—specific treatment

- If not available—prophylactic antiarrhythmic drugs
    - β-blocker
    - Amiodarone
    - Flecainide
    - Disopyramide
- Surgical resection of accessory pathway used to be done.

Note: Contraindicated in WPW syndrome—digoxin and IV verapamil due to shorten the refractory period of accessory pathway.

Why Digoxin is Avoided?

Digoxin blocks the AV node and increases the conduction through the accessory pathway. So, it increases the heart rate. It may precipitate VF.

Why PR Interval Short?

Impulse is conducted rapidly from the atria to the ventricles through the accessory pathway, causing early ventricular depolarization. So, PR interval is short.

Mechanism of Delta Wave

The accessory pathway causes early depolarization of part of the ventricle, giving rise to slow upstroke (delta wave-first portion of QRS). Then the normally conducted impulse through the AV node causes depolarization of the rest of ventricle giving rise to the rest of QRS. Delta wave is absent, if there is tachycardia, as the ventricle is excited by normal pathway.

Treatment of AF with WPW Syndrome

It is medical emergency, sudden death may occur:
- If severe symptoms-DC shock
  If not available-IV flecainide
- Radiofrequency ablation (RFA)
- *Drugs:* Amiodarne, flecainide, disopyramide, sotalol

Note: Hallmark of WPW syndrome in ECG is delta wave.

Lown-Ganong-Levine Syndrome or James Bypass Tract

In the Lown-Ganong-Levine (LGL) syndrome, the James tract 'pre-excites' the lower area of the AV node or directly to the bundle of His, avoiding the 'delay area' in the AV node, resulting in a short PR interval and normal QRS (Figs 13.9 and 13.10).

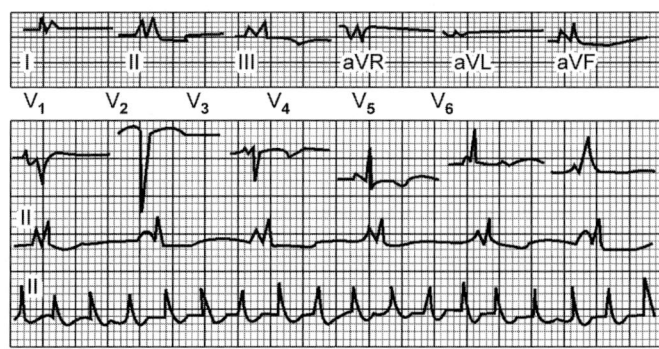

Fig. 13.9 Lown-Ganong-Levine syndrome

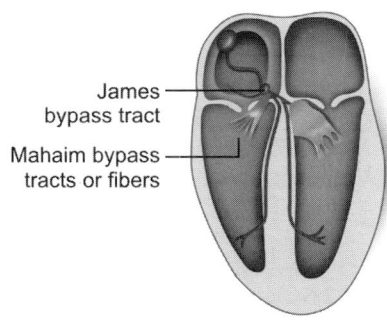

Fig. 13.10 Two types of pre-excitation syndrome. (1), Lown-Ganong-Levine (LGL), which utilizes the James bypass tract, and (2), the Mahaim bypass tract. In the LGL syndrome

ECG Criteria

- PR interval short (0.12 sec)
- QRS normal
- No delta wave.

Definition

Lown-Ganong-Levine (LGL) syndrome is a syndrome in which there is a congenital accessory pathway (James bypass tract) that arises in the atria and by pass the main region of bundle of His.

Why QRS is Normal in Lown-Ganong-Levine Syndrome?

This accessory pathway simply connects the atria to the bundle of His. It does not activate the ventricle directly. So, there is no delta wave and QRS is normal.

Note:
- Lown-Ganong-Levine (LGL) syndrome is asymptomatic
- Good prognosis
- Not treatment is necessary.

The LGL syndrome utilizes an accessory tract (James bypass tract) which joins the atrium directly to the bundle of His. The James tract bypasses the 'delay area' in the AV node. So, that conduction proceeds earlier and unchanged through the ventricles.

Mahaim Bypass Tract Syndrome

Mahaim fibers 'pre-excite' this right ventricle after the impulse has passed through the AV node, resulting in a normal PR and wide QRS.

The delay in the AV node is preserved, which result in a normal PR interval. Early excitation of the right ventricle through the Mahaim tracts results in a wide QRS resembling LBBB. No delta wave is present.

ECG Criteria

- PR interval normal
- QRS wide and
- Slurring of the QRS called delta wave present or absent.

SICK SINUS SYNDROME (FIG. 13.11) (BRADYCARDIA TACHYCARDIA)

ECG Criteria

- Bradyarrhythmias (slow arrhythmia) due to:
  - SA block, sinus arrest
  - Marked sinus bradycardia or
  - Junctional bradycardia that may alternate with various
- Tachyarrhythmias (rapid arrhythmia) due to:
  - Atrial fibrillation
  - Atrial flutter
  - Paroxysmal atrial tachycardia (PAT), etc.

Definition

Sick sinus syndrome (SSS) is a dysfunction of SA node characterized by attacks of sinus bradycardia, sinus arrest, or junctional rhythm which may lead to dizziness or syncope, followed by episodes of paroxysmal tachycardia so called tachy–brady syndrome.

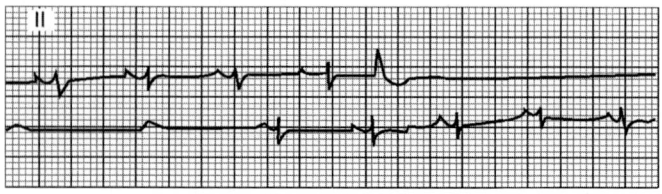

Fig. 13.11 Sick sinus syndrome

Causes of SSS

It is due to fibrosis, degenerative changes or ischemia of the SA node probable cause are:
- Elderly (due to degeneration)
- IHD
- Drugs-digoxin
- Cardiomyopathy
- Rheumatic heart disease
- Radiation
- Sarcoidosis
- Amyloidosis
- Chaga's disease
- Idiopathic.

Presentation of SSS

- Asymptomatic
- Symptomatic   Palpitation   Confusion
                     Dizziness   Angina
                     Syncope

Diagnosis of SSS

By:
- *ECG:*
  - *Sinus arrest:* Chronic and paroxysmal
  - Sinus bradycardia
  - Sinus exit block
  - Paroxysmal
    - Atrial trachycardia
    - AF
    - Atrial flutter
  - Carotid sinus hypersensitivity
  - AV block
- *Holter monitoring*
  Treatment
  - Asymptomatic
    - No treatment
    - Follow-up and avoidance and discontinuation of negative chronotropic drugs
  - Symptomatic
    - Implantation of PPM (permanent pacemaker)
    - Antiarrhythmic drugs for tachyarrhythmia.

Very Common ECG Findings

- Persistent and marked sinus bradycardia
- SA block
- Sinus arrest

- Long pause following an APC
- Chronic AF or atrial flutter with slow ventricular rate
- Carotid sinus hypersensitivity
- No stable sinus rhythm after DC shock
- Atrioventricular (AV) junctional escape rhythm
- Brady-tachyarrhythmia syndrome.

PULMONARY EMBOLISM

Pulmonary thromboembolism can cause or aggravate heart disease and is a common and serious complication of cardiac disorders.

Pulmonary embolism, pulmonary thrombosis and pulmonary infarction are related conditions.

ECG Criteria

- Sinus tachycardia (common) and other transient supraventricular arrhythmias
- P-pulmonale tall P in lead II, III, aVF
- Right bundle branch block (RBBB)— incomplete or complete
- ST depression and T wave inversion in the right precordial (V_1, V_2)
- Right axis deviation (RAD)
- S_1, Q_3, T_3 pattern
  - S in lead I
  - Q in lead III
  - T inversion in lead III (Fig. 13.12).

  Classic combination of ECG

Arrhythmias that Found in Pulmonary Embolism

As follows:
- Sinus tachycardia (most common)
- Atrial fibrillation (AF)
- Atrial flutter
- Ventricular ectopics.

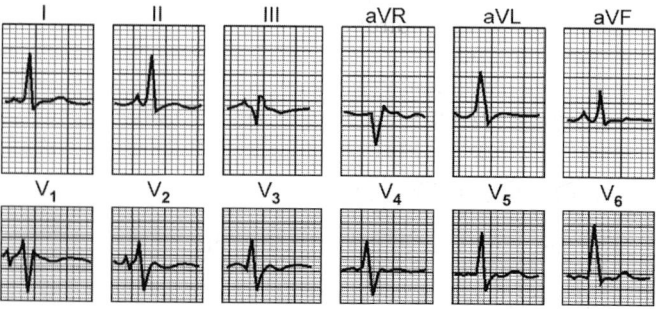

Fig. 13.12 Pulmonary embolism (S_1, Q_3, T_3)

Features of Acute Massive Pulmonary Embolism

As follows:
- Severe central chest pain
- Severe dyspnea
- Faintness or syncope
- On examination
  - Tachycardia
  - Tachypnea
  - Cyanosis
  - Wide splitting of S_2
  - Right ventricular gallop
  - Features of shock.

Note: Pulmonary embolism should be considered, if the patient present with:
- Unexplained cough
- Chest pain
- Hemoptysis
- New-onset AF or other tachycardia
- Sign of pulmonary hypertension.

Most Common ECG Findings

- P-pulmonale
- Inverted T-wave in V_1–V_3 (right ventricular strain pattern)
- Right axis deviation (RAD) with or without posterior axis deviation.

Investigation due to Diagnose Pulmonary Embolism

As follows:
- Chest X-ray
  - Oligemic lung fields
  - Enlarged pulmonary artery
  - Wedged shaped opacity due to pulmonary infarction
- ECG
- Blood gas analysis—low PaO_2, low $PaCO_2$
- If pulmonary infarction
  - ESR ↑
  - LDH ↑
  - Neutrophil leukocytosis
- *Echocardiogram:* Clot in right heart
- Spiral CT angiogram
- Magnetic resonance imaging (MRI)
- Ventilation and perfusion scan (V/Q scan)
- Pulmonary angiography.

Treatment of Pulmonary Embolism

As follows:
- High flow oxygen (60–100%)
- *Relief of pain:* Morphin or pethidine

- *Anticoagulant:* Injection heparin 10000 unit IV bolus dose followed by continous infusion 1000–2000 unit/hr
  Or, low molecular heparin-S/C
- *Oral anticoagulant:*
  - Warfarin
  - Started after 48 hours of heparin therapy
  - Heparin stopped after 5 days
  - Warfarin continuous for 6 weeks to 6 months
  - If recurrent—warfarin lifelong
- *Fibrinolytic therapy:*
  - Streptokinase 2.5 lakh unit IV infusion over 30 minutes
  - Followed by 1 lakh unit IV hourly for up to 12–72 hours
  - Or, alteplase—60 mg IV over 15 minutes
- If massive pulmonary embolism with severe hemodynamic compromise—surgical embolectomy.

DEXTROCARDIA

Definition

Dextrocardia is a congenital disorder in which the heart is located in the right side of the chest but other organs are in their usual position (Fig. 13.13).

ECG Criteria

- *P-wave:*
  - Inverted in lead I, II, aVL
  - Upright in lead III, aVF
  - Upright and equiphasic in aVR
- *QRS:*
  - Negative QRS in I, aVL
  - Upright QRS in III, aVF
- *R-wave:*
  - Tall in V_1 and diminishing
  - Progressively towards V_6
- Right axis deviation.

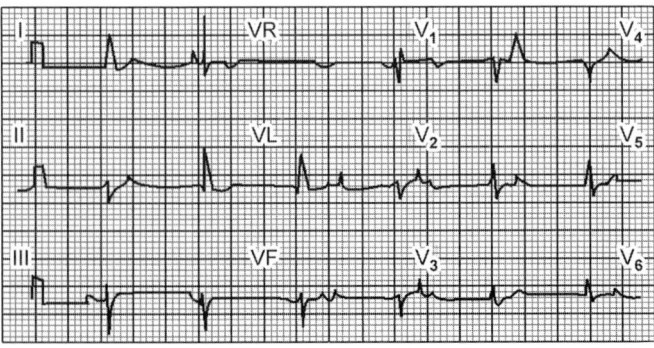

Fig. 13.13 Dextrocardia

Technical Dextrocardia

- This occur when arm electrodes placement are incorrect or reversed.
- Manifestation are similar except precordial pattern which will be normal (tall R in V_5, V_6) in this cause:
  P-wave is inverted in Lead I
  but Tall R in V_5, V_6.

Situs inversus: When there is dextrocardia with reversal of the site of viscera's (Stomach on right side, liver on left side, right lung is on the left and left lung is on the right).

Levocardia: When the heart is on the left side of the chest but there is reversal of the site of the other viscera: it is called lavocardia.

Mesocardia: When the cardiac apex is in the midline, it is called mesocardia.

Kartagener's syndrome: Characterized by:
- Dextrocardia
- Bronchiectasis
- Frontal sinusitis/Frontal sinus agenesis.

Investigation

As follows:
- Chest X-ray-heart on the right side of the chest, features of bronchiectasis
- X-ray paranasal sinus (PNS)—frontal sinusitis.

Note:
- If dextrocardia is associated with situs inversus, the heart is usually otherwise normal
- In case of isolated dextrocardia or levocardia there may also be multiple cardiac anomalies.

Association of Dextrocardia

Dextrocardia associated with:
- Pulmonary stenosis or pulmonary atresia 70–80%
- Ventricular septal defect (VSD) 60–80%
- Thermogravimetric analysic (TGA) 50–75%
- Single ventricle 15–40%
- Double outlet right ventricle (DORV) 10–18% (Double outlet right ventricle)
- Polysplenia
- Asplenia
- Kertagener's syndrome
- Tetralogy of Fallot (TOF)—Uncommon.

Clinical Importance of Situs Inversus

- Diagnosis of acute appendicitis may be missed, as appendix is on the left side
- As liver is on the left side, during liver biopsy care should be taken.

HYPERTHYROIDISM

ECG Criteria

- Sinus tachycardia (R-R> 100 bpm)
- *Arrhythmia:*
  - AF
  - Ectopic beats.

HYPOTHYROIDISM

ECG Criteria

- Low voltage ECG or tracing
- Sinus bradycardia (R-R < 60 bpm)
- T inversion.

ELECTROMECHANICAL DISSOCIATION

ECG Criteria

- P normal
- QRS normal
- T normal
- Evidence of the cause.

Definition

When heart continues to work electrically, but unable to contract. So, there will be no cardiac output, no pulse, no BP and the patient are unconscious.

Causes

- Cardiac tamponade
- Hypothermia
- Hypovolemia
- Hypoxia
- Tension pneumothorax
- Cardiac rupture
- Massive pulmonary embolism
- Electrolyte imbalance—hypokalemia
- Drug overdose—β-blocker.

Miscellaneous Conditions

Treatment

- Specific treatment of underlying cause
- Intubate and IV access
- Cardiopulmonary resuscitation (CPR).

Note: Electromechanical dissociation (EMD) is late event in cardiac arrest and indicates a poor prognosis.

EARLY REPOLARIZATION PATTERN

Definition

An early repolarization pattern (ERP) is the pattern formed by ST segment elevation (usually J point elevation) in young health individuals, particularly healthy black males (Fig. 13.14).

ECG Criteria

- The J-point ST elevation in V_4-V_6 with a small notch at the J-point (most common)
- Less common—ST elevation in V_1-V_6 concave upward
- Rarely, ST elevation in II, III, aVF.

Note:
- The early repolarization pattern resemble acute pericarditis, coronary artery spasm, an early ECG finding of acute MI
- The ERP does not produce inverted T or abnormal Q
- ST elevation in ERP is always due to J-point elevation.

JUVENILE T-WAVE PATTERN

Definition

A juvenile T-wave pattern (JTWP) is the pattern formed by deformed T-waves in leads V_1-V_3 in healthy children and young adults (Fig. 13.15).

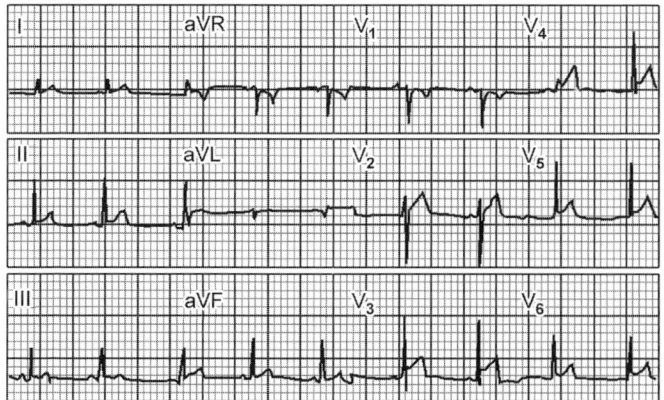

Fig. 13.14 Early repolarization pattern

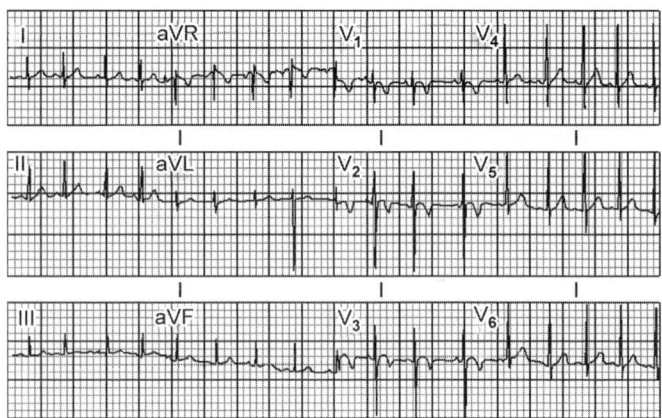

Fig. 13.15 Sinus arrhythmia with juvenile T-wave pattern

ECG Criteria

- Inverted on biphasic T in V_1-V_3 (up to Leads V_4-V_6 in some cases)
- More common in females than in males
- Frequently associated with sinus arrhythmia and high left ventricular voltage.

Note:
- It should be differentiated from other clinical conditions that produce inverted T-wave in chest leads including anterior myocardial ischemia, pulmonary embolism, myocarditis.
- Juvenile T-wave pattern (JTWP) does not produce symmetric or deep T inversion.

CARDIOMYOPATHY

Introduction

Cardiomyopathies of various causes may produce many different ECG abnormalities and cardiac arrhythmias (Fig. 13.16).

Types

- Dilated or congestive cardiomyopathy (DCM)
- Hypertrophic cardiomyopathy (HOCM)
- Restrictive cardiomyopathy (RCM).

ECG Criteria

Dilated Cardiomyopathy

- Low voltage of P-wave
- Low voltage and poor- R-progression in V_1-V_4
- Pattern of fascicular block, LBBB, RBBB are frequently seen

Miscellaneous Conditions

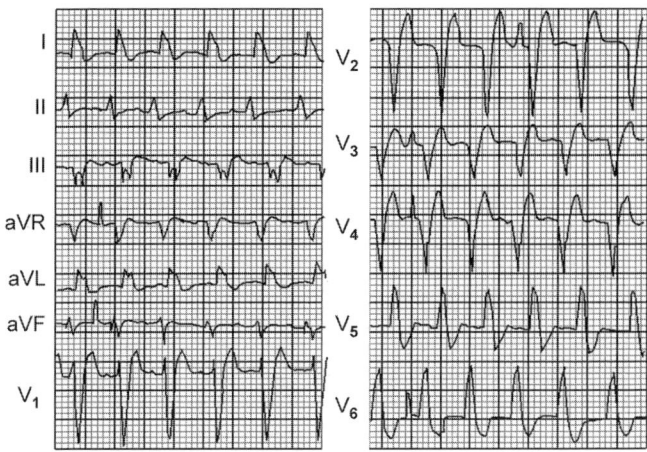

Fig. 13.16 Nonspecific intraventricular block with very broad and bizarre QRS complexes in a patient with idiopathic cardiomyopathy. Left bundle branch block is superficially simulated

- Pathological Q is infrequent
- ST depression, T inversion
- Wide QRS-T angle
- Conduction detects
- Arrhythmias.

Hypertropic Cardiomyopathies

- Left ventricular hypertrophy (LVH) or right ventricular hypertrophy (RVH)
- Intraventricular conduction defects—e.g. LAHB or left axis deviation (LAD), bundle branch block (BBB)
- Arrhythmias—ventricular common than supraventricular
- Left and/or right atrial hypertrophy
- Short PR interval
- Wolff-Parkinson-White (WPW) syndrome
- QT prolongation (QTc)
- Increased QT dispersion (QTd).

Restrictive Cardiomyopathies

- Intraventricular conduction defects with bizarre QRS
- Low voltage QRS (<10 mm) in V_1-V_4
- Poor R- progression across the V_1-V_6.

VENTRICULAR ANEURYSM

Introduction

It is an out pouching of the heart that occurs in the area of a previous myocardial infarction. It is comprised primarily of scar tissue.

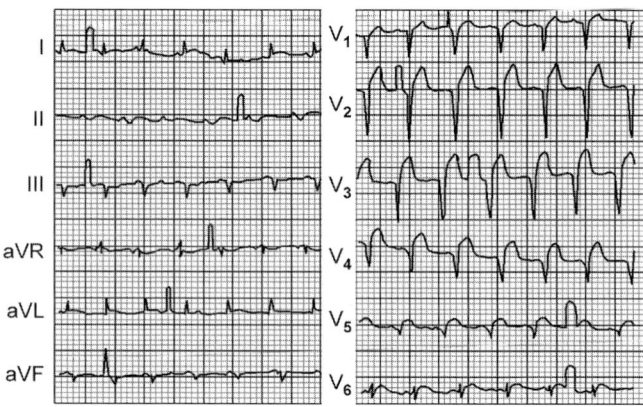

Fig. 13.17 Left ventricular aneurysm

If anterior wall is involved, the patient fails to limit his or her activity during the acute phase (Fig. 13.17).

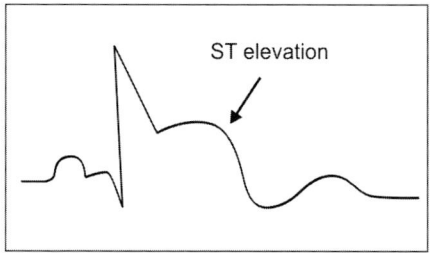

ECG Criteria

- Persistent ST elevation—in those leads representing the area of aneurysm
- ST elevation with convex upward
- ST elevation persists for weeks, months, or years.

EMPHYSEMA (FIG. 13.18)

Five most typical findings
1. Tall P in lead II, III, aVF.
2. Exaggerated atrial repolarization waves producing ≥ 0.10 mV PR and ST depression in L_2, L_3, aVF.
3. Right axis deviation in frontal plane.
4. Poor R progression in precordial leads.
5. Low voltage QRS, especially in left precordial leads.

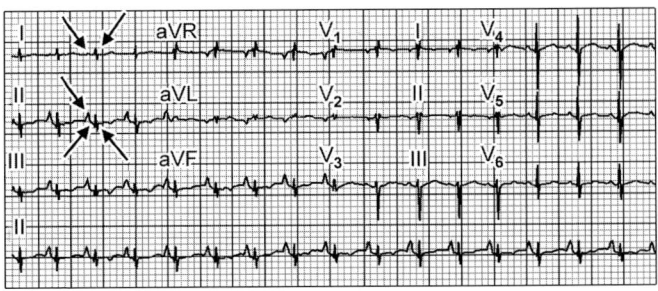

Fig. 13.18 A 12-lead ECG recording from a patient with pulmonary emphysema

ECG Criteria

Definite emphysema	Possible emphysema
• P axis > + 60° in limb lead and either	• P axis > + 60° in limb leads and either
• R and S ≤ 0.70 mv in limb leads and	• R and S ≤ 070 mV in limb leads
• R ≤ 70 mv in V_6 or SV4 ≥ RV_4	Or R ≤ 0.70 mV in V_6

Congenital Heart Diseases

VENTRICULAR SEPTAL DEFECT (FIG. 14.1)

Introduction

- Ventricular septal defect (VSD) is the most common congenital heart disease in infants and children.
- ECG findings with clinical manifestations vary markedly depending on the size of the defects, the pressure gradient between two ventricles, and the direction and magnitude of the shunt.

ECG Criteria

- Small VSD
  - ECG usually normal
  - Left ventricular hypertrophy (LVH) or even biventricular hypertrophy (BVH) (both VH)
  - Tall and peaked P in II, III, aVF and V_1-V_4

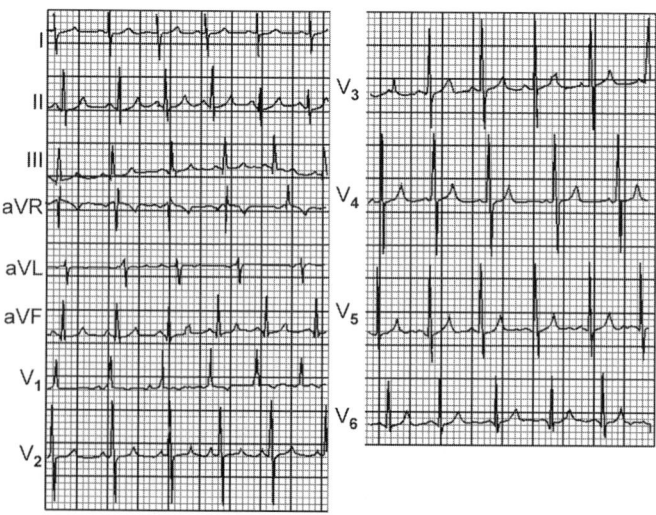

Fig. 14.1 Biventricular hypertrophy in a patient with ventricular septal defect

- In moderate size VSD
  - Both ventricular hypertrophy (BVH)
  - Tall and peaked P in II, III, aVF and V_1–V_4
  - Incompete right bundle branch block (RBBB)
- Large VSD
  - BVH, predominantly LVH with diastolic overloading pattern or RVH
  - Tall and peaked p
  - Incomplete RBBB.

ATRIAL SEPTAL DEFECT (FIG. 14.2)

Introduction

- Atrial septal defect (ASD) is the most common congenital heart disease in older children and adults
- An ostium secundum defect (ASD) is in the region of the fossa ovalis and is associated with normal AV valves.
- An ostium primun defect is located in the lower portion of the atrial septum and overlies the mitral and tricuspid valves.
- Common AV canal consists of an interatrial and an interventricular septal defect. This lesion is common in children with Down's syndrome.

ECG Criteria

In secundum type:
- Incomplete RBBB + right axis deviation (RAD) (because of RVH with a diastolic overloading pattern).
- In primum defects—Incomplete RBBB + LAD (Left axis deviation).
- Less common—tall and peaked P 1° heart block.

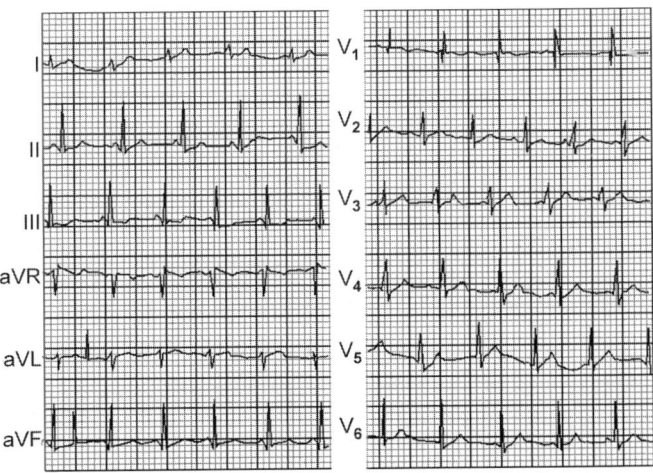

Fig. 14.2 Sinus rhythm with incomplete right bundle branch block in atrial septal defect

- In far-advanced case—BVH
- End stage of ASD—atrial fibrillation (AF).

PATENT DUCTUS ARTERIOSUS (FIG. 14.3)

Introduction

Patent ductus arteriosus (PDA) is the second most common congenital heart disease in all age groups, especially in infants and young children.

ECG Criteria

- In mild case of PDA—Normal ECG
- In large defects
  - LVH-a diastolic overloading pattern
- In severe cases
  - Both ventricular hypertrophy
  - Significant hypertension
- LAE (Left atrial enlargement)
- First degree AV block
- RBBB (occasionally).

Note:
- PDA is two times more in females than in males
- This congenital lesion is to be frequently associated with maternal rubella during early pregnancy.

TETRALOGY OF FALLOT (FIG. 14.4)

Introduction

Tetralogy of Fallot (TOF) consists of pulmonary stenosis (PS), VSD, dextroposition of the aorta and RVH. ECG findings vary

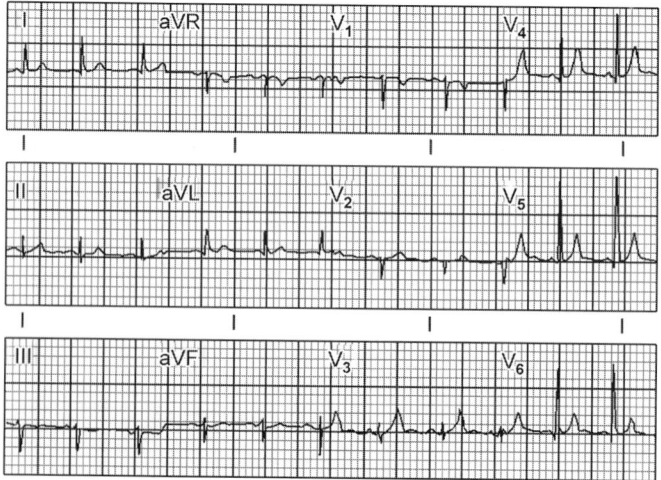

Fig. 14.3 Sinus rhythm and left ventricular hypertrophy with diastolic overloading pattern in a patient with patent ductus arteriosus

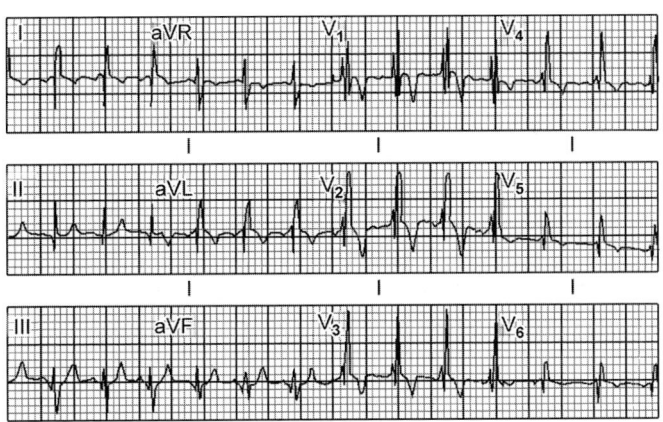

Fig. 14.4 Right bundle branch in a patient with tetralogy of Fallot associated with dextrocardia

markedly. There may be predominantly pulmonary stenosis or VSD.

ECG Criteria

- Evidence of P-pulmonale (P-congenitale)
- RBBB present, QRS broad
- RBBB present at birth, top
- Top coexist with dextrocardia, or
- RBBB associated with dextrocardia
- RBBB with marked RAD.

Note: Basically, ECG findings arise due to:
- Right atrial enlargement (RAE)
- Right ventricular hypertrophy (RVH)
- Left atrial enlargement (LAE) due to volume overload
- Possible left ventricular enlargement.

EBSTEIN'S ANOMALY (FIG. 14.5)

Introduction

Ebstein's anomaly is characterized by downward displacement of an abnormal tricuspid valve in the right ventricle. Here right ventricles get incorporated into right atrium, which becomes large, voluminous and hyperplastic called 'Atrialization of right ventricle'. Tricuspid regurgitation is commonly present but valve is not stenotic.

ECG Criteria

- Tall, peaked P-wave (Himalayan P-wave) in II, III, aVF
- RBBB: Wide (>0.12 sec) rsR' in V_1-V_4 and coving ST and inverted T. Wide deep S in V_6
- First degree AV block–PR may be 0.20 sec
- Atrial tachyarrhythmia, premature beats.

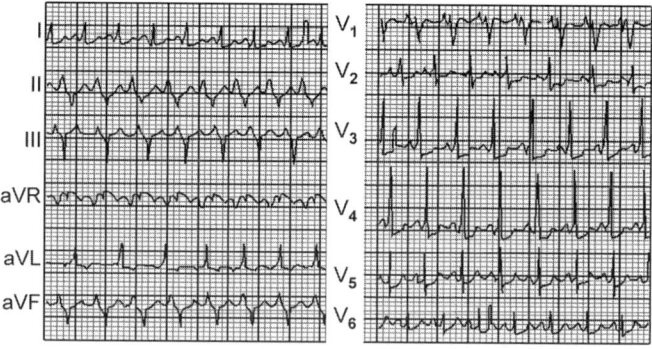

Fig. 14.5 Marked right atrial enlargement in a patient with Ebstein's anomaly associated with Wolff-Parkinson-White syndrome

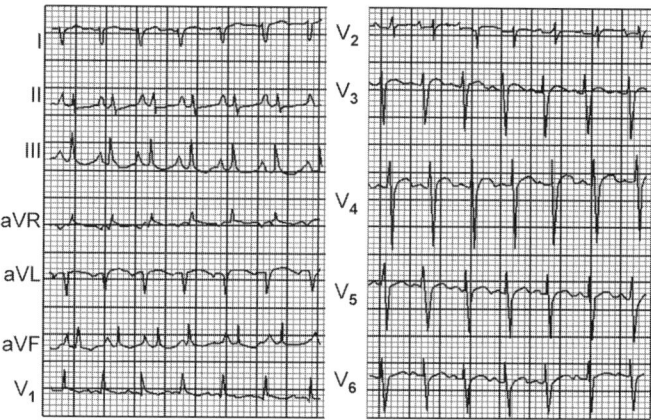

Fig. 14.6 Right ventricular hypertrophy with right atrial enlargement in a patient with pulmonic stenosis

Note:
- Ebstein's anomaly is associated with Wolff-Parkinson-White (WPW) syndrome.
- It may produce various arrhythmias.

PULMONARY STENOSIS (CONGENITAL) (FIG. 14.6)

Introduction

Pulmonary stenosis is common congenital cardiac lesion; in children and adults, it may be isolated lesion or may be associated with ASD or VSD.

ECG Criteria

- Mild or subinfundibular:
  - Normal axis (+ 40° + 60°)
  - Sharp pointed, peaked P <2.5 mm in II, V

- Tall R in V_1 or V_2
- Inverted T in V_1-V_2
- Moderate
  - Right axis deviation (RAD)
  - Sharp, pointed, tall P >2.5 mm in II, V_1
  - Tall R in V_1-V_3, R:S >1
  - Inverted T in V_1-V_2, V_4-V_5
- Severe
  - Marked RAD
  - Tall, giant P ($\geq$ 5mm) in II, V_1
  - Tall R in V_1 >20 mm in height
  - RS pattern in V_2-V_6
  - QR pattern in V_1 (severe stenosis)
  - Inverted, deep, symmetric T in V_1-V_6
  - ST depression with convexity upwards.

15

Pacemakers and Exercise Tolerance Test

PACEMAKERS

Definition: Pacemaker (PM) is an external artificial device, which gives electrical stimulation to the heart and thereby rate and rhythm of the heart is artificially controlled.

Types

- Atrificial pacemaker
  - Temporary PM (TPM)
  - Permanent PM (PPM)
- Implantable cardioverter defibrillator (ICD).

ECG Criteria

- Atrial pacing
  - Spike followed by P-wave
  - QRS normal
- Ventricular pacing (Fig. 15.1)
  - Spike followed by QRS
  - QRS-Wide (Like LBBB)
- Dual-chamber pacing
  - One spike followed by P-wave
  - Another spike-followed by wide QRS.

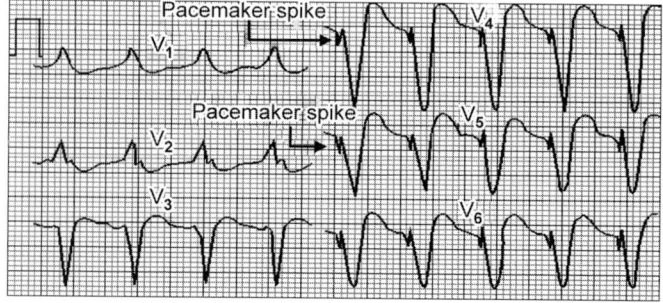

Fig. 15.1 Ventricular pacemaker

ECG Pacemaker Patterns (Fig. 15.2)

- Atrial pacing
- Ventricular pacing
- Dual-chamber pacing

Note:

- In right ventricular pacing—wide QRS looks like LBBB pattern
- In atrial or ventricular pacing, spike may not be seen in demand pacemaker
- Diagnosis of MI may be difficult in presence of pacemaker.

Pacemaker Terminology

Five-letter code of pacing modes and function (Fig. 15.3):

1st chamber paced	2nd chamber sensed	3rd mode of response
A: Atrium	A: Atrium	I: Inhibited
V: Ventricle	V: Ventricle	T: Triggered
D: Double (A+V)	D: Double (A + V)	D: Double (T + 1)
O: None	O: None	O: None (fixed-rate pacemaker)

4th : Programmable functions	5th : Antitachycardia functions
O = None	O = None
P = Simple (rate/output)	P = Pacing (Antitachycardia)
M = Multiprogrammable	S = Shock
C = Communication	D = Dual (pacing and shock) (P + S)
R = Rate responsive	

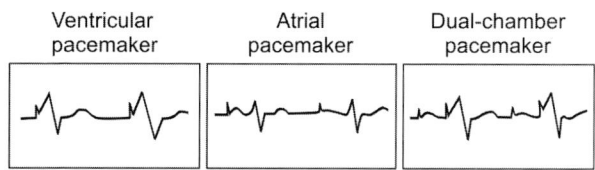

Fig. 15.2 Pacemaker patterns

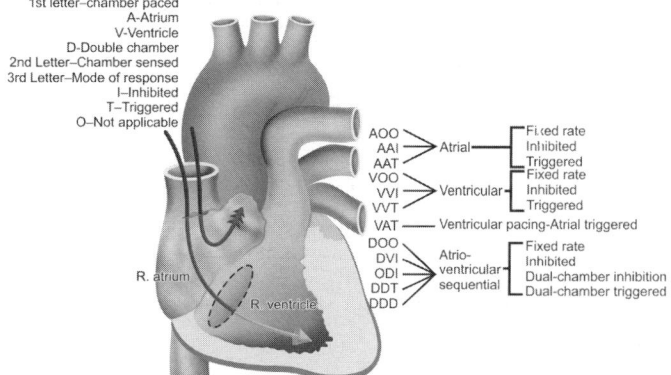

Fig. 15.3 The code system of pacemakers

Some Definitions

- *Atrial pacemaker rhythm* is a regular atrial rhythm with normal QRS initiated by an artificial pacemaker electrode placed in the right atrium. Each P-wave is initiated by an artificial pacemaker spike.
- *Demand ventricular pacemaker rhythm* is a regular ventricular rhythm initiated by an artificial pacemaker electrod placed in the right ventricular apex. The pacemaker functions by sensing the intrinsic heartbeats (there is no competition between the intrinsic heart rhythm and the pacemaker rhythm).
- *Fixed-rate ventricular pacemaker rhythm* is a regular ventricular rhythm initiated by an artificial pacemaker electrode placed in the right ventricular apex. This rhythm is independent to and competes with the basic rhythm (it does not sense the intrinsic heart rhythm).
- *Coronary sinus pacemaker rhythm* is a regular atrial rhythm with normal (narrow) QRS initiated by an artificial pacemaker electrode placed in the coronary sinus origin.
- *Atrioventricular sequential pacemaker rhythm* is a dual-chamber pacemaker rhythm initiated by two pacemaker electrodes so that the atria and the ventricles are paced sequentially.
- *Runway pacemaker (Acceleration of artificial pacing)* is the acceleration of artificial pacing at a rate faster than the preset pacing rate (ventricular fixed-rate mode in most cases).
- *Failure of cardiac capture by pacing* is the failure of an artificial pacemaker to activate the atria, ventricles, or both (more commonly the ventricles).
- *Slowing of artificial pacing* is characterized by an artificial pacing rate that is slower than the preset pacing rate.
- *Irregular artificial pacing* is characterized by irregular cardiac cycles that are stimulated by the artificial pacemaker.
- *Pacemaker hysteresis* is characterized by pacemaker escape interval (the length of the period from an intrinsic heart beat to the initial pacemaker induced beat) that is longer than the consecutively occurring pacing cycles (automatic interval).

Indications of Temporary Pacemaker (TPM)

- Acute inferior MI with second degree heart block (HB) or complete heart block (CHB)
- Acute inferior myocardial infarction (MI) with sever bradycardia with hemodynamic change
- Acute extensive anterior MI with 2° HB or CHB or new bifascicular block (LBBB or RBBB with LAHB or RBBB with LPHB)
- Patient awaiting for PPM
- After open heart surgery

- Some cases of cardiac arrest
- Severe digitalis toxicity.

Indications of Permanent Pacemaker (PPM)

- Complete heart block (CHB) with syncope or Adams-stokes syndrome and sick sinus syndrome (most common)
- Symptomatic Mobitz type-2 heart block
- Bifascicular or trifascicular block with syncope
- Carotid sinus syndrome with bradycardia
- Repeated vasovagal syndrome with bradycardia.

After MI, PPM Indications

- Acute inferior MI with CHB persisting over 2 weeks
- Anterior MI with persistent type 2 or CHB or newly acquired BBB or bifascicular block with transient type 2 HB or CHB.

Mode of PPM

- *Fixed rate*: It fires specific preset rate, regardless of patient's own heart rate.
- *Demand pacemaker*: It works when the patient's heart rate falls below a preset rate. Now, all pacemakers are demand type. Two components:
    1. *A sensing mechanism*: Designed so that the pacemaker will be inhibited, when the heart rate is adequate.
    2. *A pacing mechanism*: Designed to trigger the pacemaker when no intrinsic QRS occurs within a predetermined time period.

Pacemaker Malfunction

It may occur due to:
- Dislodgement of pacemaker wire, or
- By fibrosis around the tip of pacemaker wire.

ECG Changes

- ECG shows pacemaker spikes, but no QRS
- In other cases, no pacemaker spike is seen in ECG
- Failure to sense may occur in which pacemaker spike is inappropriate that may fall on T-wave.

Pacemaker Syndrome

It is a disorder characterized by:
- Transient hypotension
- Fatigue
- Dizziness
- Syncope
- Distressing pulsation in neck and chest.

It occurs in single-chamber pacing, which can be prevented by dual chamber pacing or by reducing the pacemaker rate so that sinus rhythm predominates.

EXERCISE TOLERANCE TEST (ETT), OR EXERCISE TESTING (FIG. 15.4)

Introduction

Exercise testing is an excellent non-invasive method for evaluating patients, diagnosing ischemic heart disease, assessing the patient's functional capacity, and selecting patients for cardiac catheterization (Fig. 15.4).

ECG Changes during Exercise Testing

- Normal ECG response to exercise:
  - Increase heart rate
  - Increase in P-wave amplitude
  - Shortening of the PR and QT intervals
  - Decrease in the R-wave amplitude
  - Shift of the QRS axis to the right
  - Depressed J-point with upsloping ST segment
  - Variable T-wave changes.
- An abnormal, positive ECG response to exercise (Fig. 15.5):
  - Depressed J points with horizontal or downsloping ST-depression greater than 1 mm, with or without angina. The greater the ST-depression, the earlier the onset of ST- depression (Stage I or stage II)
  Longer durations of ST-depression are important diagnostic criteria.

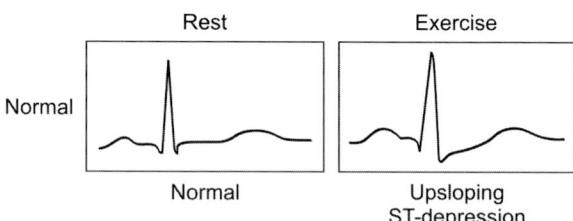

Fig. 15.4 The normal configuration of the segment at rest and during exercise

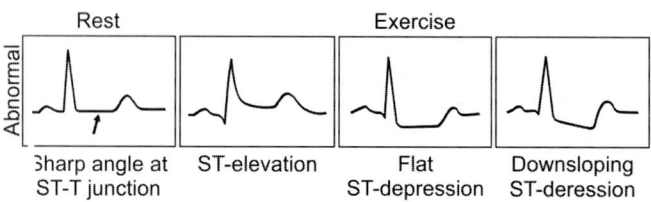

Fig. 15.5 Abnormal configuration during rest and exercise

- ST elevation >1 mm
- Increase in the R-wave amplitude
- Inversion of U-waves
- Significant arrhythmias.
• False-positive exercise tests may occur with the following:
  - Digitalis
  - Hypokalemia
  - Ventricular hypertrophy
  - BBB
  - WPW syndrome
  - Mitral valve prolapse
  - Female.

Note: Serial ECG and BP recordings are taken at each stage and continuous ECG monitoring is performed throughout the test.

ECG Interpretation of ETT

Following are the points:
- ST depression
- ST elevation
- ST alternans
- T-wave changes
- R-wave voltage (Indicate LV dysfunction)
- U-wave inversion
- Arrhythmia
- Conduction disturbances.

ST depression: Normal <1 mm.

There are four types:
1. Downslopping ST depression
   - Depression >1 mm
   - Very significant diagnostic value –95% diagnostic

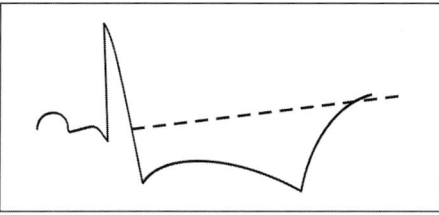

2. Horizontal ST depression
   - Good diagnostic value
   - 85% diagnostic

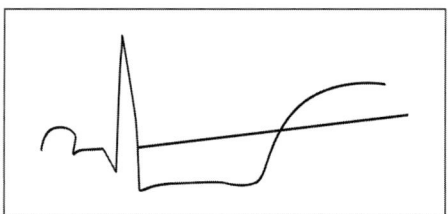

3. Slow upsloping ST depression
    - Here rate of upstroke is slow, i.e. <1 mvolt/sec
    - Significant diagnostic value
    - Have 30% false +ve

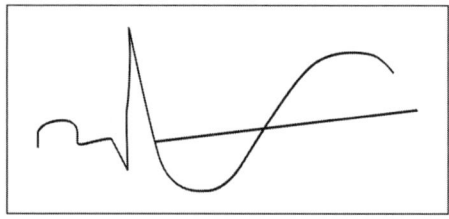

4. Rapid upsloping ST depression
    - It is a normal response to exercise or tachycardia
    - ST depression touches the baseline within <1 msec
    - No diagnostic significant

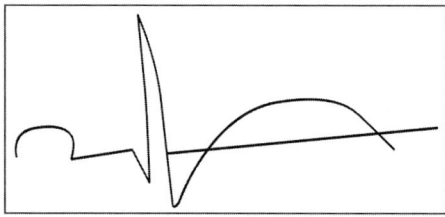

Note:
- If ST depression with chest pain—due to subendocardial infarction
- ST changes disapper within 1 minute after exercise—not significant
- If persists 3 minutes after exercise—significant value.

Features of Strongly +ve ETT

- Greater than 3 mm ST depression
- Early onset (within 3 mm) of ST depression
- Persistence (>8 mm) of ST depression during recovery phase
- Systolic BP fails to rise or fall
- Poor overall exercise duration.

16

Echocardiogram Interpretation and Diagnosis

ECG INTERPRETATION-1

The ECG shows
Sinus rhythm
Ventricular extrasystoles
Normal conduction interval,
QRS and T-waves

Interpretation
Normal ECG with VES
(Occasionally)

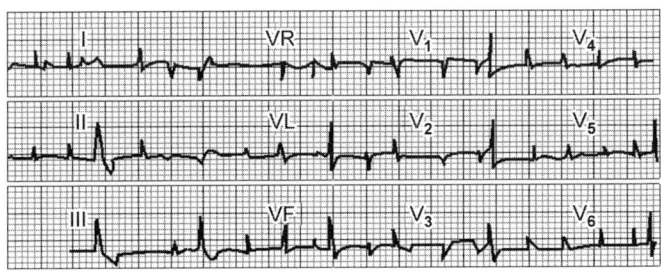

The ECG shows
Sinus rhythm; left axis deviation
ST elevation in I, aVL, $V_2 - V_5$
Q-wave in aVL, $V_2 - V_3$; deep
S in II, III, aVF

Interpretation
Acute extensive anterior MI with LAHB

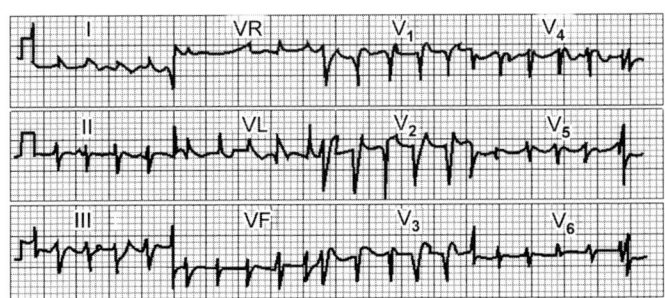

The ECG shows
Sinus rhythm
Alternate and non-conducted beats
Normal PR interval in conducted beats
Left axis deviation
Deeps in II, III, aVF; wide QRS; rSR pattern in V_1

Interpretation
Second degree (Mobitz) Type II) block with left anterior hemiblock with RBBB

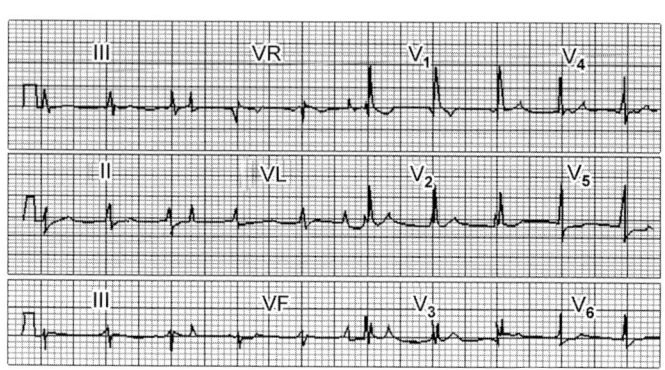

The ECG shows
Sinus rhythm; 120 beats/min
Normal PR interval; wide QRS complexes
M pattern in I, aVL, V_5, V_6

Interpretation
Sinus rhythm with LBBB

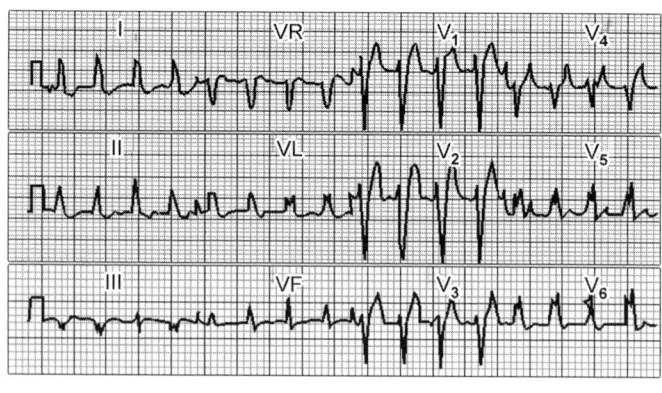

The ECG shows
Sinus rhythm; 75 beats/min
Normal PR interval: wide QRS complexes
rSR pattern in V_1, V_2 V_3; T inverted in I, II, aVF

Interpretation
Sinus rhythm with RBBB

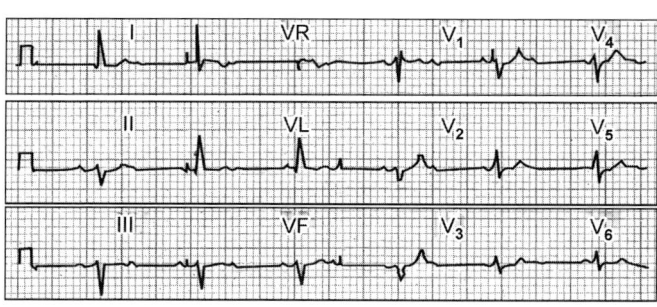

The ECG shows
No P-waves
Narrow QRS; R-R interval irregular
Rate varying between 80–180 beats/min
Normal T-wave; ST depression in $V_5 - V_6$ (for digitalis effect)

Interpretation
Atrial fibrillation with digitalis effect

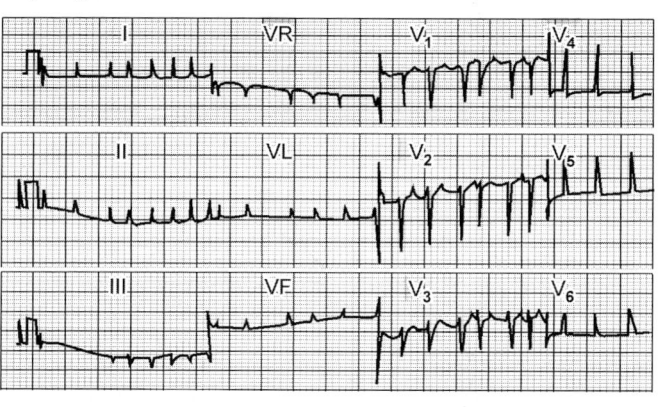

The ECG shows
No P-waves
Regular QRS (R-R) interval; Narrow QRS
Rate 180 beats/min; normal T-waves

Interpretation
Supraventricular tachycardia (SVT)

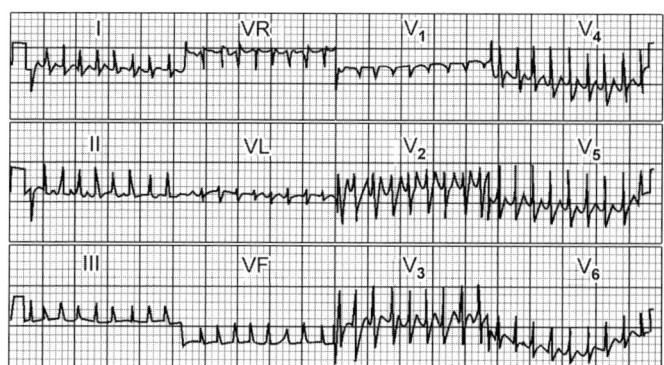

ECG INTERPRETATION-2

ECG shows:
- Atrial rate—75 bpm
- Ventricular rate—50 bpm
- Complete dissociation between P and QRS

Diagnosis: Complete heart block.

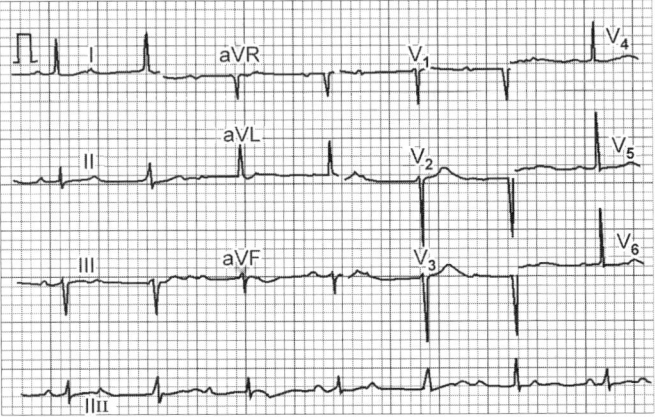

ECG shows:
- P wave—absent
- RR interval—irregular (rhythm is irregular)
- Heart rate > 100 bpm

Diagnosis: Fast atrial fibrillation

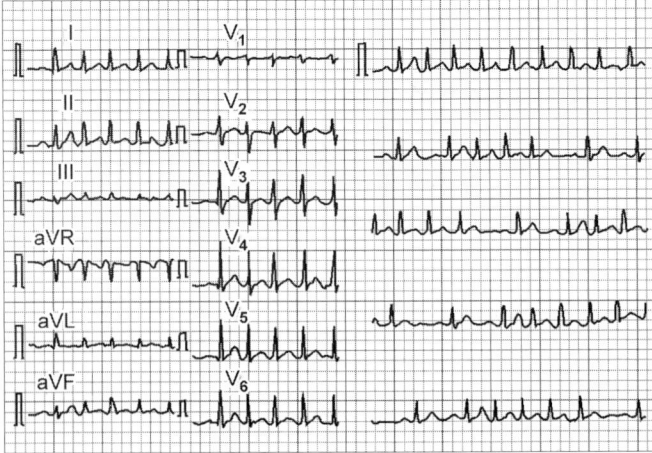

ECG shows:
- Pacemaker spike followed by QRS
- In some lead, there is no spike which indicates demand pacemaker.

Diagnosis: Demand type of ventricular pacemaker

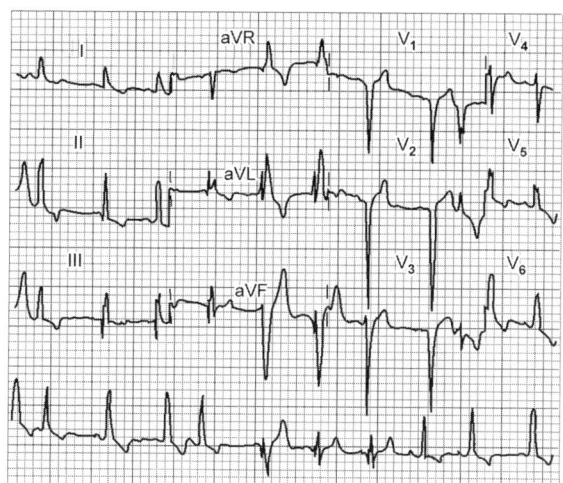

ECG shows:
- Heart rate—107 bpm
- ST elevation in V_2 - V_5 and Q in V_1 - V_5
- Q in Lead II, III and aVF

Diagnosis: Actual anterior and old inferior MI with sinus tachycardia.

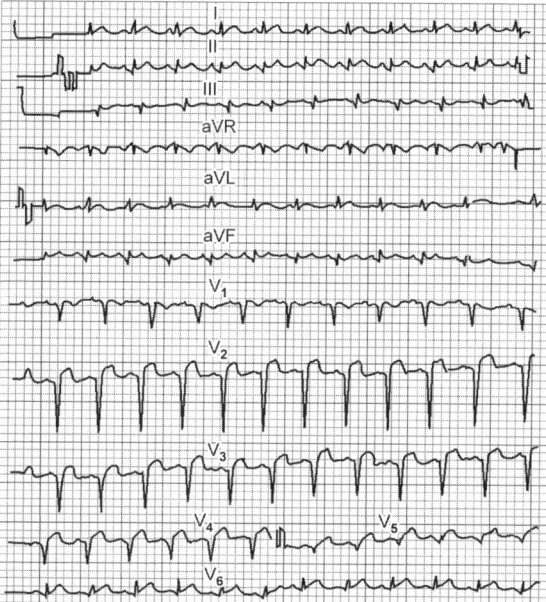

ECG shows:
- Short P-R interval
- Delta wave in V_2 - V_6
- Deep S in V_1
- Q in lead III and aVF-confuses with old inferior MI

Diagnosis: WPW syndrome type B

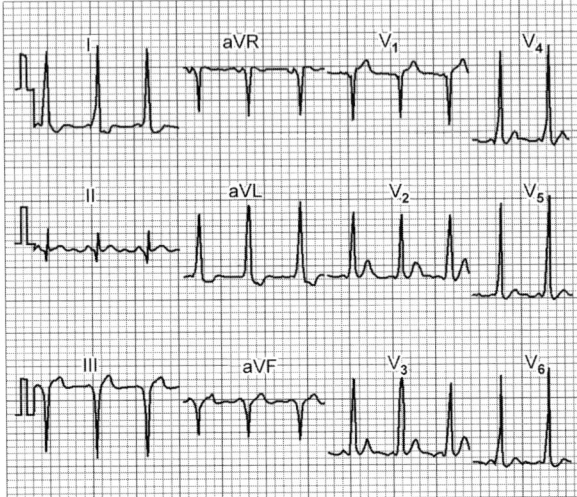

ECG shows:
- Pacemaker spike in almost all the leads

Diagnosis: Ventricular pacemaker

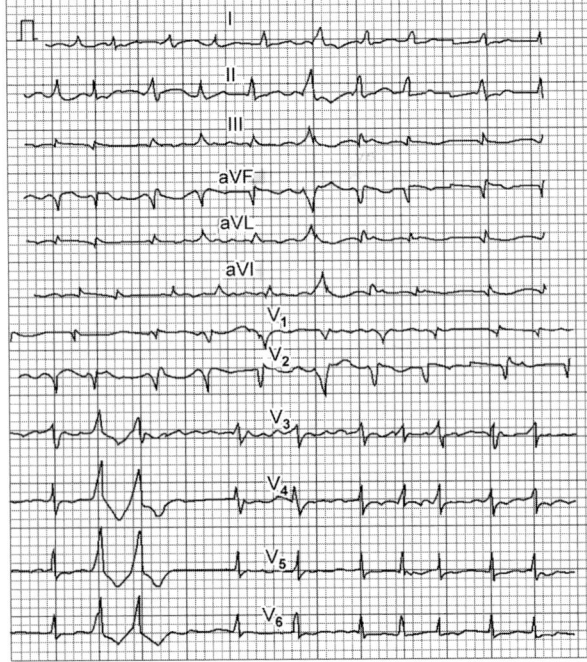

ECG shows:
- P-wave—absent
- Flutter wave in $V_1 - V_3$
- Rhythm—irregular
- Ventricular ectopics (in some leads)

Diagnosis: Atrial flutter fibrillation with multiple ventricular ectopics.

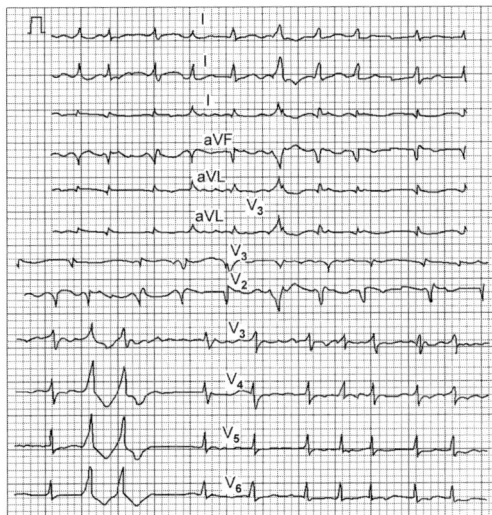

ECG shows:
- M pattern (RSR patter) in $V_5 - V_6$
- QRS—wide (0.16 second)
- Pathological Q in $V_1 - V_3$ (may be old anteroseptal MI)

Diagnosis: LBBB

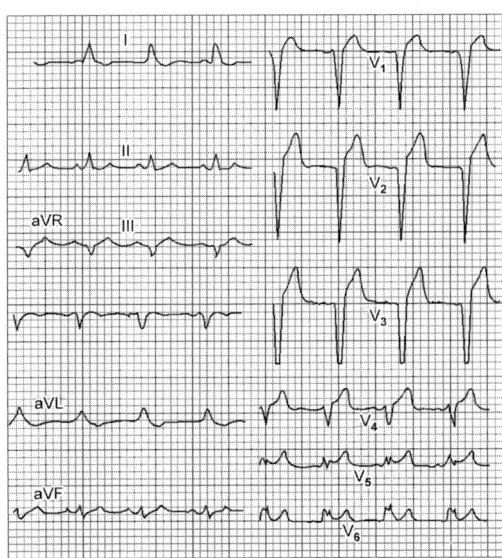

ECG shows:
- ST elevation in $V_1 - V_5$ with upward convexity
- P-absent and rhythm is irregular in II, III, aVL, aVF

Diagnosis: Acute anterior MI with paroxysmal atrial fibrillation

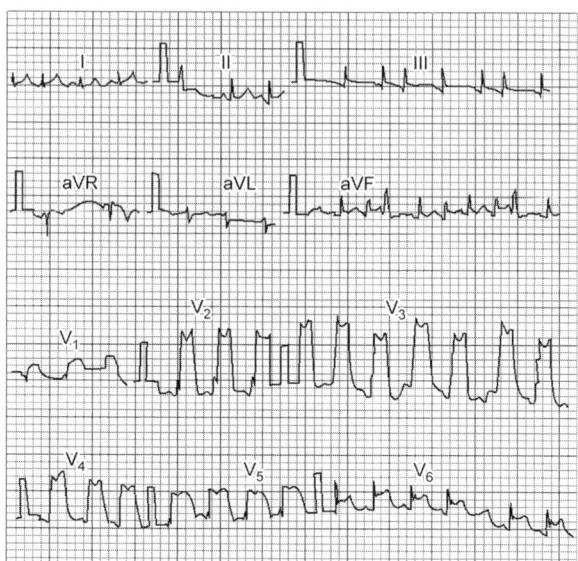

ECG shows:
- Multiple ventricular ectopics
- Tall R in lead I and deep S in Lead II, III (indicates left axis deviation)
- RSR/M-pattern in $V_1 - V_3$

Diagnosis: RBBB with LAHB with multiple ventricular ectopics.

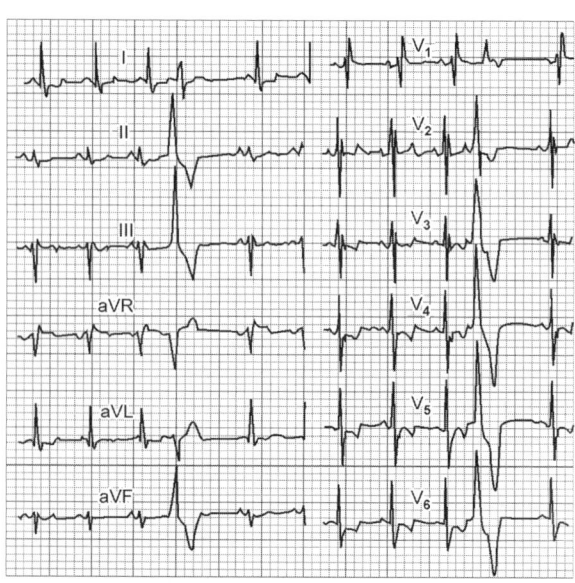

ECG shows:
- *Heart rate:* 150 bpm
- *P-wave:* Absent
- *QRS:* Normal and narrow
- Q in V_2 - V_4 with ST elevation
- Deep S in V_5 - V_6 with poor R wave progression
- Rhythm is regular

Diagnosis: AMI (Anteroseptal) with SVT.

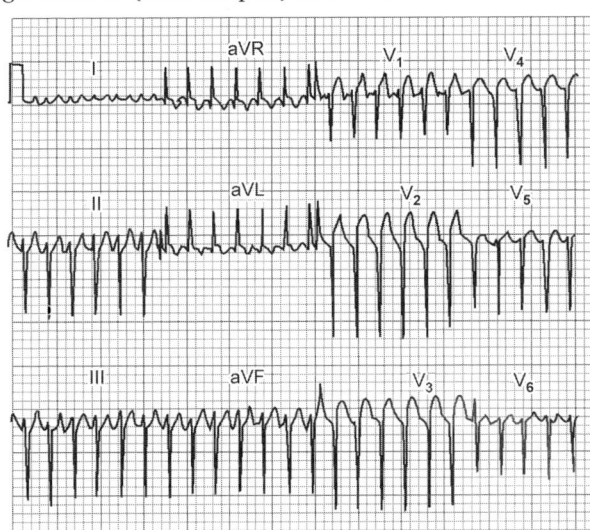

ECG shows:
- ST elevation with upward concavity in lead II, III, aVF and V_4 to V_6

Diagnosis: Acute pericarditis.

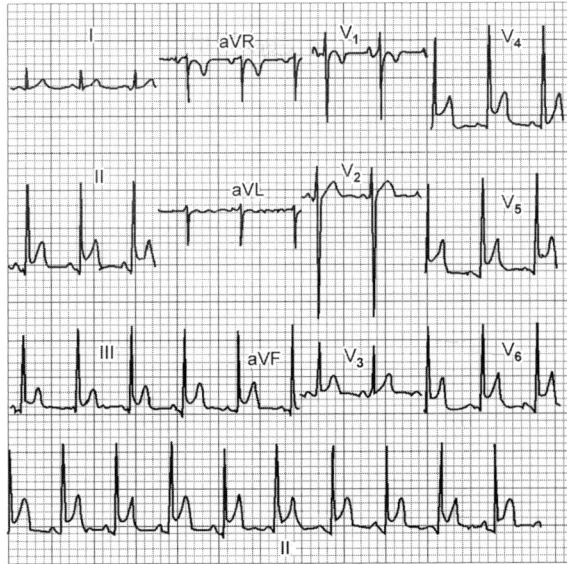

ECG shows:
- S in V_1 + R in V_6 > 35 mm
- U-wave in $V_2 - V_6$

Diagnosis: LVH with hypokalemia.

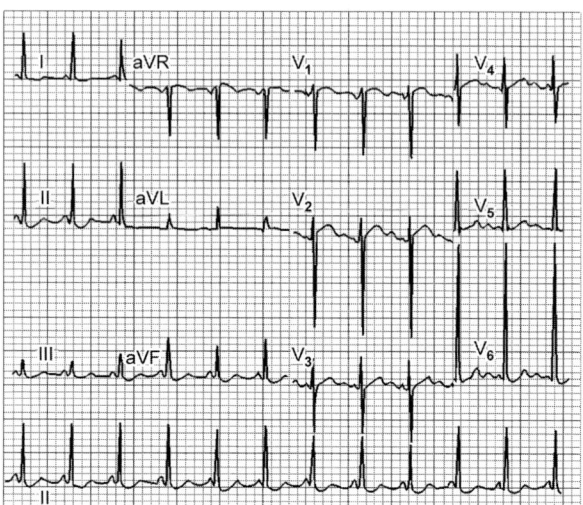

ECG shows:
- *P-wave:* Present
- *QRS, T:* Normal
- *Heart rate:* 120 bpm
- *Rhythm:* Regular
- *ST:* Elevation in V_1-V_6
- *Q-wave* – V_1-V_6

Diagnosis: Acute anterior MI with sinus tachycardia.

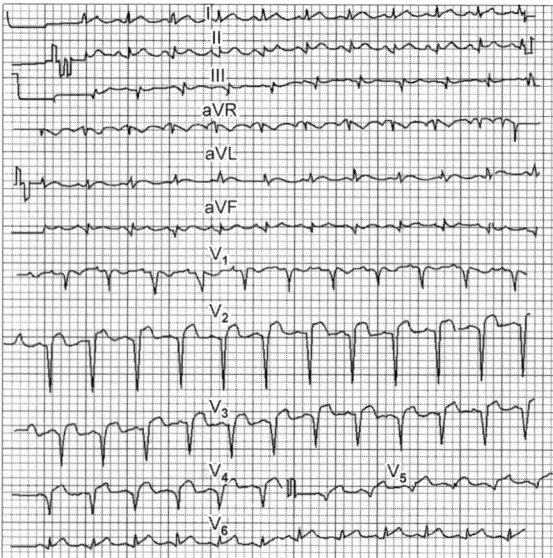

ECG shows:
- Deep S in lead I, tall R in lead III (indicates right axis deviation)
- Tall R in V$_1$ and V$_2$ with T inversion (indicates right ventricular hypertrophy)

Diagnosis: RVH with strain and LPHB.

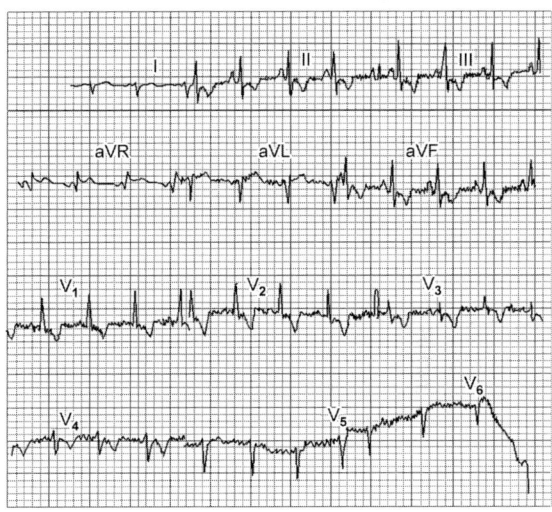

ECG shows:
- Deep S in lead I and tall R in lead III (indicates right axis deviation)
- Tall P in lead II (P-pulmonale)
- Bifid P in V$_1$ with tall upward deflection
- Tall R in V$_1$-V$_3$ with T inversion in V$_1$-V$_4$

Diagnosis: RVH + RAH.

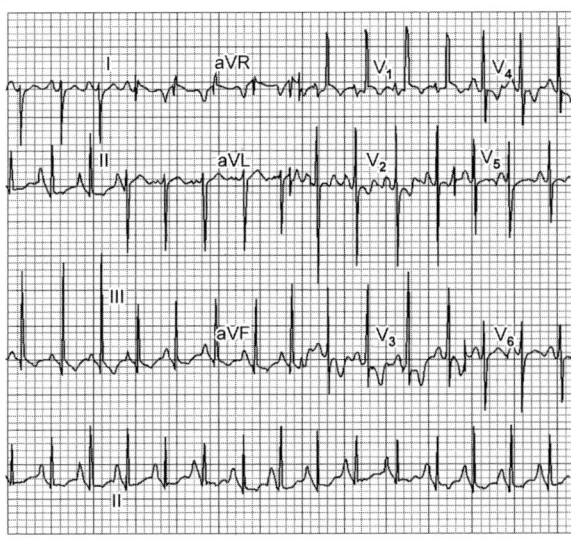

ECG shows:
- Deep S in lead I
- Deep Q and T inversion in lead III

Diagnosis: Pulmonary embolism (Typical $S_1 Q_3 T_3$ pattern).

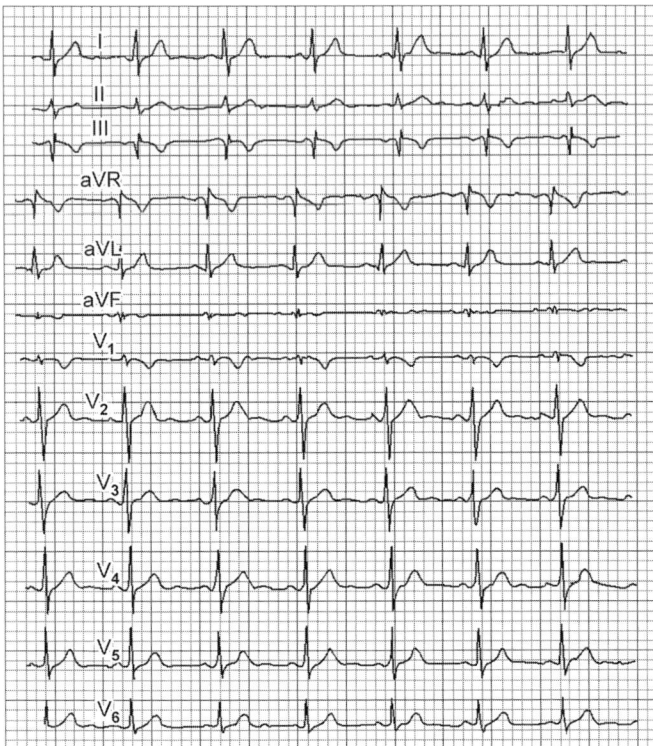

ECG DIAGNOSIS-1

Case 1

- Ventricular bigeminy
- Left atrial abnormality
- LVH by voltage criteria
- Prolonged QTC

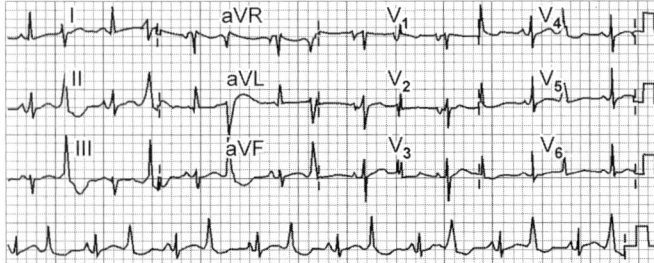

Case 2

- Sinus bradycardia
- LBBB with ST-T changes
- LAD

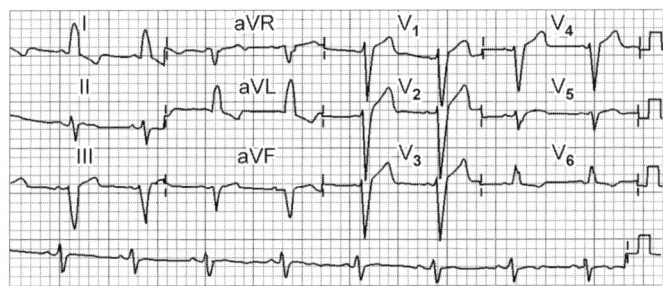

Case 3

- AF with controlled ventricular response
- Multiform VPCs
- LVH and voltage criteria
- ST-T changes

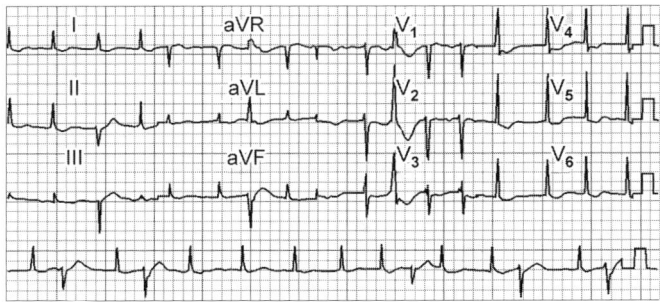

Case 4

- Sinus tachycardia
- Left bundle branch block (LBBB)
- Left-axis deviation (LAD)
- Ventricular premature complexes (VPCs)
- Atrial premature contraction (APC)

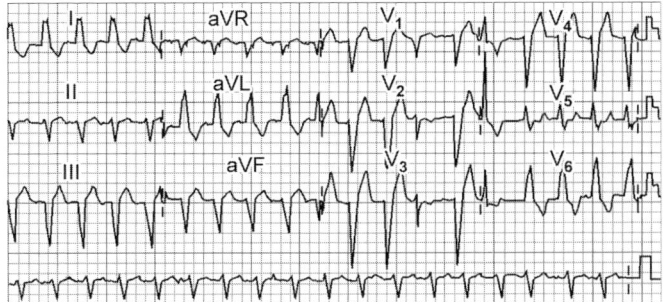

Case 5

- Sinus rhythm
- VPC
- Dual-chamber pacemaker in DDD

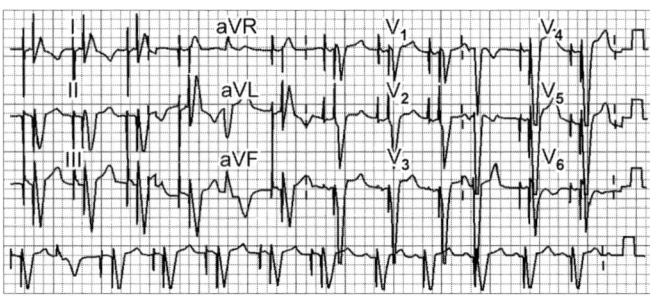

Case 6

- Atrial tachycardia with variable conduction
- Wenckebach phenomenon
- LBBB
- LVH

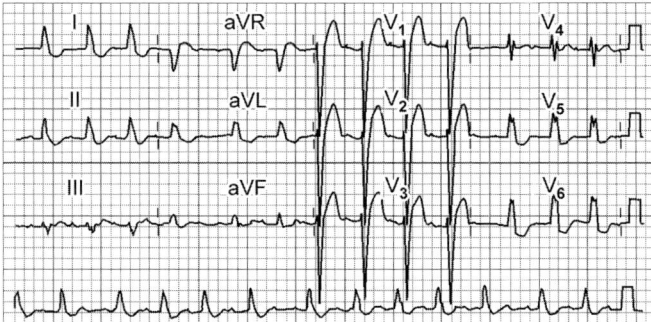

Case 7

- Sinus bradycardia
- Interpolated VPCs (Frequent)
- Inferior MI

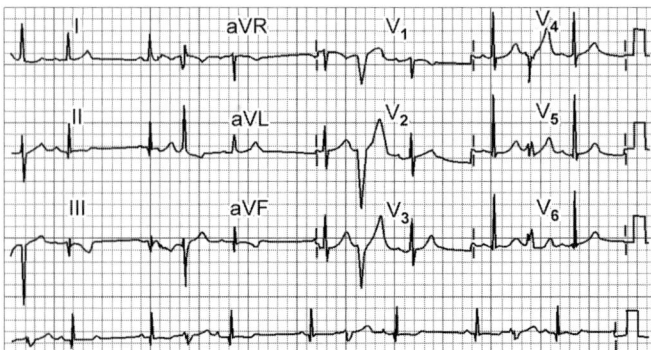

Case 8

- SVT
- Non-specific ST-T changes

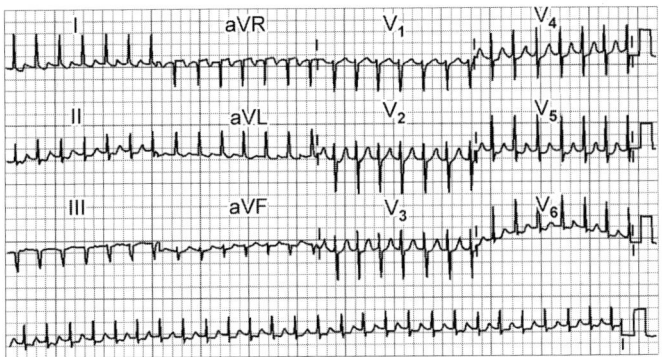

Case 9

- Sinus rhythm
- Sinus arrhythmia

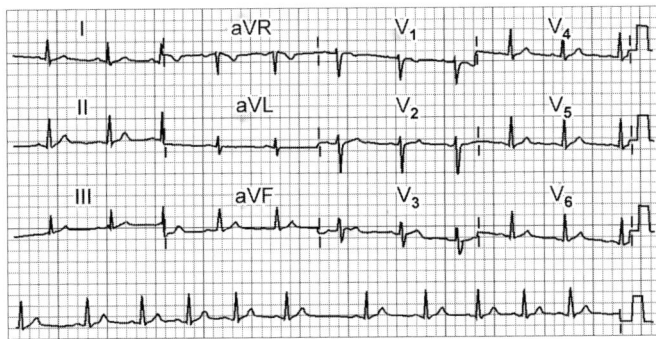

Case 10

- Sinus tachycardia
- Inferior and anterolateral MI
- Possible acute posterior MI

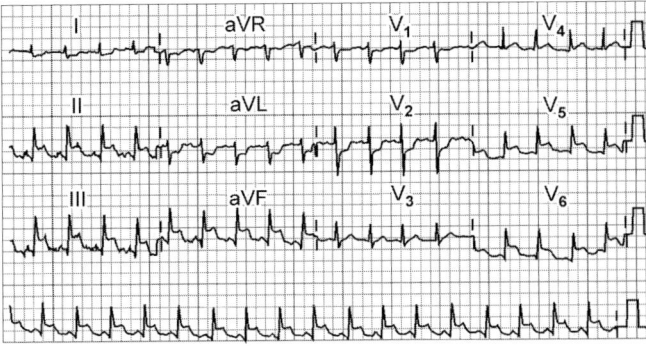

Case 11

- AF (Fast ventricular rate)
- VPC
- LAD
- LAHB/LVH
- Poor R-wave

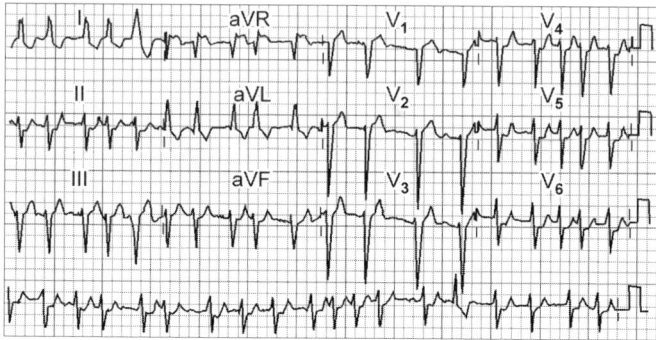

Case 12

- Complete heart block (CHB)
- Inferior MI
- Possible posterior MI

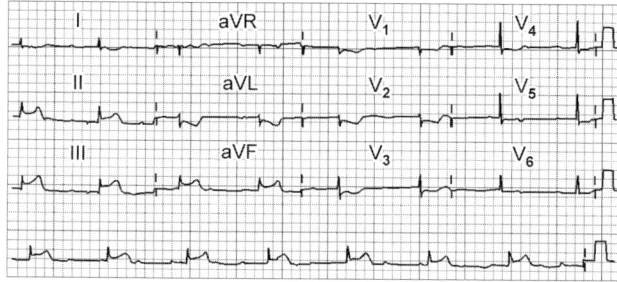

Case 13

- Ventricular tachycardia (VT)
- RAD

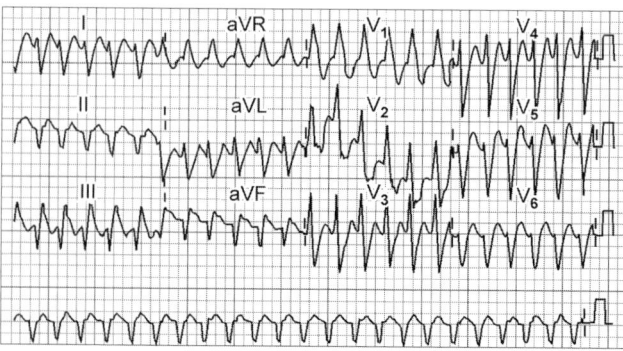

Case 14

- Ventricular tachycardia (VT)
- Left axis deviation (LAD)

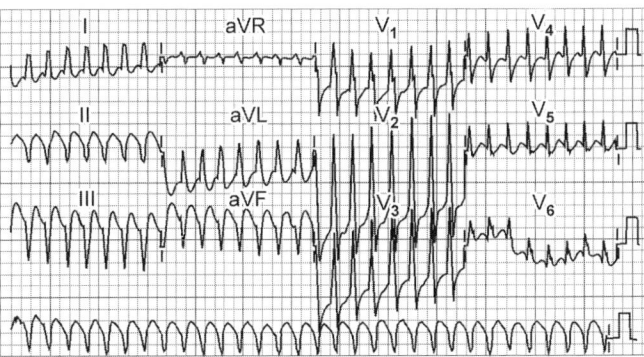

Case 15

- WPW pattern
- Sinus rhythm

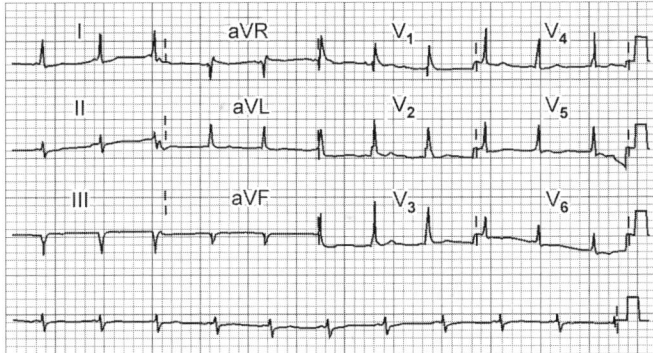

Case 16

- Atrial tachycardia, sustained
- Electrical alternans

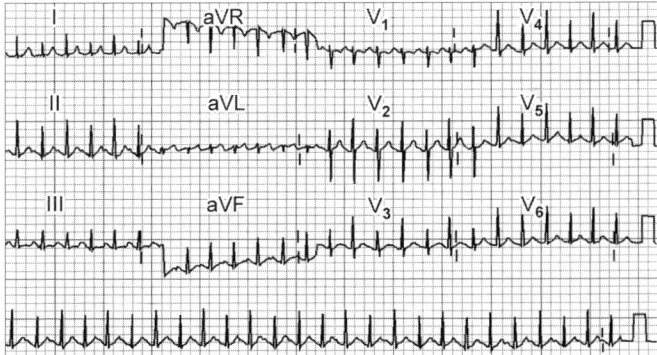

Case 17

- Sinus rhythm
- Normal variant (Age 12 years)
- Persistent juvenile T-wave pattern

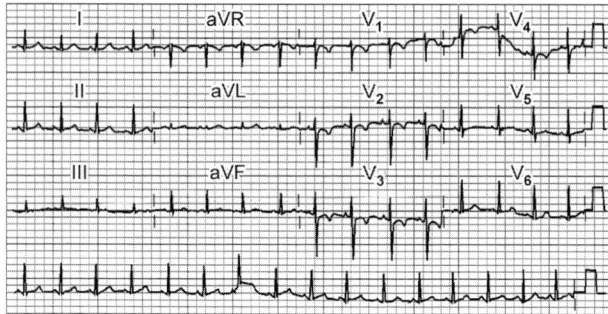

Case 18

- Sinus bradycardia
- 2 HB (Mobitz type 1)
- Inferior MI
- LVH

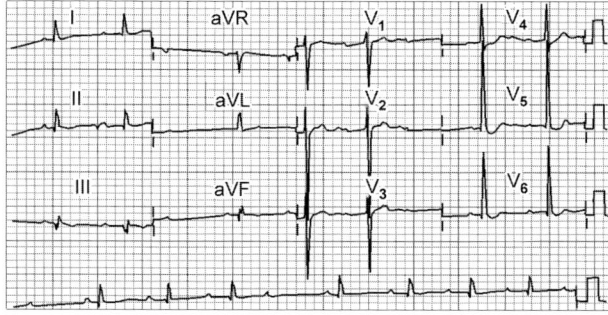

Case 19

- Ventricular pacemaker complexes
- 1° AV block
- RAD
- RVH

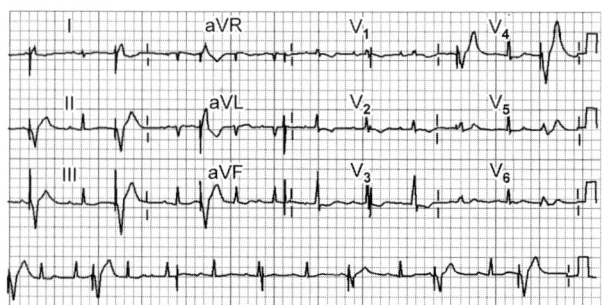

Case 20

Sinus Rhythm   VPCs
APC   LAD
LAHB   Poor R-wave

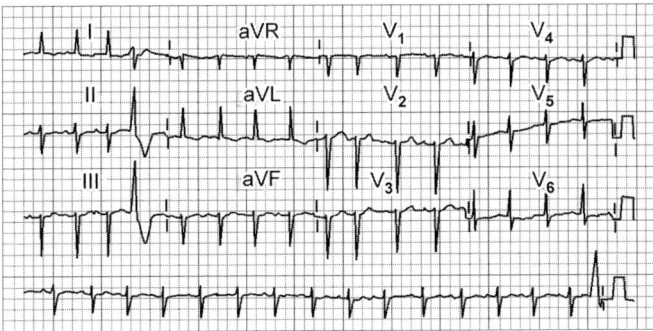

Case 21

- Accelerated AV junctional rhythm
- VPC
- RBBB

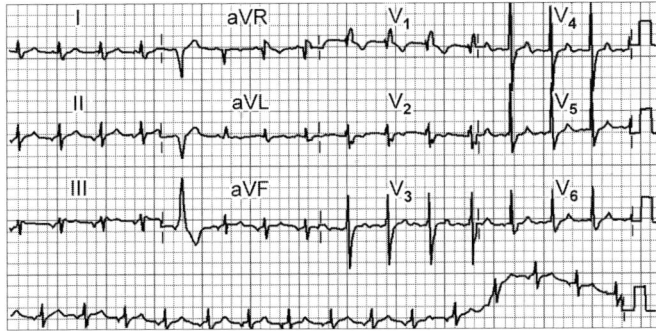

Case 22

- Atrial flutter with 4 : 1
- Incomplete RBBB

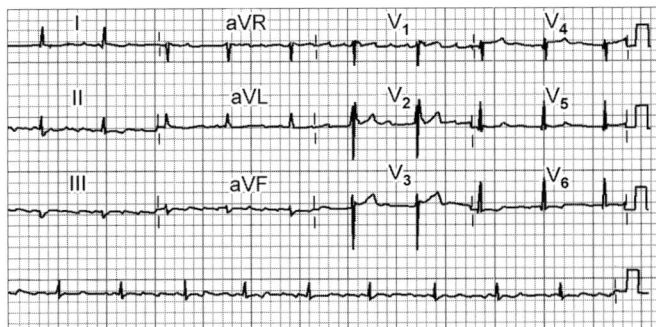

Case 23

- Accelerated AV junctional rhythm
- ST elevation—acute MI

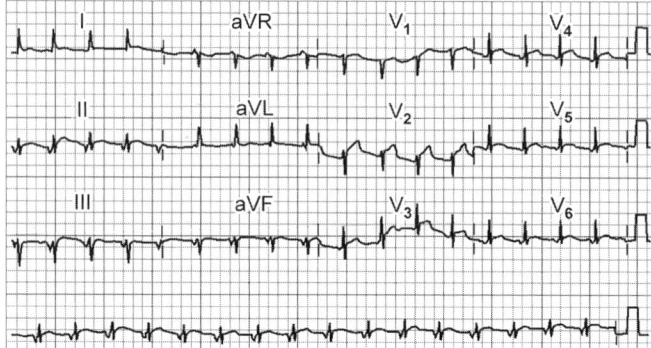

ECG DIAGNOSIS-2

Case 1

Your diagnosis
- Atrial fibrillation with
- LBBB

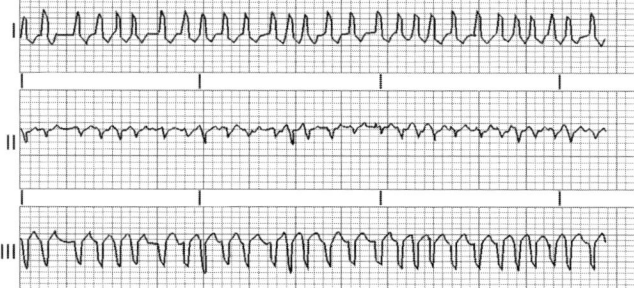

Case 2

Your diagnosis
- LBBB with
- Inferior myocardial ischemia

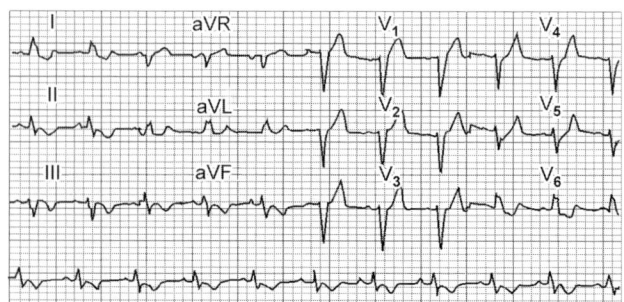

Case 3

Your diagnosis
- VPC and sustained ventricular tachycardia associated with acute inferior myocardial infarction

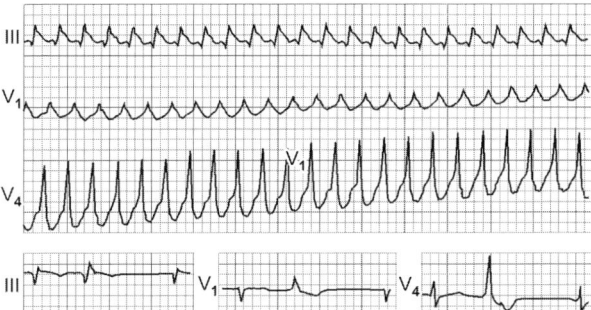

Case 4

Your diagnosis
- Right atrial enlargement (P-pulmonale) and right ventricular hypertrophy

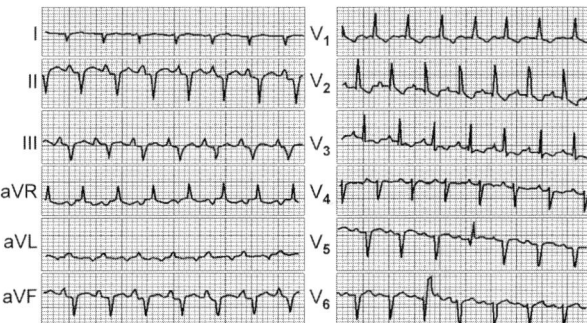

Case 5

Your diagnosis
- Atrial fibrillation associated with left ventricular hypertrophy, intermittent LBBB, and anterior myocardial ischemia.

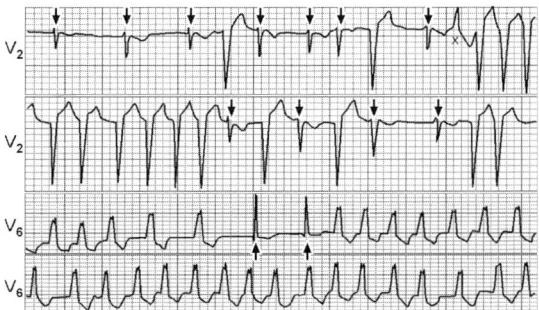

Case 6

Your diagnosis
- Sick sinus syndrome with marked sinus bradycardia, sinus arrest atrioventricular junction escape beats, APC, intermittent atrial flutter with LVH.

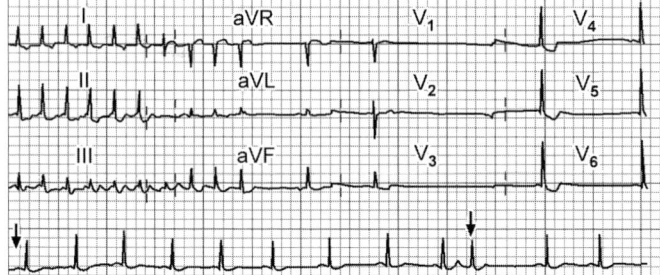

Case 7

Your diagnosis
- Intermittent Wolff-Parkinson-White syndrome.

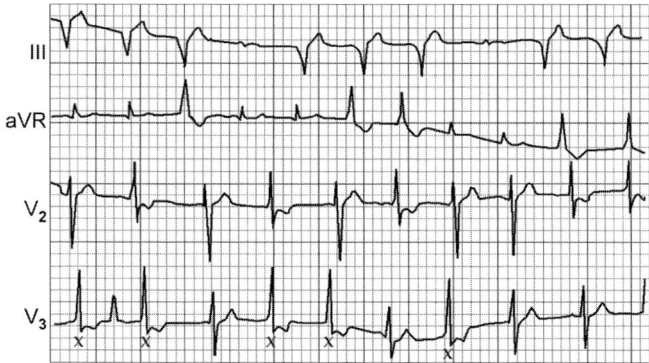

Case 8

Your diagnosis
- Parasystolic ventricular tachycardia.

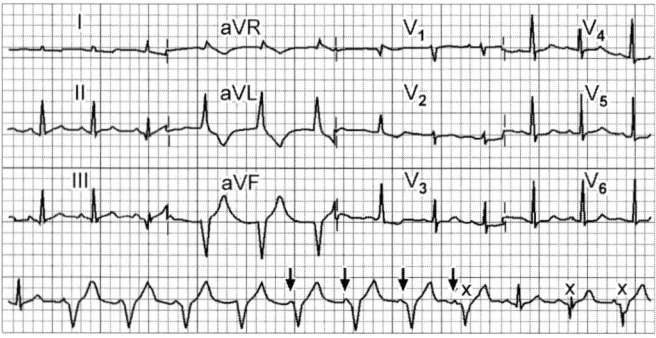

Case 9

Your diagnosis
- Sustained ventricular tachycardia.

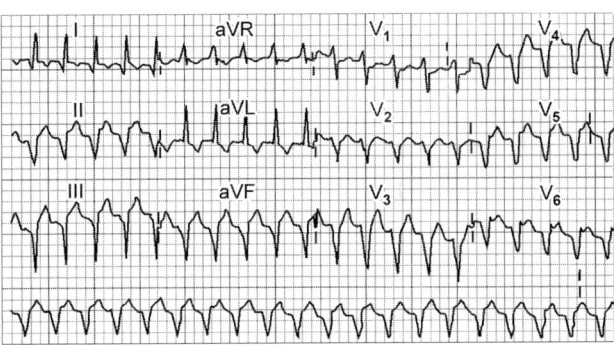

Case 10

Your diagnosis
- Atrial flutter with 1:1 atrioventricular conduction and left anterior hemiblock.

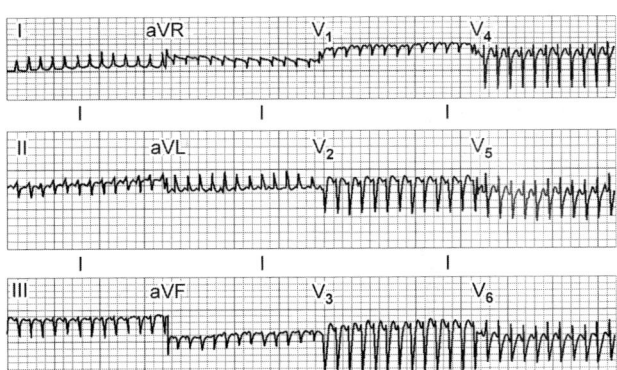

Case 11

Your diagnosis
- Sinus bradycardia with intermittent atrioventricular junctional escape rhythm producing incomplete atrioventricular dissociation.

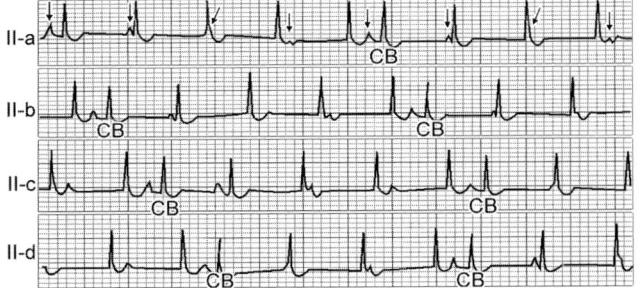

Case 12

Your diagnosis
- Non-Q-wave myocardial infarction with sinus tachycardia.

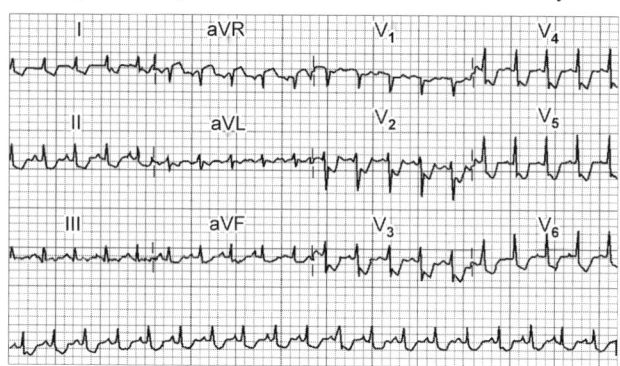

Case 13

Your diagnosis
- Bidirectional nonsustained VT and interpolated ventricular premature contractions.

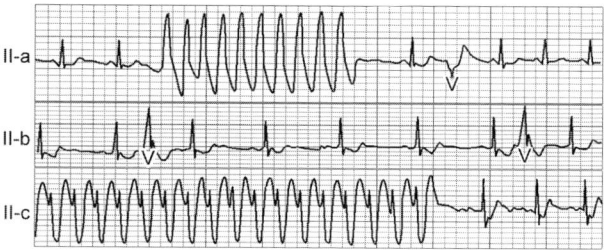

Case 14

Your diagnosis
- Sick sinus syndrome (SSS) manifested by brady-tachyarrhythmia syndrome consisting of marked sinus bradycardia, sinus arrest and intermittent atrial fibrillation, atrioventricular junctional escape beat with VPC.

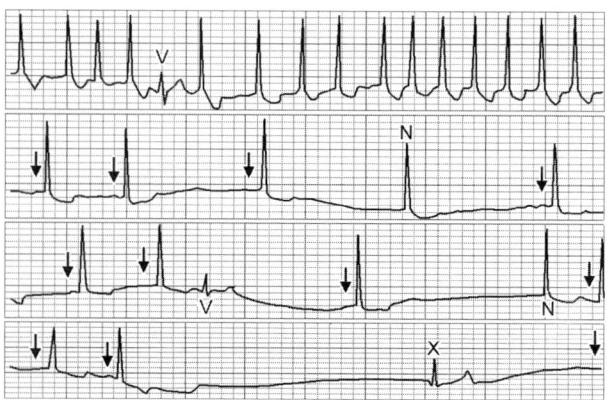

Case 15

Your diagnosis
- Ventricular premature contraction with ventricular group beats leading to nonsustained ventricular tachycardia.

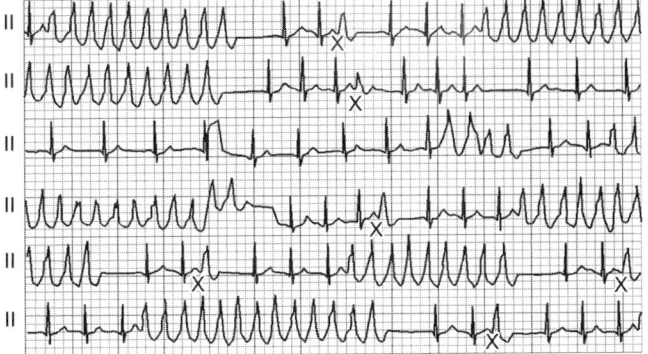

Case 16

Your diagnosis
- Ventricular flutter

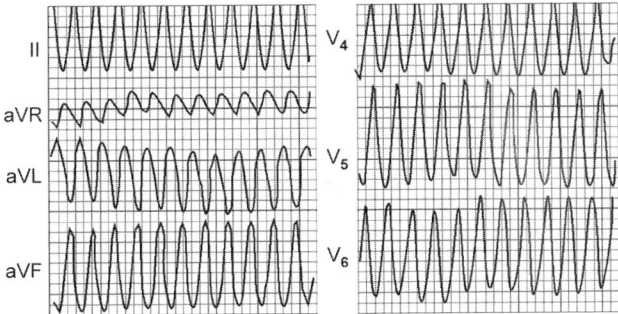

Case 17

Your diagnosis
- Torsade de pointes due to quinidine toxicity.

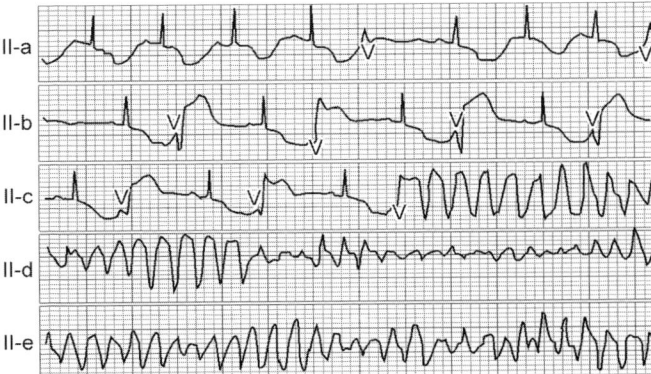

Case 18

Your diagnosis
- Malfunctioning pacemaker manifested by run away pacemaker and pacemaker electrode malposition.

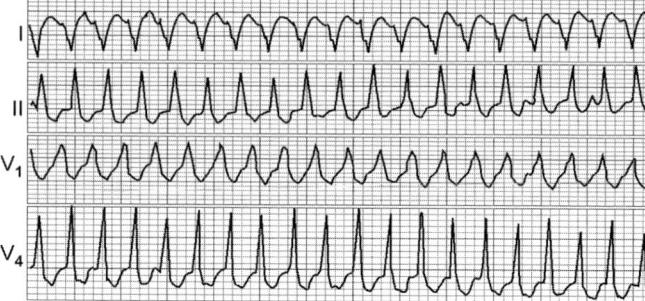

Case 19

Your diagnosis
- Malfunctioning pacemaker manifested by slowing of artificial pacing.

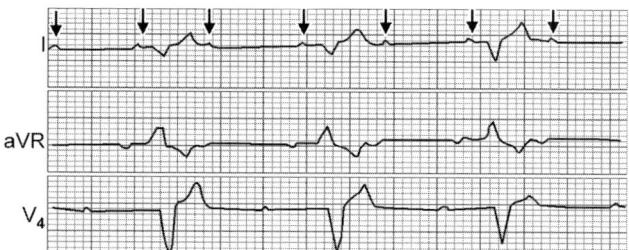

Case 20

Your diagnosis
- Central nervous system disorder subarachnoid hemorrhage (prolonged QT interval, broad and inverted T wave).
- LVH and anteroseptal MI.

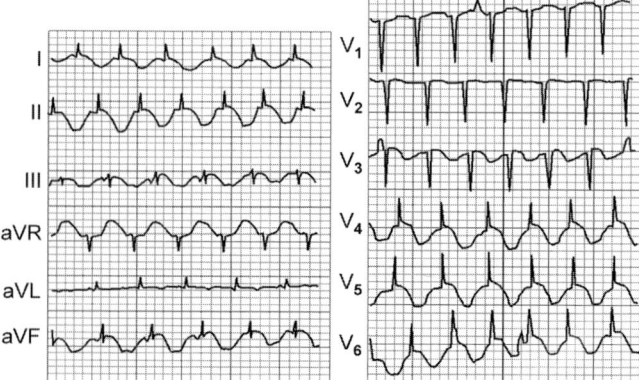

Glossary

Aberrantly: Being conducted abnormally (usually through the ventricular conduction system).

Accelerated atrial rhythm (AAR): Tachyarrhythmia caused by an increase of automaticity in atrial pacemaking cells.

Accelerated junctional rhythm (AJR): Tachyarrhythmia caused by an increase of automaticity in the pacemaking cells of the His bundle.

Accelerated rhythm: An increase in a particular cardiac rhythm above its normal limit.

Accelerated ventricular rhythm (AVR): Tachyarrhythmia caused by an increase of automaticity in pacemaking cells of the bundle branches and their fascicles.

Action potential: The electrical potential recorded from within a cell as it is activated by an electrical current or impulse.

Acute coronary syndrome: Clinical symptoms suggestive of acute myocardial ischemia/infarction of sufficient severity for an individual to seek emergency care.

Aerobic metabolism: The intracellular method for converting glucose into energy that requires the presence of oxygen and produces enough energy to nourish the myocardial cell and also cause it to contract.

Anaerobic metabolism: The intracellular method for converting glucose into energy that does not require oxygen, but produces only enough energy to nourish the cell.

Angina: Angina pectoris, precordial pressure, or pain caused by cardiac ischemia or lack of blood flow to the heart muscle.

Angioplasty: A procedure using a balloon-tipped arterial catheter to break up atherosclerotic plaques.

Anterior infarction: An infarction in the distribution of the LAD, involving primarily the middle and apical sectors of the anterior-septal quadrant of the LV.

Antidromic tachycardia: An RJT of the AV bypass vanity produced by macro–re-entry in which the causative impulse recycles sequentially through an accessory AV-bypass pathway, a ventricle, the AV node and an atrium.

Apical infarction: An infarction in the distribution of any of the major coronary arteries, involving primarily the apical sectors of the posterior–lateral and inferior quadrants of the LV.

Arrhythmia: Any cardiac rhythm other than regular sinus rhythm.

Ashman phenomenon: Aberration in the intraventricular conduction of an impulse that completes a short cardiac cycle following a long cycle because the long cycle results in delay of repolarization.

Asystole: A pause in the cardiac electrical activity with neither atrial nor ventricular waveforms present on the ECG.

Atherosclerosis: A thickening of the inner arterial wall caused by the deposition of fatty substances.

Atrial fibrillation: The tachyarrhythmia at the rapid end of the flutter/fibrillation spectrum, produced by macro-re-entry within multiple circuits in the atria and characterized by irregular multiform F-waves.

Atrial flutter: The tachyarrhythmia at the slow end of the flutter/fibrillation spectrum, produced by macro-re-entry within a single circuit in the atria and characterized by regular, uniform F-waves.

Atrial rhythm: A rhythm with a rate of <100 beats/min, and with abnormally directed P waves (indicating origination from a site in the atria other than the sinus node) preceding each QRS complex.

Atrioventricular (AV) block: A conduction abnormality located between the atria and the ventricles both the severity and the location of the abnormality should be considered.

Automaticity: The ability of specialized cardiac cells to achieve spontaneous depolarization and function as pacemakers to form new cardiac- activating impulses.

AV dissociation: A condition of independent beating of the atria and ventricles, caused either by block of the atrial-activating impulse in the AV junction or by interference with conduction of the atrial-activating impulse by a ventricular impulse.

Cardiac pacemaking and conduction system: Groups of modified myocardial cells strategically located throughout the heart and capable of forming an electrical impulse and/or of conducting impulses particularly slowly or rapidly.

Carotid sinus massage: Manual stimulation of the area of the neck that overlies the bifurcation of the carotid artery to increase parasympathetic of the carotid artery to increase parasympathetic nervous activity.

Collateral blood supply: The perfusion of an area of myocardium via arteries that have developed to compensate for an obstruction of one of the principal coronary arteries.

Compensatory pause: The long cycle length (pause) following a premature beat (PB) completely "compensates" for the short cycle length preceding the PB. This is identified when the interval between the beginning of the P-wave of the sinus beats preceding and following a PB is equal to two PP intervals of sinus beats not associated with PBs.

Concordant precordial negative: A term describing abnormally wide QRS complexes that are predominatly negative in all six of the precordial leads.

Concordant precordial positive: A term describing abnormally wide QRS complexes that are predominately positive in all six of the precordial leads.

Constrictive pericarditis: Thickening of the pericardium caused by chronic inflammation and resulting in interference with myocardial function.

Cor-pulmonale: An acute or chronic pressure overload of the right side of the heart, caused by increased resistance to blood flow through the lungs.

Degree: A measure of the severity of AV block.

Depolarization: The transition in which there becomes minimal difference between the electrical charge or potential on the inside versus the outside of the cell. In the resting state, the cell is polarized, with the inside of the cell markedly negative in comparison to the outside. Depolarization is then initiated by a current that alters the permeability of the cell membrane, allowing positively charged ions to cross into the cell.

Einthoven triangle: An equilateral triangle composed of limb leads I, II, and III that provide an orientation for electrical information from the frontal plane.

Electrical cardioversion: Use of transthoracic electrical current to terminate a re-entrant tachyarrhythmia, such as those in the atrial flutter/fibrillation spectrum.

Electrocardiogram (ECG): The recording made by the electrocardiogram, depicting the electrical activity of the heart.

Emphysema: A pulmonary disease in which the alveoli are destroyed and the lungs become overinflated.

Epicardial injury: Transmural ischemia or pericardial irritation causing deviation of the ST segments of the ECG.

Escape rhythms: Rhythms that originate from sites in the pacemaking and conduction system other than the sinus node, after a pause created by the failure of either normal sinus impulse formation or AV impulse conduction.

Fine fibrillation: Either minute f waves or no atrial activity at all in any of the ECG leads.

First degree AV block: Conduction of atrial impulses to the ventricles with PR intervals of >0.21s.

Hyperacute T-waves: T-waves directed toward the ischemic area of the left ventricular epicardium that can be identified in leads involved with the ischemic area by an increased positive amplitude.

Hypertrophic cardiomyopathy: A condition in which cardiac performance is decreased because of decreased contraction capability of the thickened myocardium.

Infarct expansion: Partial disruption of the myocardial wall in the area of a recent infarction that results in thinning of wall and dilation of the involved chamber.

Infranodal block: AV block that occurs distal to or below the AV node, and, therefore, within either the common bundle or in both the RBB and LBB.

Interior infarction: An infarction in the distribution of the posterior descending coronary artery, involving primarily the basal and middle sectors of the inferior quadrant of the LV, but often extending into the posterior aspect of the right ventricle.

Intrinsicoid deflection: The time interval between the beginning of the QRS complex and the peak of the R-wave; this represents the time required for the electrical impulse to travel from the endocardial to the epicardial surfaces of the ventricular myocardium.

Ischemia: An insufficiency of blood flow to an organ that is so severe that it disrupts the function of the organ; in the heart, ischemia is often accompanied by precordial pain and diminished contraction.

Junctional premature beat (JPB): A P wave and QRS complex produced by an impulse that originates in the AV node or His bundle and appears before the expected time of the next P wave and QRS complex generated from the sinus node.

Junctional rhythm: A rhythm with a rate of <100 beats/min, with an inverted P-wave direction visible in the frontal-plane leads and normally appearing QRS complexes. The P-waves may precede or follow the QRS complexes, or may be obscured because they occur during the QRS complexes.

Lateral infarction: An infarction in the distribution of a diagonal or marginal coronary artery, involving primarily the basal and middle sectors of the anterior-superior quadrant of the LV.

Left coronary dominance: An unusual coronary artery anatomy in which the PDA is a branch of the LCX.

Lone fibrillation: Atrial fibrillation occurring in an individual who shows no evidence of cardiac disease.

Low voltage: A total amplitude of the QRS complex that < 0.70 mv in all limb leads and <1.0 mv in all precordial leads.

Macro-re-entry: Recycling of an impulse a circuit that is large enough for its own activation to be represented on the surface ECG.

Micro-re-entry: The recycling of an impulse around a circuit that is too small for its own activation to be represented on the surface ECG.

Mobitz type I (type-I): A pattern of AV block in which there are varying PR intervals. This pattern is typical of block within the AV node, which has the capacity for wide variation in conduction time.

Mobitz type II (type II): A pattern of AV block in which there are constant PR intervals despite varying RP intervals. This pattern is typical of block in the ventricular Purkinje system, which is incapable of significant variations in conduction time.

Monomorphic VT: VT with a regular rate and consistent QRS-complex morphology.

Monomorphic: A single appearance of all QRS complexes.

Multifocal atrial tachycardia: A rapid rhythm produced by increased automaticity in pacemaking cells located at multiple sites within the atria.

Myocardial infarction: Death of myocardial cells as a result of failure of the circulation to provide sufficient oxygen to restore metabolism after the intracellular stores of glycogen have been depleted.

Myocardial ischemia: A reduction in the supply of oxygen to less than the amount required by myocardial cells to maintain aerobic metabolism.

Myocardial perfusion: The flow of oxygen and nutrients into the cells of the heart muscle.

Myocardial rupture: Complete disruption of the myocardial wall in the area of a recent infarction resulting in leakage of blood out of the involved chamber.

Myxedema: Severe hypothyroidism characterized by a decreased metabolic state and inelastic edema, dry skin and hair, and loss of mental and physical vigor.

Necrosis: Death of a living tissue; termed an infarction when it is caused by insufficient supply of oxygen via the circulation.

Non-sustained VT: VT of <30 s duration.

Orthorhombic tachycardia: An RJT of the AV bypass variety produces by macro-re-entry in which the impulse recycles sequentially through the AV node, a ventricle, an accessory AV- bypass pathway, and an atrium.

Osborn waves: Abnormal ECG waveforms caused by hypothermia.

Pacemaker: A cell in the heart or an artificial device that is capable of forming or generating electrical impulse.

Pacemaker cells: Specialized cardiac cells that are capable of automaticity.

Palpitation: A sensation felt in the chest as a result of the stronger ventricular contraction following a prolonged cardiac cycle.

Paroxysmal atrial tachycardia (PAT): A tachyarrhythmia, commonly caused by digitalis toxicity, in which a rapid atrial rhythm is accompanied by failure of some of the atrial impulses to be conducted through the AV node to the ventricles.

Paroxysmal: A term referring to an arrhythmia of sudden occurrence.

Pericardial tamponade: Filling of the pericardial sac with fluid, which restricts the relaxation of the cardiac chambers.

Polymorphic VT: VT with a regular rate but frequent changes in QRS-complex morphology.

Post-ischemic T-waves: T-waves directed away from the ischemic area of the left ventricular myocardium when the ischemic process is resolving either from infarction or to reperfusion.

Posterior infarction: Infarction in the distribution of the LCX, involving primarily the basal and middle sectors of the posterior-lateral quadrant of the LV.

Pressure or systolic overload: A condition in which a ventricle is forced to pump against an increased resistance during systole.

QT interval: The time from the onset of the QRS complex to the end of the T-wave. This interval represents the time from the beginning of ventricular activation to the completion of ventricular recovery.

QTC interval: The corrected QT interval; it represents the duration of activation and recovery of the ventricular myocardium; the correction is applied by using a formula that takes into consideration the ventricular rate.

Reciprocal: A term referring to deviation of the ST segments in the opposite direction from that of their maximal deviation.

Re-entrant junctional tachyarrhythmia (RJT): Any of the tachyarrhythmias (RJTs) that are present either normally or abnormally between the atria and the ventricles.

Re-entry circuit: A circular course traveled by a cardiac impulse, created by re-entry, and having the potential for initiating premature beats and tachyarrhythmias.

Re-entry or reactivation: Passage of the cardiac electrical impulse for a second time or even greater number of times through a structure such as the AV node or the atrial or ventricular myocardium as the result of a conduction abnormality in that area of the heart normally. The cardiac electrical impulse after its initiation in specialized pacemaking cells spreads through each area of the heart only once.

Refractory period: The period following electrical activation during which a cardiac cell cannot be reactivated.

Reperfusion: The restoration of blood circulation to an organ or tissue upon reopening of a complete obstruction to blood flow.

Repolarization: The transition in which the inside of the cell becomes markedly positive in relation to the outside. This condition is maintained by a pump in the cell membrane, and it is disturbed by the arrival of an electrical current.

Rheumatic heart disease: Active or inactive disease of the heart resulting from rheumatic fever and myocardium or by scarring of the valves that reduces the functional capacity of the heart.

Right coronary dominance: The usual coronary artery anatomy in which the PDA is a branch of the RCA.

Sick sinus syndrome: A term that is loosely used clinically to describe any abnormally low sinus rate. These bradyarrhythmias are more likely to be caused by increased parasympathetic nervous activity than by disease in the sinus node.

Sinoatrial (SA) node: A small mass of tissue situated in the superior aspect of the right atrium, adjacent to the entrance of the superior vena cava. It functions as the dominant pacemaker, which forms the electrical impulses that are then conducted throughout the heart.

Stokes-Adams attacks: Syncopal episodes caused by periods of cardiac arrest.

Stunned myocardium: A region of myocardium consisting of cardiac cells that are using anaerobic metabolism and are therefore ischemic and incapable of contraction, but which are not infarcted.

Sustained VT: VT of ≥ 30 s duration or requiring an intervention for its termination.

Sympathetic tone: The relative amount of sympathetic nervous activity as compared with the amount of parasympathetic activity.

Tachycardia-bradycardia syndrome: A condition in which both rapid and slow cardiac rhythms are present. The rapid rhythms tend to appear when the rate slows abnormally, whereas the slow rhythms are prominent immediately after the sudden cessation of a rapid rhythm.

Third-degree AV block: Failure of conduction of any atrial impulses to the ventricles. This is often referred to as complete AV block.

Thrombosis: The formation or presence of a blood clot within a blood vessel.

Tombstoning: Severe demand ischemia that obscures the transition from QRS to ST-segment to T-wave.

Torsades de pointes: A variety of ventricular tachycardia resulting from prolongation of the ventricular recovery time. The term is French for turning of the points or turning of the direction of the QRS complex alternately between positive and negative.

Transmural: Involving the full thickness of the myocardial wall.

Trifascicular block: An intraventricular conduction abnormality involving the RBB both the anterior and posterior fascicles of the LBB.

Unifascicular block: An intraventricular conduction abnormality involving only one of the three principal fascicles of the intraventricular Purkinje system.

Vagal maneuver: An intervention that increases parasympathetic activity in relation to the amount of sympathetic activity.

Vasovagal reaction (reflex): Sudden slowing of the heart rate either from decreased impulse formation (sinus pause) or decreased impulse conduction (AV block), resulting from increased activity of the sympathetic nervous system. The slowing of the cardiac rhythm is accompanied by peripheral vascular dilation.

Vasovagal syncope: Loss of consciousness caused by a vasovagal reaction. Consciousness is almost always regained when the individual falls into a recumbent position, because this results in increased venous return to the heart.

Ventricular aneurysm: The extreme of infarct expansion, in which the ventricular wall becomes so thin that it bulges outward (dyskinesia) during systole.

Ventricular fibrillation: Rapid and totally disorganized ventricular activity without discernible QRS complexes or T waves in the ECG.

Ventricular flutter/fibrillation: The spectrum of ventricular tachyarrhythmias that lack discernible QRS complexes or T waves in the ECG. These tachyarrhythmias produce ECG effects that range from gross undulations to no discernible electrical activity.

Ventricular flutter: Rapid, organized ventricular activity without discernible QRS complexes or T-waves in the ECG.

Ventricular premature beat: A QRS complex produced by an impulse originating from the ventricles and appearing before the expected time of the next QRS complex generated from the sinus node or other basic underlying rhythm.

Ventricular tachycardia: A rhythm originating distal to the branching of the common bundle, with a ventricular contraction rate of ≥ 100 beats/min.

Volume or diastolic overload: A condition in which a ventricle becomes filled with an increased amount of blood during diastole.

Wenckebach sequence: The classic from of type I AV block, which would be expected to occur in the absence of autonomic influences on either the SA or AV nodes.

PACEMAKER

Artificial cardiac pacemakers: Devices capable of generating electrical impulses and delivering them to the myocardium.

Biventricular pacemaker: A pacemaker that paces both the right and left ventricles. Atrial pacing is also included unless the patient has chronic atrial arrhythmias that would prevent atrial pacing.

Cardiac resynchronization therapy (CRT): Use of biventricular pacing to synchronize ventricular activation and contraction.

Defibrillation: Termination of either atrial or ventricular fibrillation by an extrinsic electrical current.

Demand mode: A term describing an artificial pacemaking system with the ability to sense and be inhabited by intrinsic cardiac activity.

Dual-chamber pacemaker: A pacemaker that includes both atrial and ventricular pacing.

Fixed-rate pacing: Artificial pacing with the capability only to generate an electrical impulse, without sensing of the heart's intrinsic rhythm.

Oversensing: Abnormal function of an artificial pacemaker in which electrical signals other than those representing activation of the myocardium are sensed and inhibit impulse generation.

Pacemaker artifacts: High-frequency signals appearing on an ECG and representing impulses generated by an artificial pacemaker.

Pacemaker mediated tachyarrhythmia: A rapid heart rate occurring with a dual-chambered pacing system, using intrinsic VA conduction and artificially paced AV conduction.

Pacemaker syndrome: A reduction in cardiac output caused by activation by an artificial pacemaker that does not produce an optimally efficient sequence of myocardial activation.

Pacemaker-induced tachyarrhythmia: A rapid heart rate produced by an artificial pacemaker. A paced impulse occurring when the myocardium is vulnerable to induction of a re-entrant circuit because it is just emerging from total refractoriness.

Pacing electrodes: Electrodes that, in contrast with the electrodes used to record the ECG, are designed to transmit an electrical impulse to the myocardium. In pacing systems with sensing capability, these electrodes also transmit the intrinsic impulses of the heart to the pacemaking device.

Pulse generator: A device that produces electrical impulses as the key component of an artificial pacing system.

Single-chamber pacemaker: A pacemaker with one lead pacing and sensing one cardiac chamber.

Suggested Reading

1. Barbara Aehlert. ECGs Made Easy, 4th edition. Elsevier, 2011.
2. Chung Edwark K. Poket Guide to ECG Diagnosis, 1st edition. Oxford University Press, 1997.
3. Dune Marvin I, Lipman Bernard S, Lipman-Massie. Clinical Electrocardiography, 8th edition. Yearbook Medical Publishers Inc, 1989.
4. Gold Berger Ary L, Gold Berger Emanuel. Clinical Electrocardiography, a simplified Approach, 7th edition. Elsevier, 2006.
5. Goldman MJ, Goldchlager N. Principles of Clinical Electrocardiography, 13th edition. Lange Medical Book, 1989.
6. Hampton John R. The ECG made Easy, 5th edition. Churchill Livingstone, 1997.
7. Julian DG, Cowan JC, McLenachan JM. Cardiology, 9th edition. Elsevier Ltd, 2009.
8. Lipman Bradford C, Lipman Bernard S. ECG Pocket Guide, 1st edition. Jaypee Brothers Medical Publishers Ltd, 1990.
9. Luthra A. ECG Made Easy, 3rd edition. Jaypee Brothers, 2007.
10. Schamroth Leo. An Introduction to Electrocardiography, 7th edition. Black Well Science Ltd, 1990.
11. Wagner SG. Marriott's Practical electrocardiography, 11th edition. Lippincott W and W, 2001.

Index

Page numbers followed by *f* refer to figure and *t* refer to table.

A

Abdominal pain 196
Aberrant ventricular conduction 105, 106, 115
Acetylcholine 9
Activated cell 19*f*
Adrenaline 81
Aerobic metabolism 265
Alcohol 81
Amylnitrate 81
Anaerobic metabolism 265
Anemia 81
Angina 265
Anorexia 196
Antidromic tachycardia 265
Anti-ischemic therapy 194
Anti-thrombotic therapy 194
Aortic incompetence 72
Aortic stenosis 69
Apical infarction 265
Arrhythmia 62, 76, 196, 216, 265
   mechanisms of 79
   supraventricular 90
Ashman phenomenon 117, 117*f*, 265
Asystole, characteristics of 141
Atherosclerosis 266
Atria conducting system 6
Atrial activation 23
Atrial arrhythmia 102, 196, 197
Atrial dissociation 102
Atrial ectopic 87*f*
   beat 86
   causes of 87
   types of 88
Atrial enlargement 63*f*, 64*f*
   causes of 44, 67
   left 65, 66
   right 66, 230*f*
Atrial escape rhythm 102
Atrial extrasystoles 87
Atrial fibrillation 81, 95, 102, 110*f*, 111, 111*f*, 112*f*, 114, 115, 115*f*, 116, 116*f*, 129*f*, 141*f*, 216, 258, 259, 266
   causes of 112
   classical 108
   complication of 113
   fast 242
   in elderly patient, causes of 112
   in young patient, causes of 112
   treatment of 114
   types of 111
Atrial flutter 76, 81, 95, 102, 107, 108, 108*f*, 109, 110*f*, 111*f*, 114, 216, 266
   causes of 108
   fibrillation 115*f*
   management of 109
Atrial hypertrophy 63, 66*f*
   left 64, 65, 65*f*, 66*f*
   right 63, 64*f*, 65, 66*f*
Atrial pacemaker rhythm 234
Atrial pacing 232
Atrial parasystol 102
Atrial premature 87
   beats 76
   contraction 87, 87*f*, 102, 105, 105*f*
   frequent 105*f*
Atrial rhythm 76, 266
   accelerated 265
   left 102
   right 102
Atrial septal defect 65, 112, 227, 227*f*
Atrial standstill 102
Atrial tachycardia 81, 97, 97*f*, 99, 102, 106, 106*f*, 109, 195*f*, 252, 255
   causes of 98
   slow 102
Atrial thythm 104
Atrioventricular block 106, 142, 143, 146, 147, 266
   advanced 116, 116*f*, 141*f*
   causes 146, 148
   first degree 146*f*, 267
   locations of 142*f*
   third-degree 270
   treatment 147, 148

Atrioventricular dissociation 154
    causes 154
    type of 154f
Atrioventricular sequential pacemaker rhythm 234
Atrium, right 3
Atropin 81
Augmented unipolar limb leads 13
Autorhythmicity 8
Axis deviation 38
    left 39f
    right 39f
    types 38

B

Bartter's syndrome 200
Bicarbonate 199
Bifascicular block, treatment of 161
Bigeminy ves 122
Biochemical cardiac markers 193
Biventricular hypertrophy 74, 74f, 226f
    causes of 74
Biventricular pacemaker 272
Brady arrhythmias 78
Bradycardia
    causes of 83
    tachycardia 214
Brain tumors 204
Bundle branch block 2, 115
    causes
        complete left 157
        complete right 155
    complete left 157, 158f
    complete right 155, 156f
    diagnosis, complete left 157
    incomplete
        left 158, 159f
        right 156, 157f, 227f
    intermittent 161
        left 162f
    left 17, 44 187, 188f, 223f
    treatment, complete left 158
Bundle branch, right 79, 229f
Butler-Leggett formula 71

C

Caffeine 81
Calcium effect 201
Calibration 26
Calibration, diagram of 26f
Cardiac arrest
    in systole 197
    rhythms 141
Cardiac capture by pacing, failure of 234
Cardiac causes 112
Cardiac cell 8, 18
Cardiac pacemakers, artificial 272
Cardiac pacemaking 266
Cardiac resynchronization therapy 272
Cardiac rhythm 76
    description of abnormal 79
    genesis of abnormal 79
Cardiac rupture 220
Cardiac surgery 151
Cardiac tamponade 220
Cardiopulmonary surgery 112
Cardiomyopathy 17, 44, 47, 98, 156, 222
    types 222
Carotid sinus massage 266
Central nervous system disorder 204, 264
Cerebrovascular accident 204
    pattern 204, 205f
Chagas disease 151
Chaotic ventricular rhythm 139
Chest
    electrode placed incorrectly 17
    infection, acute 112
    leads 17
        electrode placement of 16f
    wall
        deformity of 17
        thick 30, 47
Coarctation of aorta 69
Collagen disease 151
Collateral blood supply 266
Concordant precordial
    negative 266
    positive 266
Conduction defects 77
Conduction system 7t, 78f
    anatomy of 78
    physiology of 78
    portion of 5
Confusion 196
Congenital disorder 218
Congenital heart disease 112, 156, 226
Congenital syndrome 134
Conn's syndrome 200

Constrictive pericarditis 266
   chronic 30, 47, 81, 112
Cor pulmonale, chronic 156
Coronary arterial anatomy,
   normal 5*f*
Coronary artery 5, 167
   disease 2, 112
      diffuse 47
   left 4, 5
   right 4
   spasm 52, 179, 179*f*
Coronary blood flow
   impaired 57*f*
   severe impaired 58*f*
Coronary circulation 4
Coronary dominance
   left 268
   right 270
Coronary heart disease 52
Coronary insufficiency 51*f*, 57*f*
Coronary occlusion 189
Coronary sinus pacemaker
   rhythm 234
Coronary syndrome, acute 190,
   191, 194*f*, 265
Corpulmonale 112, 266
Couplet ventricular extrasystole
   123*f*
Cushing's syndrome 200
Cyanosis 217

D

Deflection, negative 20*f*
Delirium 196
Depolarization 18
Depression 196
Dextrocardia 17, 71, 218, 218*f*,
   219, 229*f*
Diarrhea 196
Diastolic overload 72, 73
   causes 72
Digitalis effect 195, 195*f*
Digitalis toxicity 195
Digoxin 212
   toxicity 58*f*, 98, 195, 196
      extracardiac effect of 196
   toxicity, treatment of 196
Dilated cardiomyopathy 30, 222
Downward deflection 20*f*
Dresslers syndrome 61, 189
Drowsiness 196
Drugs electrolytes effect 195
Dual-chamber pacemaker 252,
   272
Dual-chamber pacing 232

E

Early reinfarction 189
Early repolarization 221
   pattern 221*f*
   syndrome 61
Ebstein's anomaly 229, 230*f*
Ectopic beat 86, 86*f*, 87
Ectopic tachycardia 99
Ectopic, types of 86
Einthoven triangle 267
Eisenmenger's syndrome 71, 74
Electrical axis, determination
   of 37*f*
Electrical cardioversion 267
Electrocardiogram 1, 51, 60-62
   clinical value of 2
   complexes 24*f*
   deflection, normal 22*f*
   measurements, normal 27
   normal 22
   paper 26, 26*f*
   standardization of 30
Electrocardiographic complexes
   23*f*
Electrocardiographic phase 172
Electrode placement 11
Electrolyte
   disturbance 203
   effect 195
   imbalance 87
Electromechanical dissociation
   220
   causes 220
   treatment 221
Emphysema 2, 30, 47, 224, 267
Endocarditis 151
Endocardium 4
Endocrine cause 200
Epicardial injury 267
Epicardium 4
Epilepsy 154
Escape rhythm 151, 267
Exercise testing 236
Exercise tolerance test 232, 236
Extensive anterior
   infarction 180*f*
   myocardial infarction 179

F

Fascicular block, left
   anterior 158
   posterior 160
Fever 81
Fine ventricular fibrillation 137*f*

G

Giant T-wave inversion 50f
Gitelman's syndrome 200
Glucose with insulin 199
Gynecomastia 196

H

Haemophilus influenzae 206
Hallucination 196
Heart 13
    activation, sequence of 8
    anatomy of 3
    block 142
        causes of 143
        classification 143
        complete 150, 150f, 242, 254
        determination of complete 151
    conductive system of 6, 6f
    disease 120
        organic 87
    failure 81
    junctional tissues of 6
    nerve supply of 8
    rate, determination of 28, 29f
    rhythm of 31, 62
    sound-S1 152
    wall, layers of 4
Heat stroke 204
Hemiblock 143
    left
        anterior 143, 158, 159f
        posterior 143, 160, 160f
Hexaxial reference system 15, 15f, 35f
Hyperacute T-waves 267
Hypercalcemia 201, 203
Hyperkalemia 2, 47, 51, 51f, 197, 203
    causes of 199
    ECG changes in 198f
    features of 199
    on heart, effect of 197
Hypermagnesemia 202, 203
Hypertension 67, 112
Hypertensive heart disease 52
Hyperthyroidism 220
Hypertrophic cardiomyopathy 69, 74, 267
Hypertrophy 63
Hypertropic cardiomyopathies 223
Hypocalcemia 202, 202f, 203
Hypokalemia 2, 49f, 112, 199, 203, 220
    causes of 200
    ECG changes in 200f
    effects of 200
    on heart, effects of 200
Hypomagnesemia 202, 203
Hyponatremia 112
Hypothermia 2, 30, 47, 204, 220
    ECG changes in 204f
Hypothyroidism 47, 220
Hypovolemia 220
Hypoxia 220

I

Idiopathic cardiomyopathy 223f
Idioventricular rhythm 47
    accelerated 131
Impulse formation and conduction 7
Infarction 163, 163f, 164f, 166
    anterior 265
    inferior 182, 183f
    lateral 268
    posterior 269
    size 189
Infiltrative disease 151
Insufficient myocardial perfusion 164
Intra-atrial block 77, 142
Intra-his block 142
Intraventricular block 77, 142
    nonspecific 223f
Irregular rhythm, cause of 31, 62
Ischemia 164f, 165, 167, 267
    diffuse anterior 181f
    injury, acute 163f
Ischemic heart disease 98

J

James bypass tract 212
Junctional arrhythmias 196
Junctional premature
    beat 268
    contraction 88, 88f
    types 88
Junctional rhythm 88, 268
    accelerated 92, 92f, 265
Junctional tachyarrhythmia, re-entrant 269

K

Kartagener's syndrome 219
Katz-Wachtel phenomenon 75

L

Left axis deviation, causes of 40
Left ventricular hypertrophy 73
    causes of 68
    diagnosis of 68
Lev's disease 150
Levocardia 219
Liddle's syndrome 200
Limb leads 13*f*
    standard 11t
Lown-Ganong-Levine syndrome 212, 213
Lutembacher's syndrome 66
Lyme's disease 151

M

Mahaim bypass tract syndrome 214
Massive pulmonary embolism 220
    acute 217
Mesocardia 219
Minnesota criteria 188
Mitral incompetence 72
Mitral regurgitation 69
Monomorphic ventricular tachycardia 130, 130*f*
    causes of 128
Multifocal atrial tachycardia 91, 91*f*, 95, 102, 268
Multifocal chaotic atrial tachycardia 76
Multifocal ventricular
    extrasystole 121*f*
    premature contractions 127*f*
Muscle cells 7
Myocardial disease 67
Myocardial infarction 44, 60, 163-165, 167, 172, 268
    acute 207
        anterior 188*f*
        diaphragmatic 182*f*
    anterior 180, 181*f*
    anterolateral 180, 181, 181*f*, 182*f*
    electrocardiographic evolution of 173*f*
    high lateral 182, 183*f*
    inferoposterolateral 185
    old 165
    posterior wall 184, 185*f*
    subacute 165
Myocardial injury 163-165
Myocardial ischemia 163, 165*f*, 166, 168, 190, 268
    acute 57*f*
    inferior 258
Myocardial perfusion 268
Myocardial rupture 268
Myocarditis 112
Myocardium 2, 4
    normal 165
Myxedema 30, 268

N

Narrow complex tachycardia, causes of 81
Nausea 196
Neck vein 152
Necrosis 163
Nicotine 81
Nodal ectopic
    beat 86
    low 86*f*
Nodal rhythm 88, 89*f*
    causes of 89
Noncardiac cause 112
Nonconducted atrial premature contraction 105
Nonparoxysmal junctional tachycardia 92
Nonrespiratory sinus arrhythmia 83
Nonsustained ventricular tachycardia 127

O

Obesity 30, 47
Obstructive pulmonary disease
    chronic 17, 32, 41, 176, 207
    ECG changes in chronic 208*f*
Orthorhombic tachycardia 269
Osborn waves 269

P

Pacemaker 47, 232, 269, 272
    artifacts 272
    cells 7, 269
    code system of 233*f*
    induced tachyarrhythmia 272
    malfunction 235
    mediated tachyarrhythmia 272
    patterns 233*f*
    sites 85*f*
        of heart 85
    syndrome 235, 272
    temporary 234

terminology 233
types 232
Pacing electrodes 272
Parasympathetic stimulation 9
Parasystolic ventricular tachycardia 260
Paroxysmal atrial
 fibrillation, causes of 113
 tachycardia 76, 93, 107f, 269
Paroxysmal SVT, types of 97
Patent ductus arteriosus 72, 228, 228f
P-congenitale 63
Pericardial effusion 30, 47, 207
 ECG changes in 208f
Pericardial rub 206
Pericardial tamponade 269
Pericarditis 205
 acute 112, 206, 207
 causes of 206
 ECG changes in 205f
 management 207
Permanent pacemaker 235
Phenothiazines tricyclics 171
Pleural effusion, left-sided 17
P-mitrale 64, 65
 causes of 65
Pneumonia 112
Pneumothorax, left-sided 17
Polymorphic ventricular tachycardia 130, 130f
Postinfarction syndrome 61
Postmyocardial infarction syndrome 189
Potassium effect 197, 199
Potential pacemakers of heart 79
P-pulmonale 63, 65
 cause of 65
PR segment depression, causes of 54
Precordial leads placement 16
Pre-excitation syndrome 209
 types of 209, 213f
Psychotropic drugs 171
Pulmonary circulation 4
Pulmonary embolism 112, 156, 216, 216f, 250
 diagnose 217
 treatment of 217
Pulmonary emphysema 225f
Pulmonary hypertension 71
Pulmonary stenosis 71, 230, 230f
Pulse generator 272
P-wave
 abnormal 42
 absent 43
 inverted 43
 normal 42
 small 43
 variable 43

Q

QRS axis 33
 deviation 38f
QRS complete 25, 46f
QRS complex
 abnormal 46, 47
 normal 46
QRS rhythm 102
QRS tachycardia, wide 78
QRS vector, determination of 35
QRS, causes of low voltage 47
QT interval 54
 abnormalities of 55
 causes of
  long 55
  short 55
 long 55
Quinidine
 effects 196
 therapy 197f
Q-wave
 causes of pathological 44
 infarction 186
 normal 44
 pathological 44

R

Renal tubular necrosis 200
Repolarization syndrome 61f
Residual ischemia 189
Respiratory sinus arrhythmia 83
Resting cell 18f
Restrictive cardiomyopathies 223
Rheumatic heart disease 98, 270
 chronic 112
Rhythm
 accelerated 265
 primary disorders of 76
Right axis deviation, causes of 41
Right ventricular hypertrophy
 causes of 71
 diagnosis of 71
Romhilt-Estes scoring system 69
R-on-T phenomenon 123, 124f
Runway pacemaker 234
R-wave
 abnormal 45, 46f
 normal 45, 45f
 progression 17

causes of 17
normal 17

S

Salbutamol 81
Shock 81, 217
Sick sinus syndrome 81, 98, 112, 214, 214f, 260, 262, 270
    causes of 215
    diagnosis of 215
Single muscle cell 19f
Single-chamber pacemaker 272
Sinoatrial block 2, 142-144, 144f
    causes 144
    diagnosis 144
    treatment 145
Sinoatrial node 270
Sinus 99
    arrest 76, 145
    arrhythmia 76, 83, 83f, 85, 222f, 253
    bradycardia 76, 82, 82f, 83, 252, 256, 261
    bradycardia, causes of 82
    pause 145, 145f
    premature beats 76
    rhythm 62, 76, 80, 105f, 107f, 127f, 227f, 228f, 253
        characters of 31
        normal 80, 80f
    standstill 145
    tachycardia 76, 80, 80f, 81, 216, 248, 253
        causes of 81
        pathological, causes of 81
Situs inversus 219, 220
ST and T changes, causes of 171
ST depression
    causes of 60
    downward sloping 58f
    horizontal 57
    junctional 57f
    sagging 58f
ST segment
    abnormal 56
    elevation, causes of 60
    normal 56
Staphylococcus aureus 206
Stokes-Adams attacks 153, 154, 270
Stokes-Adams syndrome treatment 154
Stunned myocardium 270
Subendocardial infarction 185, 186f
Subendocardial ischemia 177
    diffuse 177f
Subepicardial injury 178, 178f
Subepicardial ischemia 177
    diffuse 178f
Supraventricular tachycardia
    causes of 94
    classification of 96
    complication of 95
Sympathetic nerves 9
Sympathetic tone 270
Systemic circulation 4
Systemic hypertension 69
Systolic overload 72
    cause 72

T

Tachyarrhythmia 77, 80
Tachycardia 81, 217
    bradycardia syndrome 270
    causes of broad complex 81
    re-entrant 99
    supraventricular 93, 93f, 95, 96f
Tachypnea 217
Technical dextrocardia 219
Tension pneumothorax 220
Tetralogy of Fallot 71, 228, 229f
Thoracic surgery 112
Thrombolysis 189
Thyroid medications 81
Thyrotoxicosis 81, 112
Torsade-de-pointes 133, 133f, 197, 270
    causes of 133
    management of 134
Toxic arrhythmia 198
Transmural infarction 187f
Transmural myocardial infarction 186
Tricuspid regurgitation 65, 71
Tricuspid stenosis 65
Trifascicular block 271
Trigeminy ventricular extrasystole 122f
T-wave
    abnormal 48
    inversion, causes of secondary 51f
    normal 48
    pattern, juvenile 52, 221, 222f

U

Unifascicular block 271
Unifocal ventricular extrasystole 122f
Unipolar limb leads 14f

U-wave
    abnormal 52, 53*f*
    normal 52, 52*f*

V

Vagal maneuver 271
Valvular disease, multiple 74
Valvular supravalvular 69
Vasovagal reaction 271
Vasovagal syncope 271
Vaughan William classification 198*f*
Vena cava, superior 78
Ventricle, right 3
Ventricular activation time 24, 27, 73
Ventricular aneurysm 184, 223, 271
    left 224*f*
Ventricular arrhythmia 90, 196, 197
Ventricular conducting system 6
Ventricular diastolic overload, left 73
Ventricular ectopic
    beat 86
    causes of 119
    multiple 245
Ventricular enlargement, left 75
Ventricular escape rhythm 139
Ventricular extrasystole 118, 118*f*, 120
    interpolated 120*f*
    triplet 123*f*
Ventricular fibrillation 135, 136*f*, 137, 271
    causes of 136
    coarse 137*f*
    treatment of 138
    types of 137
Ventricular flutter 135, 135*f*, 271
Ventricular hypertrophy 44, 47, 67
    left 17, 67, 67*f*, 71, 73, 75, 228*f*
    right 69, 70*f*, 156, 230*f*
Ventricular myocardial infarction, right 186, 187*f*
Ventricular pacemaker 232*f*, 244
    complexes 256
    rhythm, fixed-rate 234
    type of 243
Ventricular pacing 232
Ventricular parasystole 138, 138*f*
Ventricular premature
    beat 271
    complex 120
    contraction 118, 162*f*
Ventricular rhythm, accelerated 265
Ventricular septal defect 72, 226, 226*f*
Ventricular systolic overload, left 72*f*
Ventricular tachycardia 47, 125, 125*f*, 254, 255, 271
    bidirectional 129, 129*f*
    cause of 125, 128
    classification of 126, 130
    sustained 127, 261
    treatment of 131
Ventriculophasic sinus arrhythymia 84
Visual disturbance 196
Voltage tracing, low 30
Vomiting 196

W

Wall myocardial infarction, acute extensive anterior 50*f*
Wandering atrial pacemaker 76, 89, 89*f*
Wandering pacemaker 89, 90
    causes of 90
Wave intervals, abnormalities of 42
Wenckebach phenomenon 143
Wenckebach sequence 271
Wide complex tachycardia, causes of 131
Wolff-Parkinson-White syndrome 47, 71, 112, 176, 209, 209*f*, 210, 210*f*, 223, 230*f*, 244, 260
    treatment of 211